**The Official
Rails-to-Trails
Conservancy
Guidebook**

W9-BML-153

Rail-Trails
Midwest Great Lakes

Rail-Trails Midwest: Great Lakes

1st EDITION 2009
  7th printing 2014

Copyright © 2009 by Rails-to-Trails Conservancy

Front and back cover photographs copyright © 2009 by
  Rails-to-Trails Conservancy
All interior photographs by Rails-to-Trails Conservancy

Maps: Tim Rosner, Gene Olig and Lohnes+Wright
Map data courtesy of: Environmental Systems Research Institute
Cover design: Lisa Pletka and Barbara Richey
Book design and layout: Lisa Pletka
Book editors: Laura Shauger, Jennifer Kaleba and Wendy Jordan

ISBN 978-0-89997-467-5

Manufactured in the United States of America

Published by: **Wilderness Press**
                  Keen Communications
                  PO Box 43673
                  Birmingham, AL 35243
                  (800) 443-7227; FAX (205) 326-1012
                  info@wildernesspress.com
                  www.wildernesspress.com

Visit our website for a complete listing of our books and for ordering
information.

Distributed by Publishers Group West

Cover photos: Glacial Drumlin State Trail *(main image);* Monon Trail *(upper
                    left);* Lakelands Trail State Park *(lower right);* Sam Vadalabene
                    Great River Road Bike Trail *(back cover)*

Title page photo: Pere Marquette Rail-Trail

SAFETY NOTICE: Although Wilderness Press and Rails-to-Trails Conservancy
have made every attempt to ensure that the information in this book is accurate
at press time, they are not responsible for any loss, damage, injury, or inconve-
nience that may occur to anyone while using this book. You are responsible for
your own safety and health while in the wilderness. The fact that a trail is described in this book does not mean that it will be safe for you. Be aware that trail
conditions can change from day to day. Always check local conditions, know
your own limitations, and consult a map.

About Rails-to-Trails Conservancy

Headquartered in Washington, D.C., Rails-to-Trails Conservancy (RTC) fosters one great mission: to protect America's irreplaceable rail corridors by transforming them into multiuse trails. Its hope is that these pathways will reconnect Americans with their neighbors, communities, nature and proud history.

Railways helped build America. Spanning from coast to coast, these ribbons of steel linked people, communities and enterprises, spurring commerce and forging a single nation that bridges a continent. But in recent decades, many of these routes have fallen into disuse, severing communal ties that helped bind Americans together.

When RTC opened its doors in 1986, the rail-trail movement was in its infancy. While there were some 250 miles of open rail-trails in the United States, most projects focused on single, linear routes in rural areas, created for recreation and conservation. RTC sought broader protection for the unused corridors, incorporating rural, suburban and urban routes.

Year after year, RTC's efforts to protect and align public funding with trail building created an environment that allowed trail advocates in communities all across the country to initiate trail projects. These ever-growing ranks of trail professionals, volunteers and RTC supporters have built momentum for the national rail-trails movement. As the number of supporters multiplied, so too did the rail-trails. By the turn of the 21st century, there were some 1100 rail-trails on the ground, and RTC recorded nearly 84,000 supporters, from business leaders and politicians to environmentalists and healthy-living advocates.

Americans now enjoy more than 15,000 miles of open rail-trails. And as they flock to the trails to commune with neighbors, neighborhoods and nature, their economic, physical and environmental wellness continue to flourish.

In 2006, Rails-to-Trails Conservancy celebrated 20 years of creating, protecting, serving and connecting rail-trails. Boasting more than 100,000 members and supporters, RTC is the nation's leading advocate for trails and greenways.

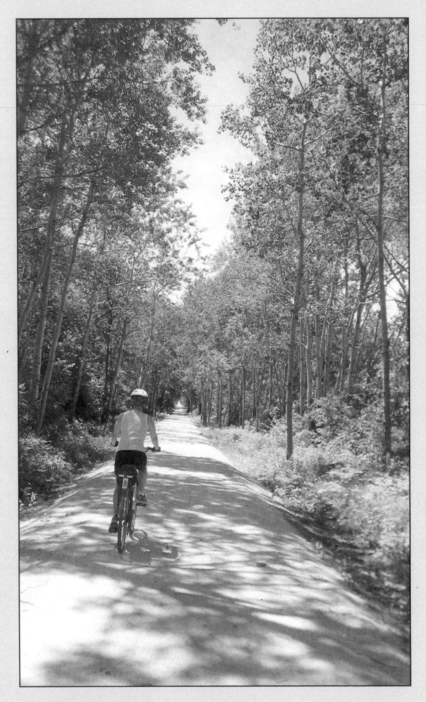

Ahnapee State Park Trail in Wisconsin

Foreword

Dear Reader:

For those of you who have already experienced the sheer enjoyment and freedom of riding on a rail-trail, welcome back! You'll find *Rail-Trails Midwest: Great Lakes* to be a useful and fun guide to your favorite trails, as well as an introduction to pathways you have yet to travel.

For readers who are discovering, for the first time, the adventures you can have on a rail-trail, thank you for joining the rail-trail movement. Since 1986, Rails-to-Trails Conservancy has been the No. 1 supporter and defender of these priceless public corridors. We are excited to bring you *Rail-Trails Midwest: Great Lakes* so you, too, can enjoy this region's rail-trails.

Built on unused, former railroad corridors, these hiking and biking trails are an ideal way to connect with your community, with nature, and with your friends and family. I've found that rail-trails have a way of bringing people together, and as you'll see from this book, there are opportunities in every state you visit to get on a trail. Whether you're looking for a place to exercise, explore, commute or play—there is a rail-trail in this book for you.

So I invite you to sit back, relax, pick a trail that piques your interest—and then get out, get active and have some fun. I'll be out on the trails, too, so be sure to wave as you go by.

Happy Trails,
Keith Laughlin
President, Rails-to-Trails Conservancy

Midwest: Great Lakes

CANADA
Lake Superior
Wisconsin
see page 281
Lake Michigan
see page 123
Michigan
Lake Huron
Milwaukee
Chicago
Detroit
Lake Erie
Cleveland
Iowa
Ohio
see page 7
Illinois
Indiana
Columbus
Indianapolis
see page 197
see page 83
Cincinnati
St Louis
West Virginia
Louisville
Missouri
Kentucky
Tennessee
Memphis
N
rails·to·trails conservancy

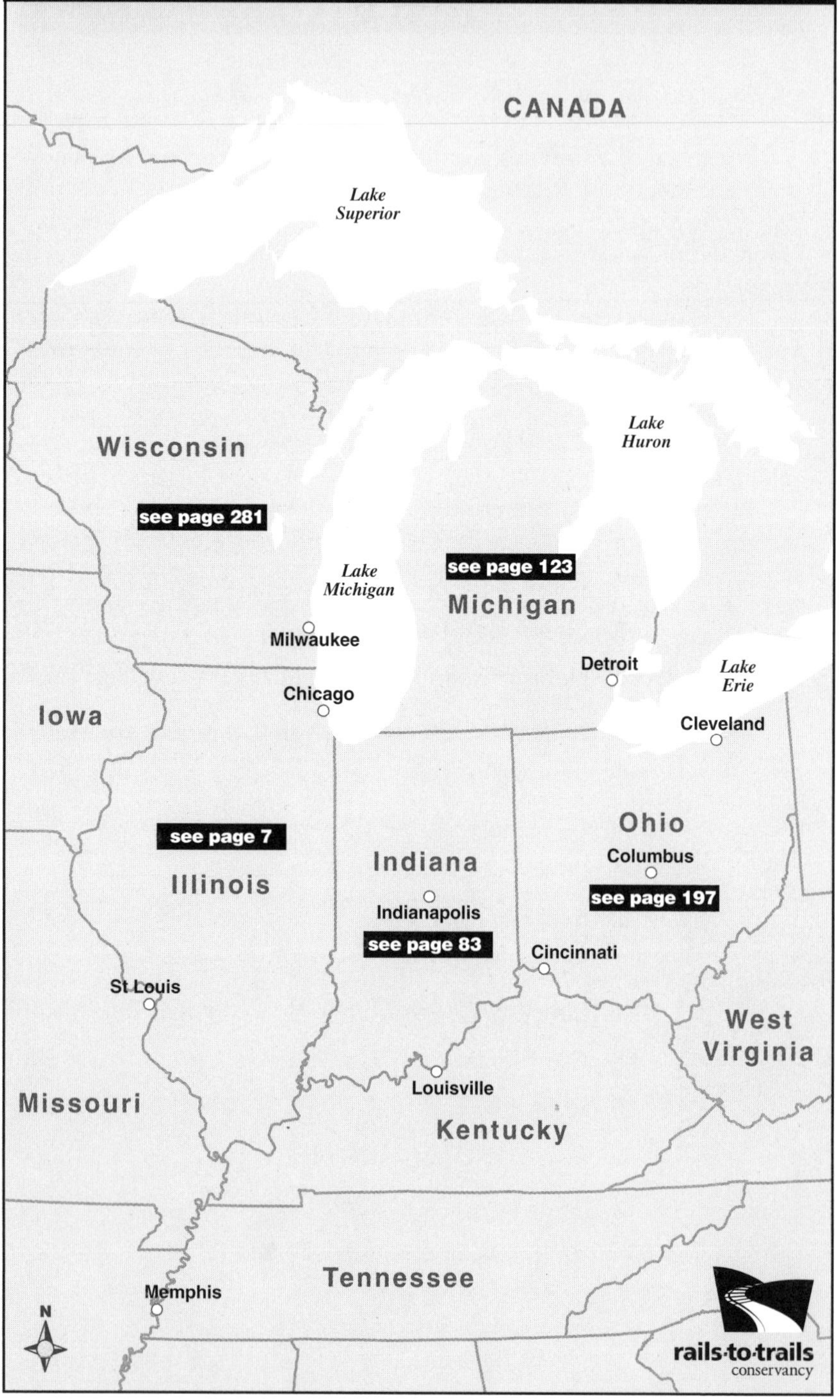

Contents

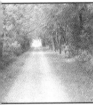

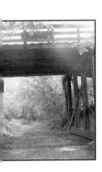

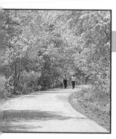

INDIANA   83

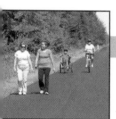

MICHIGAN   123

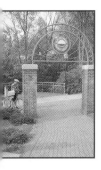

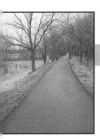

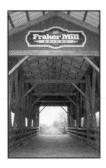

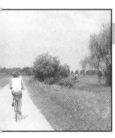

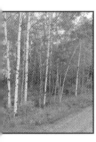

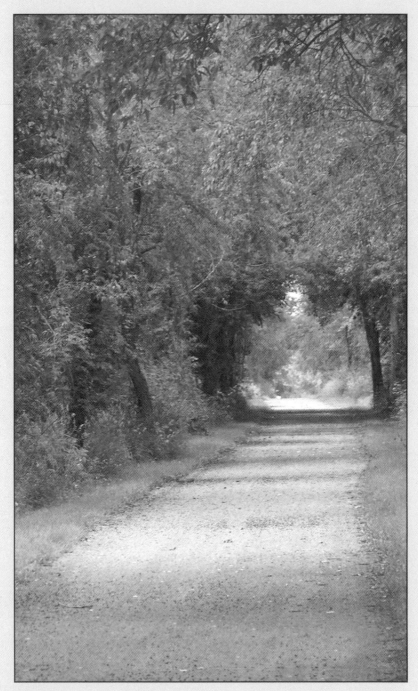

Rock Island Trail State Park in Illinois

INTRODUCTION

The Midwest was a hub of activity in the railroading heyday, resulting in thousands of miles of rail corridor stretching out like spokes on a wagon wheel toward the Pacific and Atlantic coasts, down to the Gulf of Mexico and up into neighboring Canada. As railroads fell into disuse, they left behind thousand of miles of corridor and, of course, potential trails.

Today, the Great Lakes region of the Midwest boasts 381 rail-trails, and Wisconsin and Michigan are constantly vying for the most rail-trail miles of all 50 states and the more than 1500 rail-trails across the United States (Wisconsin has converted 1591 miles of rail-trail; Michigan, 1573).

Rail-Trails Midwest: Great Lakes showcases 113 diverse rail-trails in Illinois, Indiana, Ohio, Michigan and Wisconsin, each serving as a window into the world the railroad once served. Visit the 61-mile Illinois Prairie Path, for instance, which links suburban neighborhoods outside Chicago and was sparked by a 1963 letter to the editor of the *Chicago Tribune*. Named to the Rails-to-Trails Conservancy's Rail-Trail Hall of Fame in 2008, the Illinois Prairie Path is a true elder statesman of the rail-trail movement.

Find out how a rail-trail can be a bustling city playground in Indianapolis, Indiana, on the 15-mile Monon Trail. Trailside living has never been as cool or as easy as it is on the mighty Monon. Rail-trails make for great family destinations. Make your vacation a bike-and-beach combo on the Pere Marquette Rail-Trail that offers 34 miles of easy riding, beaches and trailside fun.

Take a trip back in time on Ohio's 11-mile Holmes County Trail; it shares its corridor with the local Amish who run their horse-and-buggies on an adjacent path. The two communities—Amish and "English"—have worked together to make the trail an amenity but also a bridge between cultures.

Discover new "olde" worlds on the 23-mile Sugar River State Trail tucked into an area of Wisconsin dubbed "America's Little Switzerland." Your trip back in time takes you over 14 bridges, including one covered bridge that will have everyone reaching for their cameras.

No matter which route in *Rail-Trails Midwest: Great Lakes* you decide to try, you'll be touching on the heart of the community that helped build it and the history that first brought the rails to the region.

What is a Rail-Trail?

Rail-trails are multiuse public paths built along former railroad corridors. Most often flat or following a gentle grade, they are suited to walking, running, cycling, mountain biking, inline skating, cross-country skiing, horseback riding and wheelchair use. Since the 1960s, Americans have created more than 15,000 miles of rail-trails throughout the country.

These extremely popular recreation and transportation corridors traverse urban, suburban and rural landscapes. Many preserve historic landmarks, while others serve as wildlife conservation corridors, linking isolated parks and establishing greenways in developed areas. Rail-trails also stimulate local economies by boosting tourism and promoting trailside businesses.

What is a Rail-with-Trail?

A rail-with-trail is a public path that parallels a still-active rail line. Some run adjacent to high-speed, scheduled trains, often linking public transportation stations, while others follow tourist routes and slow-moving excursion trains. Many share an easement, separated from the rails by extensive fencing. There are more than 115 rails-with-trails in the U.S.

HOW TO USE THIS BOOK

*R*ail-Trails Midwest: Great Lakes provides the information you need to plan a rewarding rail-trail trek. With words to inspire you and maps to chart your path, it makes choosing the best route a breeze. Following are some of the highlights.

Maps

You'll find three levels of maps in this book: an **overall regional map**, **state locator maps**, and **detailed trail maps**. The Midwest region includes Illinois, Indiana, Michigan, Ohio and Wisconsin. Each chapter details a particular state's network of trails, marked on locator maps in the chapter introduction. Use these maps to find the trails nearest you, or select several neighboring trails and plan a weekend hiking or biking excursion. Once you find a trail on a state locator map, simply flip to the corresponding page number for a full description. Accompanying trail maps mark each route's access roads, trailheads, parking areas, restrooms and other defining features.

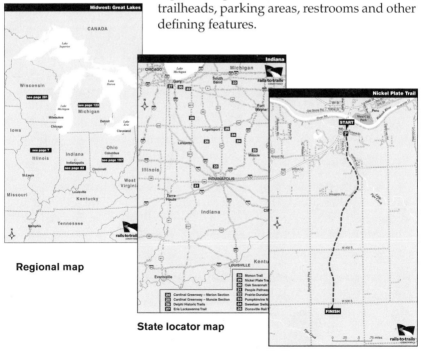

Regional map

State locator map

Trail map

Trail Descriptions

Trails are listed in alphabetical order within each chapter. Each description leads off with a set of summary information, including trail endpoints and mileage, a roughness index, the trail surface and possible uses.

The map and summary information list the trail endpoints (either a city, street or more specific location), with suggested points from which to start and finish. Additional access points are marked on the maps and mentioned in the trail descriptions. The maps and descriptions also highlight available amenities, including parking and restrooms, as well as such area attractions as shops, services, museums, parks and stadiums. Trail length is listed in miles.

Each trail bears a roughness index rating from 1 to 3. A rating of 1 indicates a smooth, level surface that is accessible to users of all ages and abilities. A 2 rating means the surface may be loose and/or uneven and could pose a problem for road bikes and wheelchairs. A 3 rating suggests a rough surface that is only recommended for mountain bikers and hikers. Surfaces can range from asphalt or concrete to ballast, cinder, crushed stone, gravel, grass, dirt or sand. Where relevant, trail descriptions address alternating surface conditions.

All rail-trails are open to pedestrians, and most allow bicycles, except where noted in the trail summary or description. The summary also indicates wheelchair access. Other possible uses include inline skating, mountain biking, hiking, horseback riding, fishing and cross-country skiing. While most trails are off-limits to motor vehicles, some local trail organizations do allow ATVs and snowmobiles.

Trail descriptions themselves suggest an ideal itinerary for each route, including the best parking areas and access points, where to begin, your direction of travel, and any highlights along the way. The text notes any connecting or neighboring routes, with page numbers for the respective trail descriptions. Following each description are directions to the recommended trailheads.

Each trail description also lists a local contact (name, address, phone number and website) for further information. Be sure to call these trail managers or volunteer groups in advance for updates and current conditions.

Key to Map Icons

Parking

Drinking water

Bathrooms

Trail Use

Rail-trails are popular routes for a range of uses, often making them busy places to play. Trail etiquette applies. If passing other trail users on your bicycle, always try to pass on the left with an audible warning such as a bike-mounted bell or a polite but firm, "Passing on your left!" For your safety and that of other trail users, keep children and pets from straying into oncoming trail traffic. Keep dogs leashed, and supervise children until they can demonstrate proper behavior.

Cyclists and inline skaters should wear helmets, reflective clothing, and other safety gear, as some trails involve hazardous road crossings. It's also best to bring a flashlight or bike- or helmet-mounted light for tunnel passages or twilight excursions.

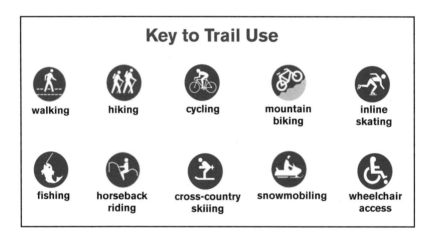

Key to Trail Use

walking   hiking   cycling   mountain biking   inline skating

fishing   horseback riding   cross-country skiing   snowmobiling   wheelchair access

Learn More

While *Rail-Trails Midwest: Great Lakes* is a helpful guide to available routes in the region, it wasn't feasible to list every rail-trail in New England, and new rail-trails spring up each year. To learn about additional rail-trails in your area or to plan a trip to an area beyond the scope of this book, log on to the Rails-to-Trails Conservancy home page (www.railstotrails.org) and click on the Find a Trail link. RTC's online database lists more than 1400 rail-trails nationwide, searchable by state, county, city, trail name, surface type, length, activity and/or keywords regarding your interest. A number of listings include photos and reviews from people who've already visited the trail.

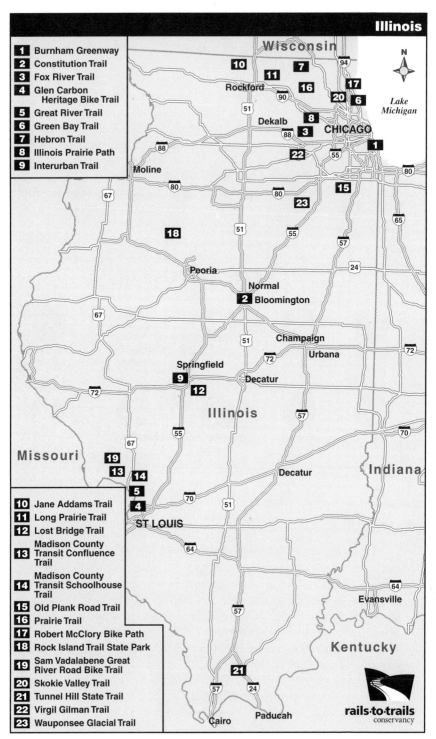

Illinois

1 Burnham Greenway
2 Constitution Trail
3 Fox River Trail
4 Glen Carbon Heritage Bike Trail
5 Great River Trail
6 Green Bay Trail
7 Hebron Trail
8 Illinois Prairie Path
9 Interurban Trail

10 Jane Addams Trail
11 Long Prairie Trail
12 Lost Bridge Trail
13 Madison County Transit Confluence Trail
14 Madison County Transit Schoolhouse Trail
15 Old Plank Road Trail
16 Prairie Trail
17 Robert McClory Bike Path
18 Rock Island Trail State Park
19 Sam Vadalabene Great River Road Bike Trail
20 Skokie Valley Trail
21 Tunnel Hill State Trail
22 Virgil Gilman Trail
23 Wauponsee Glacial Trail

Wisconsin

Rockford
Dekalb
CHICAGO
Lake Michigan
Moline
Peoria
Normal
Bloomington
Champaign
Urbana
Springfield
Decatur
Illinois
Missouri
ST LOUIS
Decatur
Indiana
Evansville
Kentucky
Paducah
Cairo

rails·to·trails
conservancy

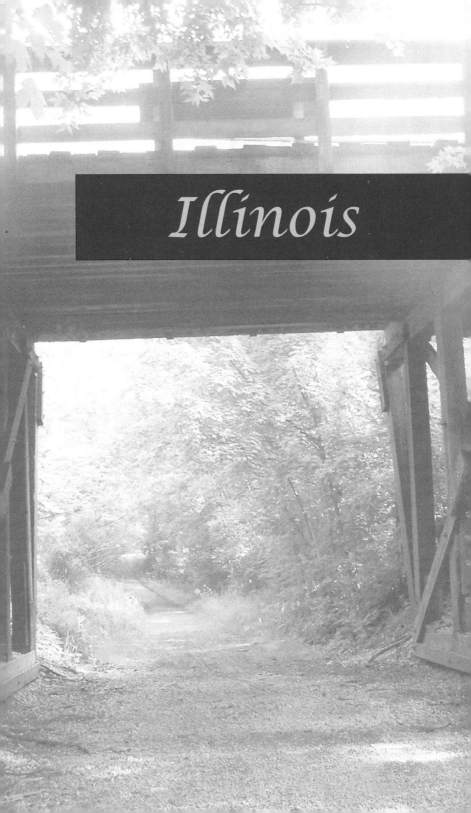

Illinois

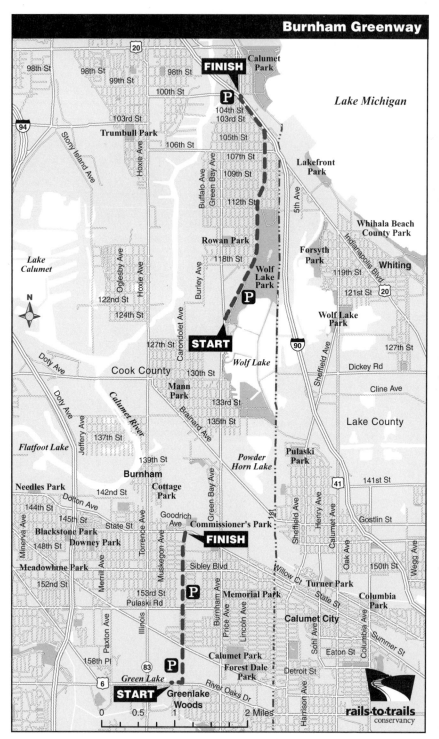

Burnham Greenway

Lake Michigan

Lake County

Cook County

rails·to·trails
conservancy

Burnham Greenway

The Burnham Greenway is composed of two trails—Burnham Greenway North and Burnham Greenway South—that run along a former railroad corridor between Chicago and Lansing, Illinois. There are plans to extend and connect these short sections, which will create 11 miles of trail through some of this urban environment's best natural areas. Until that point, however, it is best to treat these as two separate trips.

Burnham Greenway North stretches 2.75 miles from Wolf Lake to 104th St. The lake, which straddles the state line between Illinois and Indiana, has a parking area and playgrounds, as well as access to swimming, fishing and biking. Wolf Lake and other neighboring lakes are believed to be among the most biologically diverse places in the Midwest. Wolf Lake is home to the endangered lake sturgeon and the threatened banded killifish; and its wetlands are inhabited by three species of endangered heron, plus the rare yellow-headed blackbird. So impressive is this area that more than 150 experts in botany, zoology and related ecological fields gathered here to identify and record organisms living in the lake and surrounding forest, prairie and marshland. The undertaking revealed the extraordinary biodiversity of green pockets that have survived within the urban and industrial landscape south of Chicago.

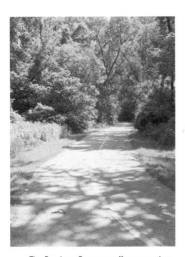

The Burnham Greenway offers more than just bicycling–birding, botany and other zoological pastimes are popular here.

Heading north from Wolf Lake, you will travel through a populated urban area where locals frequently use the path to walk or bike to and from grocery stores. It's a wonderful example of a path that doubles as a

Location
Cook County

Endpoints
Northern portion:
Wolf Lake to
104th Street in
Hegewisch

Southern portion:
Greenlake Woods
to Commissioner's
Park in Calumet
City

Mileage
5.25

**Roughness
Index**
1

Surface
Asphalt

neighborhood transportation corridor, with housing, restaurants and small grocery stores nearby. There are a few road crossings that require careful crossing, but all crossings are well marked.

Burnham Greenway South covers 2.5 miles between Greenlake Woods and Commissioner's Park. If you are arriving by car, start at Greenlake Woods, which has the only parking. The trail here is pleasant and well traveled, passing baseball fields and many neighborhoods. It ends at Commissioner's Park, which features a playground and skate park.

DIRECTIONS

To reach Wolf Lake (the Burnham Greenway North trailhead) just outside Hegewisch, IL, from Interstate 90 east/Interstate 94 east, take the exit for Indianapolis Blvd./US Highways 12/20/41 south and take a slight left on South Indianapolis Blvd./ US 12 E/ US 20 E/ US 41 south. Bear right at South Avenue B and turn right at East 106th Street. Turn left on South Avenue O, travel on South Avenue O for 2.4 miles, then turn left again at South Wolf Lake Avenue. Upon entering the park, turn left onto the first road that leads into the parking lot. The trailhead is on the left about a half mile ahead along the park road.

To reach Greenlake Woods (the Burnham Greenway South trailhead) west of Calumet City, from I-94 exit at US Route 6 and head east. Turn north on Torrence Avenue and then turn right into the trailhead parking lot.

Contact: Forest Preserve District of Cook County, Illinois
536 North Harlem Avenue
River Forest, IL 60305
(800) 870-3666
www.fpdcc.com/tier3.php?content_id=68&file=map_68i

Constitution Trail

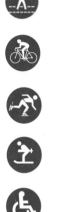

The Constitution Trail is so named because it was dedicated on the 200th birthday of the U.S. Constitution, September 17, 1987. Plans for the trail are as lofty as its name: The 5.4-mile asphalt trail is the north-south spine of a developing trail system covering 20-plus miles between the "twin cities" of Normal and Bloomington, Illinois. While this trail makes a great outing any time of year, take the locals' advice and try some cross-country skiing along the corridor in winter.

Begin your ride at the Atwood Wayside trailhead in Bloomington (the official beginning is 0.2 mile south at East Grove Street). This stretch of the trail is lined with trees and travels through well-kept Bloomington neighborhoods.

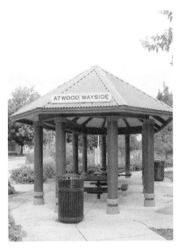

History and neighborhood convenience combine on the Constitution Trail.

Almost 2 miles into your journey, look for the Allers Wayside trailhead and signs for the 4.1-mile spur trail heading east. Along this commercial corridor are the Shoppes at College Hill and the corporate headquarters of State Farm Insurance. Tipton Trails Prairie Park, at mile 3 of the spur trail, features a fishing pond, basketball courts and a nature area with a large expanse of rare native prairie grassland. From the park, head north through a quiet neighborhood before entering a wonderful stretch shaded with a beautiful tree canopy. Cardinals, robins, mourning doves and golden finches flit through the treetops, while squirrels, butterflies and brightly colored wildflowers are visible closer to the ground.

Back on the main north-south trail from the Allers Wayside trailhead heading north again, the trail emerges

Location
McLean County

Endpoints
Atwood Wayside in Bloomington to Kerrick Road in Normal

Mileage
9.5 (including 4.1-mile East-West Spur)

Roughness Index
1

Surface
Asphalt

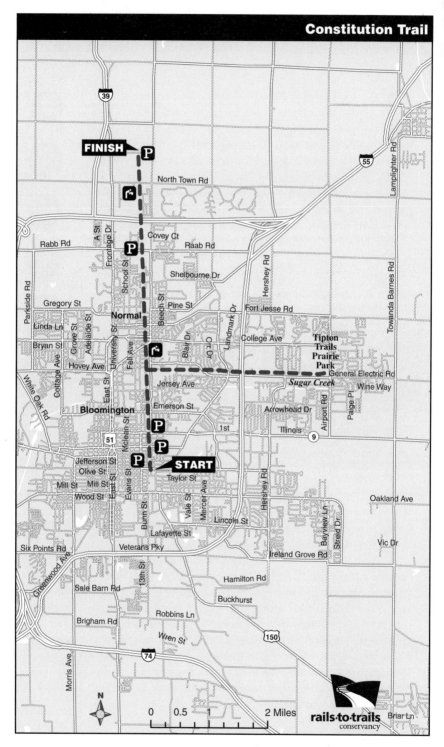

FINISH P

North Town Rd

P Covey Ct

Rabb Rd Raab Rd

A St

Frontage Dr

School St

Shelbourne Dr

Hershey Rd

Parkside Rd

Gregory St

Pine St

Beech St

Fort Jesse Rd

Towanda Barnes Rd

Lamplighter Rd

39

55

Normal

Linda Ln

Bryan St

Hovey Ave

Grove Ave

Adelaide St

Cottage Ave

White Oak Rd

Fell Ave

University Ave

East St

Blair Dr

Orr Dr

Landmark Dr

College Ave

Tipton Trails Prairie Park

General Electric Rd

Wine Way

Paige Pl

Airport Rd

Bloomington

Jersey Ave

Emerson St

Sugar Creek

Arrowhead Dr

51

McLean St

P

P

P **START**

1st

Illinois

9

Jefferson St

Olive St

Mill St Mill St

Wood St

East St

Evans St

Bunn St

Taylor St

Vale St

Mercer Ave

Hershey Rd

Lincoln St

Bayview Ln

Streid Dr

Oakland Ave

Vic Dr

Six Points Rd

Lafayette St

Veterans Pky

Ireland Grove Rd

Greenwood Ave

Morris Ave

13th St

Sale Barn Rd

Hamilton Rd

Buckhurst

Brigham Rd

Robbins Ln

Wren St

74

150

N

0   0.5   1   2 Miles

rails·to·trails
conservancy

Briar Ln

from the trees and enters the town of Normal right at the police station. Cross the active railroad tracks at the dedicated crossing and look for the downtown area on the right. Home to Illinois State University, Normal is a charming college town, and this area is full of colorful storefronts and hip eateries and pubs.

Leaving the quaint downtown, the rail-trail meanders through suburban neighborhoods and past larger housing complexes that appear to be rentals for the college crowd. Constitution Park sits on the east side of the trail, just under 4 miles from the start in Bloomington. A huge, open field dominates the area, which also features a playground, water fountain and parking lot. An interpretive sign commemorates the location of the historic Empire Machine Works. In 1870, William Flagg, a prominent early citizen, built his factory to produce mowers, reapers and other agricultural implements that he could easily ship out on the Illinois Central Gulf Railroad. In 1848, Flagg was involved in a lawsuit over patent rights and retained the services of a young lawyer from Springfield named Abraham Lincoln. In spite of his success in defending Flagg, Lincoln refused more than $10 for his services.

The final mile of Constitution Trail takes you under Interstate 55 and past a few more housing developments interspersed with some farm fields. There are also two gravel-processing facilities along this stretch. On the horizon, a row of large silos signals the northern trailhead and conclusion of the Constitution Trail at Kerrick Road.

DIRECTIONS

To reach the Atwood Wayside trailhead in Bloomington, take Interstate 55 to the West Market Street exit and head east for 1.8 miles. Turn right on North Main Street, go two blocks and then turn left onto East Jefferson Street. Turn left again on North Robinson Street and look for the trailhead on the right.

The Normal endpoint is accessed from I-55 by taking the North Main Street exit and driving north for 1 mile. Turn right onto Kerrick Road and look for the trailhead on the right after a half mile.

Contact: Town of Normal
Parks and Recreation
611 South Linden Street
Normal, IL 61761
(309) 454-9540
www.normal.org/Gov/ParksAndRec/Facilities/
ConstitutionTrail.asp

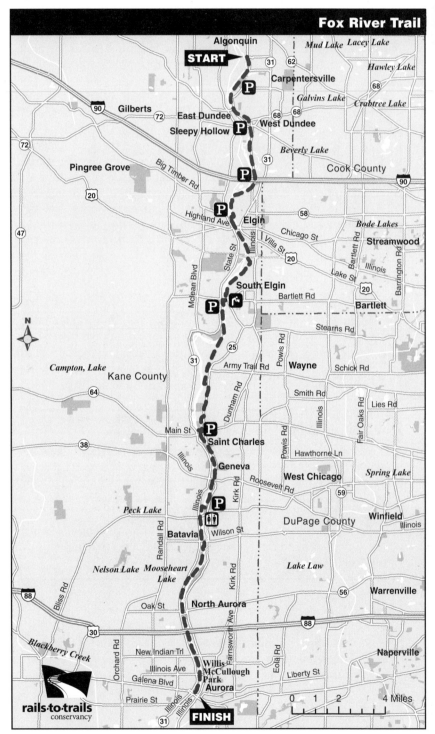

Fox River Trail

Fox River Trail

The Fox River Trail, built on the former Chicago, Aurora and Elgin Railroad line, features 32 miles of spectacular biking, hiking and cross-country skiing along the scenic Fox River. The path can be challenging here and there, but the extra effort is rewarded with some impressive scenery along the trail and in the charming small towns.

As the Fox River Trail meanders south from Algonquin, it closely follows its namesake river and at times there is a pathway on both sides of the river. While this is a nice amenity and there are plenty of signs along the trail, it also increases the potential for confusion; consult a map before heading out for a longer trip.

There is an upside to bouncing back and forth across the river—the bridges. These six bridges (some specifically for bicyclists and pedestrians) are perfect spots for taking photos. The bridges vary in form and function, from trestle to pedestrian, allowing the user to experience the Fox River from many different viewpoints.

Location
Kane and McHenry counties

Endpoints
Algonquin to Aurora

Mileage
32

Roughness Index
2

Surface
Asphalt, crushed stone and concrete

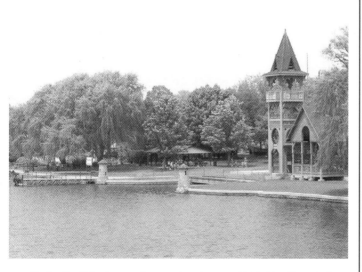

The Fox River Trail crisscrosses its namesake waterway, and is ideal for either a short walk or a serious bicycle ride.

15

The Fox River Trail draws a lot of visitors (including wildlife and birds like bald eagles, herons and woodpeckers) and many of the towns along the way feature good restaurants, cafes, bike shops and souvenir shops. (Best yet, no one will bat an eye at spandex bike shorts.)

Small parks that dot the landscape throughout the trail are perfect for small family picnics or a well-earned break. There are local fishing haunts, too. So whether for a leisurely stroll, a hard cycling workout, a picnic in the park or just a relaxing day of fishing, the Fox River Trail offers plenty of options to make your day.

DIRECTIONS

To reach the Algonquin trailhead from State Route 31, travel toward Algonquin and turn east on State Route 62. From there, head north on North Harrison Street. Look for the Riverfront Park parking lot approximately a quarter mile ahead.

To access the Aurora trailhead from Interstate 88 (Ronald Reagan Memorial Tollway), exit onto State Route 31 in Aurora and head south. Willis McCullough Park is on the left in approximately 1 mile.

Contact: Kane/Kendall Council of Mayors
41W011 Burlington Road
St. Charles, IL 60175
(630) 584-1170

Glen Carbon Heritage Bike Trail

The 11-mile Glen Carbon Heritage Trail (a.k.a. the MCT Heritage Bike Trail) is part of more than 85 miles of rail-trails managed by Madison County Transit (MCT), which also runs busses equipped with bike racks for passenger convenience. The feel of the trail is a mix of suburban and rural, and the many people on the trail demonstrate that diversity. Spandex-clad athletes whiz past people from the neighborhood out for a leisurely stroll. Children often use the trail to get to Citizen's Park or Miner Park. It serves as the heart of an integrated transportation system that can be a model for communities in Illinois and beyond.

The flat, chip-and-seal surface is good for jogging, so many runners signed up for the Chicago Marathon use the trail as a training ground. And if people-watching gets tiresome, there's always bird-watching; the best times to spot the more reclusive creatures are in the earliest hours of sunrise and at dusk.

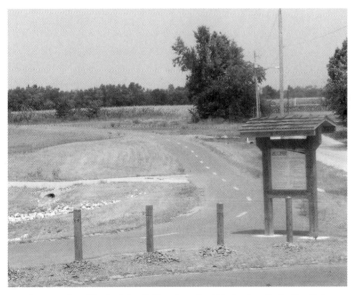

Long stretches of farmland dotted with parks and neighborhoods make the Glen Carbon Heritage Bike Trail a pleasure for all trail users.

Location
Madison County

Endpoints
Meridian Rd. and W. Main St. in Glen Carbon to Kuhn Station Road in Edwardsville

Mileage
11

Roughness Index
2

Surface
Asphalt and gravel

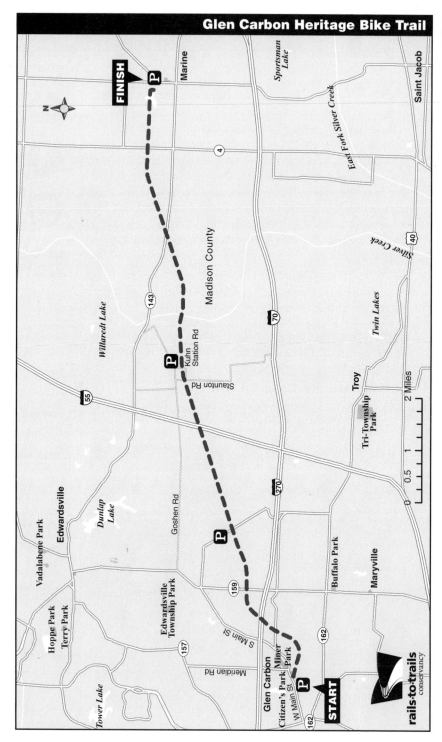

Glen Carbon Heritage Bike Trail

Start the trail in Citizen's Park in Old Town Glen Carbon, where you can also pick up the Nickel Plate Trail (page 101). Several blocks east is Miner Park, which has restrooms, and there are always trail maps and displays at the trailheads. Be sure to bring your camera for a photo of the 340-foot Silver Creek Railroad Trestle in town. The majority of the trail stretches out through farmland on either side, farmhouses dotting the landscape, especially as it approaches the Kuhn Station Road trailhead to the northeast.

DIRECTIONS

To the Glen Carbon trailhead at Meridian Road and West Main Street, take Interstate 255 to Glen Carbon, then follow Interstate 270 east for 2 miles. Next, take State Route 157 south for 1 mile and turn left on West Main Street. Look for the trailhead on the right in 1 mile.

To access the Kuhn Station Road trailhead, take Interstate 55 to State Route 143 and follow that east for 0.3 mile. Take Staunton Road south just over 0.75 mile and then follow Goshen Road another 0.75 mile east. Finally, turn south on Kuhn Station Road and look for the trailhead just ahead.

Contact: Madison County Transit
One Transit Way
Granite City, IL 62040
(618) 874-7433
www.mcttrails.org

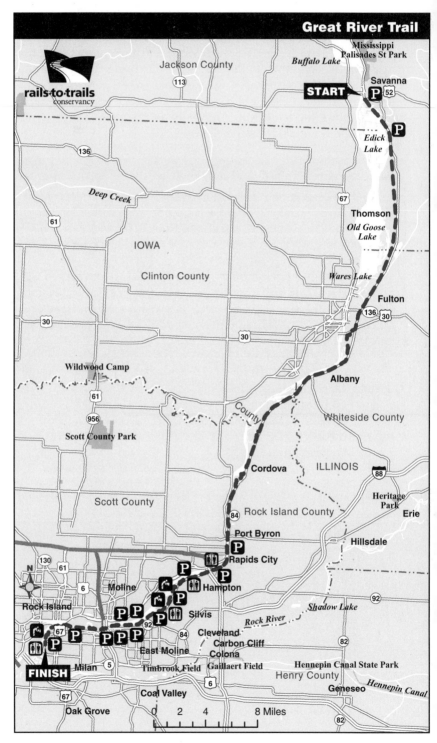

Great River Trail

Great River Trail

The Great River Trail is a breathtaking journey along 60 miles of the Mississippi River. The route is a mixture of paved rail-trail, small-town sidewalks, dedicated bike lanes on the street and a stretch of road shoulder along the Great River Road. The Great River Trail begins in Savanna and travels south through many small river towns with traditions still steeped in the quintessential culture of the Mississippi River. There are many opportunities for antiques, sumptuous catfish dinners and viewing the boats and barges. If you stop for a spell, the friendly locals will chat to you about the river and how it has . . . and hasn't . . . changed.

Starting in Savanna, in the north, the Great River Trail is a nicely paved, secluded trail, but soon after the two bridges south of town the trail ends and a 1.1-mile section of road begins. The road section is on State Route 84 and prone to heavy rush-hour traffic. Back on the trail you travel through a beautiful section that is sometimes

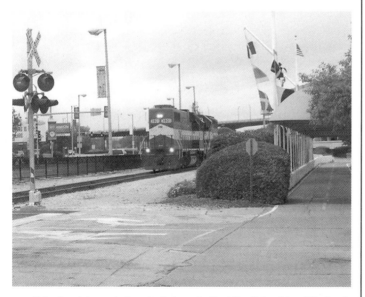

Railroads and rivers make for a classic duo on the Great River Trail as it hugs 60 miles of the mighty Mississippi.

Location
Carroll, Rock Island and Whiteside counties

Endpoints
Savanna to Rock Island

Mileage
60

Roughness Index
1

Surface
Asphalt and crushed stone

21

secluded and quiet and other times parallels Route 84. North of Albany, at mile 25, there is a second, short road section, again Route 84. The trail picks back up just south of town.

Through Cordova, near mile 35, the route follows quiet streets. Be sure to watch for the green bike signs that mark this section. After less than 2 miles, the rail-trail picks up again and closely follows Great River Road for 4 miles into Port Byron, a charming river town visible from the trail's riverbank course. Most of the corridor here is shared with an active rail line, offering a fine example of a safe rail-with-trail relationship.

Three miles downriver is Rapids City. You will see numerous blue herons, gulls and waterfowl in and over the water here. In town, there is a stone monument next to the trail offering a prayer from Native Americans for both the trail and its users.

After another 3 miles, the trail quickly cuts underneath Interstate 80, then through the town of Hampton, past lovely riverfront homes. A large public park on the south side of town has a great wooden playground and makes a wonderful rest stop. Shortly after leaving the park, the trail climbs to the top of a levee wall, where it stays for quite a while. Just ahead on the left, the John Deere manufacturing plant, with row after row of shining new farm equipment, marks the beginning of the trail's urban section. Traveling on top of the levee affords great views of the bridges over the river connecting the Quad Cities.

From Hampton, it is only 5.5 miles to the city of Moline. Follow the bike route signs to navigate through the city and return to the trail on the other side. The Quad City Convention and Visitors Bureau, right off the trail, is a pleasant place to stop. This stretch follows a slough of the river, across which you can see historic Rock Island. The Rock Island Arsenal (operated here by the U.S. Army) was a Union army prison camp during the Civil War.

Leaving downtown Moline, the trail stays up on the riverbank and crosses under the Centennial Bridge as you enter the city of Rock Island, whose industrial area dominates the landscape for most of the final 7.5 miles from Moline. When you ride into Sunset Park, the large marina and extensive river views provide a fitting end to this scenic trail.

DIRECTIONS

To reach the Savanna trailhead from State Route 84 (Great River Road), take US Route 50 (Chicago Street) west and turn left on Broderick Drive. The trailhead is on the left.

The Cordova trailhead is on Main Avenue. From State Route 84 (Great River Road) turn west on Main Avenue and then take a left on 11th Street. The parking lot is in the park on the right. You will not see the trail; from the parking lot, head left (north) on 11th Street, turn left again on 2nd Avenue, and then look for the green bike route signs.

To reach the Rock Island trailhead from Interstate 280, take State Route 93 (Centennial Expressway) to the Sunset Lane exit. Turn left on Sunset Lane and look for the trailhead on the right at Sunset Park.

Contact: Quad Cities Convention and Visitors Bureau
2021 River Drive
Moline, IL 61265
(800) 747-7800 or (563) 322-3911
www.visitquadcities.com/site/page.php?page_id=67&section=forvisitors

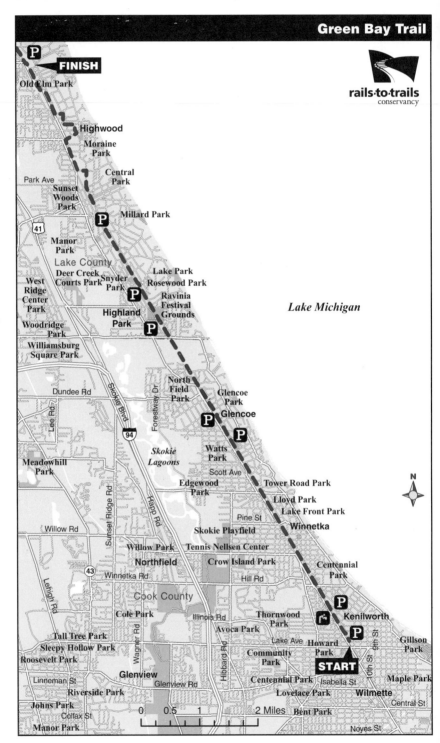

Green Bay Trail

rails·to·trails
conservancy

FINISH
Old Elm Park

Highwood
Moraine Park
Central Park
Park Ave
Sunset Woods Park
41
Millard Park
Manor Park
Lake County
Deer Creek Courts Park
West Ridge Center Park
Snyder Park
Lake Park
Rosewood Park
Ravinia Festival Grounds
Woodridge Park
Highland Park
Williamsburg Square Park

Lake Michigan

Dundee Rd
Skokie Blvd
Forestway Dr
North Field Park
Glencoe Park
Glencoe
94
Lee Rd
Meadowhill Park
Skokie Lagoons
Watts Park
Scott Ave
Edgewood Park
Tower Road Park
Lloyd Park
Lake Front Park
Winnetka
Sunset Ridge Rd
Happ Rd
Pine St
Willow Rd
Skokie Playfield
Willow Park
Tennis Nellsen Center
Northfield
Crow Island Park
Centennial Park
43
Winnetka Rd
Hill Rd
Lehigh Rd
Cook County
Cole Park
Illinois Rd
Thornwood Park
Kenilworth
Wagner Rd
Avoca Park
Tall Tree Park
Sleepy Hollow Park
Roosevelt Park
Hibbard Rd
Lake Ave
Howard Park
Community Park
START
Gillson Park
Linneman St
Glenview
Glenview Rd
Centennial Park
Isabella St
Maple Park
Riverside Park
Lovelace Park
Wilmette
Johns Park
Colfax St
Bent Park
Central Ave
Manor Park
Noyes St

N

0   0.5   1   2 Miles

Green Bay Trail

Stretching through North Shore towns such as Kenilworth, Winnetka, Highland Park and Lake Bluff, the 16-mile Green Bay Trail runs parallel to Chicago's Metra commuter rail line along a corridor flanked by restaurants, shops, community parks and beautiful homes. Because the rail-with-trail stays generally within a mile of Lake Michigan, you can take any number of on-road side trips for beachfront views of the lake.

The trail is suitable for even the youngest of riders, although the route does travel on some sidewalks and on a very small stretch of residential road in Kenilworth. In addition, the surface alternates between asphalt and crushed limestone.

This is a true multipurpose trail. Commuters take the trail to train stations along the way, bikes are allowed on the Metra in limited numbers (children under 16 must be accompanied by an adult when bringing a

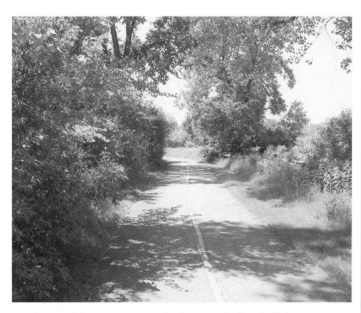

From your daily commute to your weekend excursion, the Green Bay Trail serves up pretty pathways, music venues and beaches.

Location
Cook and Lake counties

Endpoints
Wilmette to Highland Park

Mileage
16

Roughness Index
2

Surface
Asphalt and crushed stone

bicycle), and residents and tourists alike use the trail for exercise and car-free travel between communities.

From the southern trailhead in Wilmette, you immediately experience the fresh air and beachfront atmosphere that is comfortably juxtaposed with the business and commuter traffic. The trail itself, paved and very well maintained here, travels through upscale neighborhoods with well-manicured homes and lawns.

Nearing Highland Park, you may find people flocking to Ravinia, one of Chicagoland's best music venues. An open-air, covered pavilion features symphony, dance and pop concerts, while smaller indoors theaters showcase chamber music performances and dance recitals.

Yet another park at mile 8 has benches overlooking the trail. You may have just as much fun taking a break to watch the passers-by as you do traveling the trail itself.

By the time you reach the northern trailhead at St. John's Ave., you will appreciate the nearby restrooms, public telephones, playgrounds and parks built to service the rail line. Another bonus of the adjacent train: If you're too tired to do the return trip, you can easily hop on a Metra train back to the start of your trip.

DIRECTIONS

To get to the Wilmette trailhead, take Interstate 94 to Exit 34 (Lake Avenue) and head east for just over 2 miles to Green Bay Road. Head north on Green Bay and make an immediate right on Forest Avenue. You will see the trail crossing Forest Avenue, where there is limited parking. Additional parking can be found in any one of the many Metra parking lots that run parallel to the trail. These stations also offer restrooms, water fountains and telephones.

To access the Highland Park trailhead, take US Route 41 to Highland Park and head east on Deerfield Road. After about a half mile, turn left on Central Avenue and follow it for just over a half mile. Turn south on St. John's Avenue and continue for a quarter mile to the Metra parking lot on the right, which doubles as trail parking.

Contact: Northern Illinois Planning Commission
400 West Madison Street
Chicago, IL 60606
(312) 454-0400

Hebron Trail

Open to runners, walkers, bikers, horseback riders and equestrians, the rustic and rural Hebron Trail provides the perfect nature escape. (The trail does include a very small section of road that crosses an active rail line, but it is a lightly used county road. However, the tracks are a little bumpy, so it's best to dismount and walk over the tracks if you're on a bike.)

Only a couple miles from the Illinois-Wisconsin border, this route sees many users from both sides of the state line. Since the trail attracts many types of users, brush up on your trail etiquette and call out when passing equestrians, or if you are passing on snowmobiles.

Starting from Church Street, this quiet and peaceful trail cuts through the rural and heavily wooded outskirts of Hebron until the trees succumb to fields of corn and other local agriculture. Toward the trail's end, the trees begin to return, providing plenty of opportunities

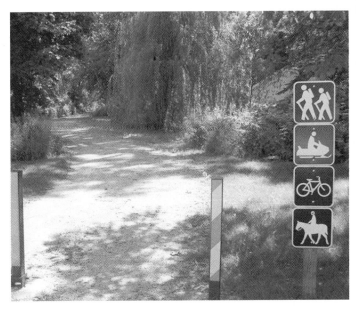

A trip on the Hebron Trail offers a quiet respite from the typical daily bustle.

Location
McHenry County

Endpoints
Church Street to
Burgett Road in
Hebron

Mileage
5.2

Roughness Index
2

Surface
Crushed stone
and gravel

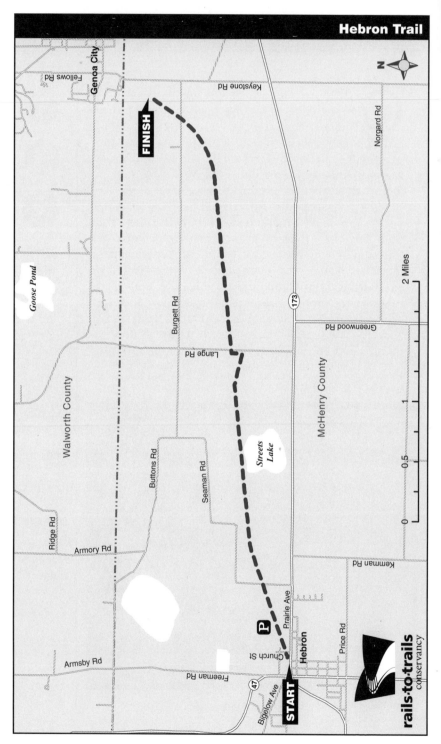

for enjoyment of the natural beauty, wildlife and birds of the tree-lined corridors.

Hikers along the trail may belong to the McHenry County Century Hikers Club, an organization that encourages people to get out and hike area trails and keep track of their mileage. When members reach 100 miles, they are officially recognized with a Century Club T-shirt. Members who log 1000 miles or more get their names on a plaque.

The corridor was originally the Kenosha Division Railroad. Spanning from Kenosha, Wisconsin, to Rockford, Illinois, the trains served as a lifeline to the outside world, hauling mail, newspapers and even milk. Out on this quiet trail, you can get a small glimpse of what life was like before cell phones, pagers and the predominance of the automobile. The Hebron Trail brings back the past while you enjoy this one-of-a-kind trail experience.

DIRECTIONS

To access the Church Street starting point, follow State Route 47 to the town of Hebron and turn east on State Route 173 (Maple Avenue). Take the first left onto Church Street and look for the trailhead parking on the right.

Contact: McHenry County Administrative Office
18410 US Highway 14
Woodstock, IL 60098
(815) 338-6223
www.mccdistrict.org/index.asp

Illinois Prairie Path

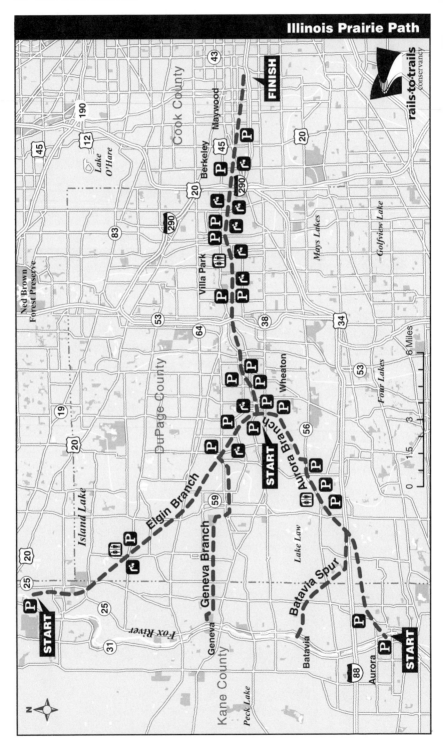

Illinois Prairie Path

The Illinois Prairie Path (IPP) is one of the country's first rail-trail conversions. It consists of five connected trail segments with three main branches that converge at Volunteer Park in Wheaton. The trail—totaling 61 miles—follows the historic path of the Chicago, Aurora and Elgin electric railroad. The railroad provided passenger service from western suburbs into downtown Chicago beginning in 1902. With the railroad in decline, many routes were transferred to bus service. The completion of the Eisenhower Expressway in 1955 spelled the end for this once-mighty railroad: By 1959 passenger and freight service on the line were finished.

A letter to the editor by noted naturalist May Theilgaard Watts in the *Chicago Tribune* in September 1963 argued for the novel idea of converting the abandoned corridor into a "footpath." That letter sparked the efforts a determined group of Chicagoans and gave rise to the unprecedented conversion of railroad to public trail.

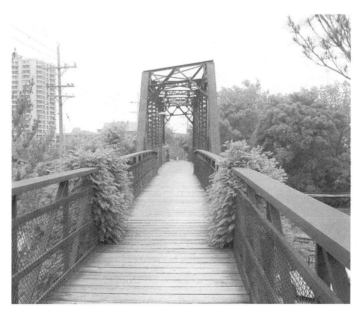

A granddaddy of the rail-trail movement, the Illinois Prairie Path is part of the Rail-Trail Hall of Fame and is one of the most popular paths in the country.

Location
Cook, DuPage and Kane counties

Endpoints
Maywood to spurs to Aurora, Batavia, Elgin and Geneva

Mileage
61

Roughness Index
2

Surface
Asphalt and crushed stone

MAIN BRANCH

The Illinois Prairie Path's 17-mile main branch is the most urban of its corridors. In Wheaton the main stem of the trail begins along city streets on bicycle-friendly extra-wide sidewalks. Distinct green trail markers shepherd you east through the lively shopping district of this college town. As you leave downtown Wheaton, Metra commuter rail tracks share the corridor, allowing you about 4 miles of rail-with-trail experience.

The trail maintains a distinct urban ambiance as it passes through the heart of the western suburbs. About midway to Maywood, in Villa Park, a lovely restored train depot houses great historical displays as well as a chance for water and restrooms. The trail ends as it hits 1st Avenue in Maywood. Parking is spotty at this end of the trail, so plan on a return trip where the *Chicago, Aurora and Elgin* once roared.

AURORA BRANCH

The 13-mile long Aurora Branch begins on the Fox River in Aurora, traveling north along the river and through a mix of commercial areas and older neighborhoods on a strip of asphalt. After 1 mile the surface changes to a hard-packed crushed stone that makes up the majority of the trail and the corridor leaves the river and moves northeast toward Wheaton. In another 5 miles, look for the trail connection on the left—this is the IPP's Batavia Branch. This 6-mile spur takes you west to the town of Batavia.

Your journey on the Aurora Branch is likely to be quiet, passing through woodlands, fields and under high-tension power lines. Wildlife finds refuge on the trail; most common are deer, rabbit and a plethora of bird species. Pay attention at just past mile 7 where the crossing at Winfield Road can be confusing. Other trails converge here, so look for the green IPP marker directly across Winfield Road.

ELGIN BRANCH

The Elgin Branch of the IPP is the 14-mile northern segment between Elgin and Volunteer Park in Wheaton. The surface of the trail is almost entirely a hard-packed crushed stone. Heading southeast from the Elgin trailhead, you immediately plunge into a lush, rural atmosphere of farm fields and pockets of trees. Near mile 4 in Wayne, between Army Trail Road and Smith Road, a steep hill climb will give pause to youngsters and road bicyclists and is not advisable for wheelchair users.

Upon cresting this hill, it is a pleasant 4-mile ride through a mixture of woodland forest and residential development to Prince Crossing Road, where the IPP connects with the 11.5-mile Great Western Trail at the trailhead facility. This trail meets up with the IPP again in Villa Park along the Main Branch between Wheaton and Maywood. Another 3 miles through similar terrain brings you to the connection with the Geneva Spur of the IPP, on the west side of the trail at Geneva Road. The spur travels 11 miles west to the elegant Chicago suburb of Geneva.

Well-manicured neighborhoods soon indicate your arrival in the town of Wheaton. Just when you think you have left the trail's remoteness behind, the Lincoln Marsh Natural Area affords an excellent bucolic diversion. With multiple overlooks and interpretive signs, the marsh presents the perfect finishing touch to a wonderful 14-mile trip. In less than 1 mile, after spanning an impressive bridge over two city streets and three active rail lines, you arrive at Volunteer Park.

DIRECTIONS

Access the Aurora trailhead by taking Interstate 88 to Farnsworth Avenue South.Go 1.1 miles. Turn right on Indian Trail, and after 1.5 miles turn left on Aurora Avenue for just under 1 mile. Take a right onto Illinois Avenue and the trailhead is on the right just before the Fox River.

To reach the Maywood endpoint from Interstate 290, take 1st Avenue North. The trail is about 0.3 mile north on the left between Quincy and Wilcox Streets. There is no parking at this trailhead.

To reach the Wheaton trailhead, take Interstate 355 to Roosevelt Road. Go west 3.6 miles. Turn right on West Street and go 0.4 mile. Make a left onto Liberty Drive. The trailhead is on the right just past a parking garage. Park on the street or in the garage.

The Elgin trailhead is on Raymond Street in Elgin. From I-90 take the State Street exit south for 2.7 miles. Turn left onto National Street and go just under a half mile then turn right onto Raymond Street. The trailhead is about 1.3 miles ahead on the right between Purify Drive and Riverview Drive.

Contact: Illinois Prairie Path
P.O. Box 1086
Wheaton, IL 60189
(630) 752-0120
www.ipp.org

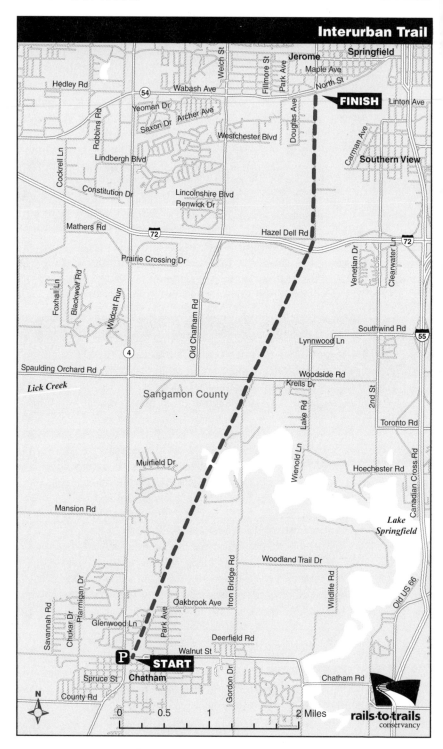

Interurban Trail

The paved 5-mile Interurban Trail, which travels north from Chatham to Illinois's state capital of Springfield along the old interurban electric rail line, provides a pleasant mix of urban and rural scenery. The Interurban is a wonderful example of a rail-with-trail, where train and trail traffic share the corridor's use. The trail serves as a great commuter route for people heading into and out of Springfield—home to more than 110,000 residents—from Chatham and surrounding communities.

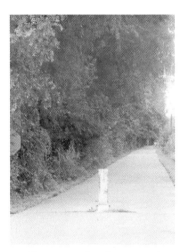

Sharing its corridor with an active rail line, the Interurban Trail is a rail-with-trail that pleasantly balances both form and function.

You will travel through standard suburban surroundings, but a certain amount of serenity not found in the suburbs prevails along this trail. Just north of Chatham, the trail skirts a paved golf cart path as it winds through the manicured greens and fairways of a beautiful golf course.

Only a quarter mile beyond the golf course is the true highlight of the Interurban Trail—Lake Springfield. The lake is visible from the Interurban, but don't be fooled by the terrain. What looks like a small amount of water from ground level is actually a vast, 4,200-acre reservoir that supplies water to residents of Springfield and surrounding areas all year.

After Lake Springfield, the trail offers views of the rural landscape dominated by fields of corn, though this setting is fleeting. Interstate 72 looms ahead, reminding you of the city yet to come, and as the trail comes to a close in Springfield, people and neighborhoods become more prevalent. As a small oasis from the bustle of

Location
Sangamon County

Endpoints
Chatham to Springfield

Mileage
5

Roughness Index
1

Surface
Asphalt

suburban and city life, the Interurban Trail is exactly the kind of useful and pleasant link you expect from a rail-trail.

DIRECTIONS

To access the Chatham trailhead from Interstate 72, take State Route 4 south for approximately 4 miles to Chatham. In Chatham, head east on Walnut Street. There is no official trail parking lot, but there are plenty of free parking spots off of Walnut. The trailhead is on the left, just past the Post Office.

To reach the Springfield trailhead from I-55, head west on East Stanford Avenue for about a mile to South Macarthur Blvd. Turn south on South Macarthur and you will dead-end into the parking lot for the trail.

Contact: City of Springfield
2500 South Eleventh Street
Springfield, IL 62703
(217) 544-1751
www.springfieldparks.org

Jane Addams Trail

Stretching almost 16.4 miles from Freeport, Illinois, north to the Wisconsin state line, the Jane Addams Trail is a natural wonder. Expect to see birds and wild animals—from exotic aerial hunters such as owls and hawks to run-of-the-mill squirrels and deer. The trail is closed every fall during deer-hunting season and snowmobiling is allowed when there are at least 4 inches of snow on the trail. (Winter users are encouraged to wear bright-colored clothing so they are visible to snowmobilers.)

The trail is named for the renowned humanitarian, reformer, and Nobel Peace Prize winner who grew up in Cedarville, less than 2 miles from the trail. The home Jane Addams was raised in and her gravesite can be visited in Cedarville.

Starting in Freeport, the crushed limestone trail enters a heavily wooded area that supports a wide variety of trees and birds—and likely some school groups as

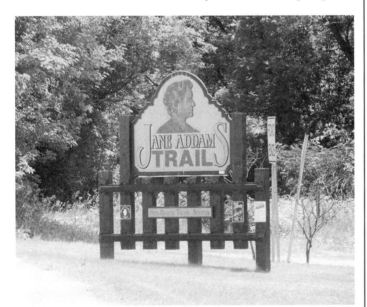

The Jane Addams Trail honors a local Nobel Peace Prize winner, and awards trail users with a nature-filled trail experience.

Location
Stephenson County (IL) and Green County (WI)

Endpoints
Fairview Rd. in Freeport to Richland Creek trailhead in Orangeville

Mileage
16.4

Roughness Index
2

Surface
Crushed stone

37

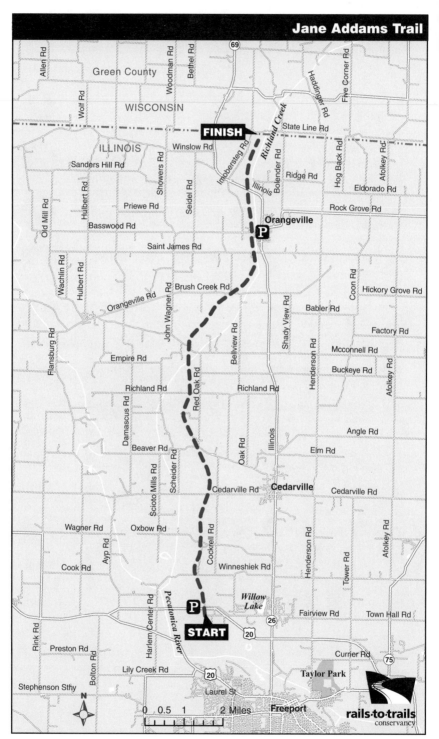

well. The natural attractions make for popular educational field trips. (Fortunately, the parking lot in Freeport can easily accommodate the school buses.)

As you travel from Freeport to Orangeville, you enjoy many nice views of some jutting rock sides and local creeks. These vistas are peppered amongst the other wooded areas and more common agricultural fields that predominate the landscape.

In the town of Orangeville, the Richland Creek trailhead provides a quiet and convenient place to end your trip. The location features a covered shelter and nearby gas station with refreshments. If you brought your camera, be sure to get a photo near the Orangeville sign to commemorate your trip.

The official end of the trail is at the Illinois–Wisconsin state line, but it is easy to miss, so pay close attention if you need to turn around at the border. The line is very close to a small, rural road leading to a quaint family farm on the left. At that road crossing, on the right side of the trail, there is a sign welcoming visitors to Illinois and the Jane Addams Trail; this is the state line.

Although the trail ends less than 3 miles north of Orangeville, your adventure can continue on Wisconsin's Southwest Commuter Path (page 357) and the 50-plus miles of rail-trail that lead to Madison.

DIRECTIONS

To access the southern trailhead in Freeport, follow State Route 26 north from US Route 20. Turn west on Fairview Road and follow it all the way to the trailhead on the left.

To access the Richland Creek trailhead in Orangeville, from State Route 26, turn right on Orangeville Road/ East 2nd Street. The trailhead is on the left at the large white shelter.

Contact: Freeport Convention and Visitors Bureau
4596 US Route 20 East
Freeport, IL 61032
(800) 369-2955
www.janeaddamstrail.com

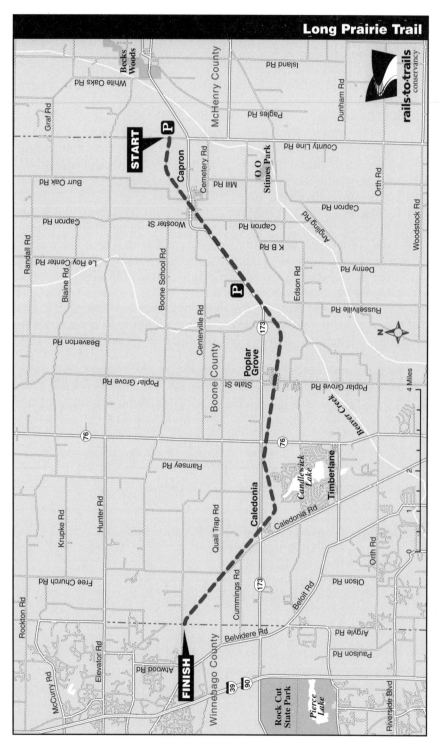

Long Prairie Trail

The Long Prairie Trail began life as a section of the Kenosha Division Rail Line in the 1850s, when most small communities in northern Illinois and southern Wisconsin were serviced by the crisscrossing tracks of the "KD" Line as it traveled from Kenosha to Rockford, Illinois. The line offered passenger service and also hauled an enormous amount of milk and ice from the dairies and lakes along the route.

Today the trail is pure prairie and legend has it the railroad gets all the credit. For years, rail cars sparked periodic blazes along the grasslands adjacent to the right-of-way. However, the native swaths of prairie grassland along the corridor adapted easily and the fires helped in their preservation.

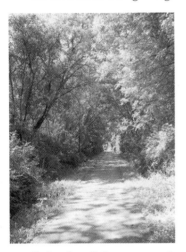

The Long Prairie Trail's name sums up the trail experience: a lovely, gently rolling and uninterrupted journey through classic prairie land.

The small villages of Capron, Poplar Grove and Caledonia are anchored by this beautiful, paved rail-trail. Starting near the town of Capron at the McHenry–Boone County Line trailhead on County Line Road, you immediately encounter an interpretive sign detailing the Potawatomi Indians' history in the area. There are many interpretive signs along the trail, with information ranging from area history to flora and fauna identification.

Traveling west, you are parallel to Illinois Route 173 for close to 2.5 miles, with immaculate and large farms providing the scenic backdrop. The trail is located in one of the most rural areas of Boone County, through open countryside, small farms and gently rolling hills that are periodically obscured by stands of trees that create a tunnel of growth around the corridor. On sunny

Location
Boone and Winnebago counties

Endpoints
County Line Road near Capron to Wyman School Road, east of Roscoe

Mileage
14.5

Roughness Index
1

Surface
Asphalt

days, you will be thankful for the shade. The trail eventually breaks from the woods and enters grasslands across which are gently rolling hills and small farms.

The next stop on the trail is Caledonia, a quaint village with well-kept streets and the kind of idyllic atmosphere that would make Norman Rockwell feel at home. Leaving the village, the trail continues another 3.75 quiet miles through forest and fields before ending at Wyman School Road. The trail's end is unceremonious: There are no facilities and no parking here. For that you'll have to head back to Caledonia—and enjoy the passing countryside one more time.

DIRECTIONS

Each village has trail parking and access.

To reach the County Line Road trailhead near Capron from Interstate 90, take US Highway 20 (Grant Highway) north for approximately 10 miles to Marengo. Turn right onto State Street (County Road 23) and go north for 10 miles. Turn left onto South Division Street (US Highway 14) and drive for just over a mile. Turn left on Brink Street (County Road 173), go 5 miles and then turn right on County Line Road. The trailhead is a half mile ahead on the left.

To reach the Randolph Street trailhead (3.75 miles before the trail's end at Wyman School Road) in Caledonia, take Interstate 90 to Riverside Blvd. and go east for 1.25 miles. Turn left onto Argyle Road and go north for 2.8 miles. Turn left onto Belvidere Road. After 0.75 mile, turn right onto West Lane Road (County Road 173) and continue for 2.4 miles. Turn right onto Caledonia Road and go 0.4 mile. Turn left on Randolph Street and look for the trailhead in two blocks.

Contact: Boone County Conservation District
603 Appleton Road
Belvidere, IL 61008
(815) 547-5432
www.boonecountyconservationdistrict.org/
longprairie.htm

Lost Bridge Trail

T he Lost Bridge Trail, jointly managed by the Springfield Park District and the village of Rochester, is one of the area's earliest and most popular multiuse trails—even for locals taking a weekday break on their lunch hour.

Well-maintained, the trail's starting point is located behind the Illinois Department of Transportation building in Springfield. This portion of the trail is not actually on a former rail corridor, but wraps partway around a beautifully landscaped and tree-lined lake near the complex.

At the lake's southwest end, the trail joins the former railroad corridor—an obvious change, as the trail becomes straight and flat as it travels through a dense tree canopy. Almost immediately, you reach a clearing and pass under Interstate 55, then plunge back into the forest. The heavy vegetation along the route makes it easy to forget how closely the trail parallels busy Route 29.

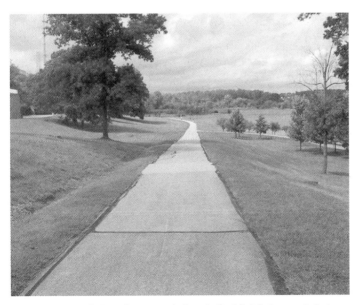

The Lost Bridge Trail actually sports two bridges; the South Fork Bridge in particular is a nod to railroad history with its trestle-style span.

Location
Sangamon County

Endpoints
Reilly Drive in
Springfield to
Walnut Street in
Rochester

Mileage
5

**Roughness
Index**
1

Surface
Asphalt

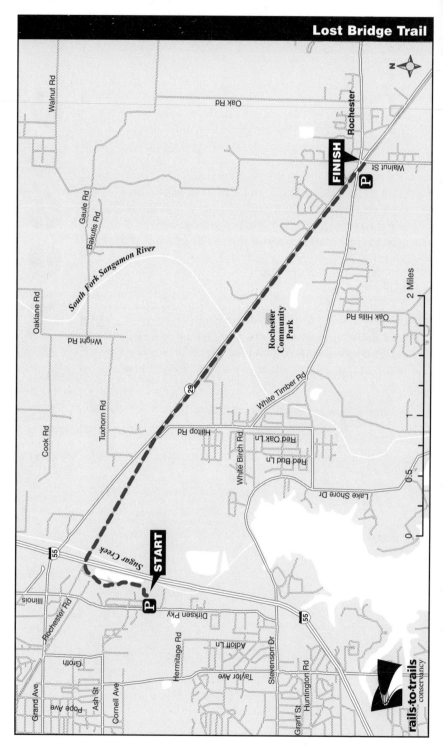

Lost Bridge Trail

Just beyond a mile from the start, the trail crosses charming Sugar Creek Bridge, which offers great views of Sugar Creek and the lush vegetation hugging its banks.

At mile 2, the trail passes beneath Hilltop Road and at mile 3 it reaches the South Fork Bridge over the South Fork of the Sangamon River. This old trestle-style span is another important remnant of the trail's railroading history; its excellent condition today is evidence of the remarkable engineering and artistry it took to build the structure. After the bridge, look closely for a paved trail connector on the south side that gives you the option of making a quick loop through Rochester Community Park.

For the final 2 miles after South Fork Bridge to the trail's end in Rochester, you pass through a short stand of trees before the landscape opens into some beautifully manicured grass fields behind one of Rochester's school facilities.

The trail may one day extend southeast from its terminus at Walnut Road to the towns of Taylorville and Pana. Until then, you must be content to walk, ride, roll, run, skate or ski back to Springfield on this suburban rail-trail gem.

DIRECTIONS

To access the Springfield trailhead on Reilly Drive, take Interstate 55 to Route 29 (South Grand Ave. east) and head west for a half mile. Turn left on South 31st Street (Dirksen Parkway) and go about 1 mile. Turn left on Reilly Drive and look for the trailhead at the far end of the parking lot.

To reach the Rochester trailhead, take Interstate 55 to Route 29 (South Grand Avenue east) and head east for 4 miles. Turn right on Walnut Street and look for the trailhead directly on the right.

Contact: Springfield Parks
2500 South 11th St
Springfield, IL 62703
(217) 544-1751
www.springfieldparks.org

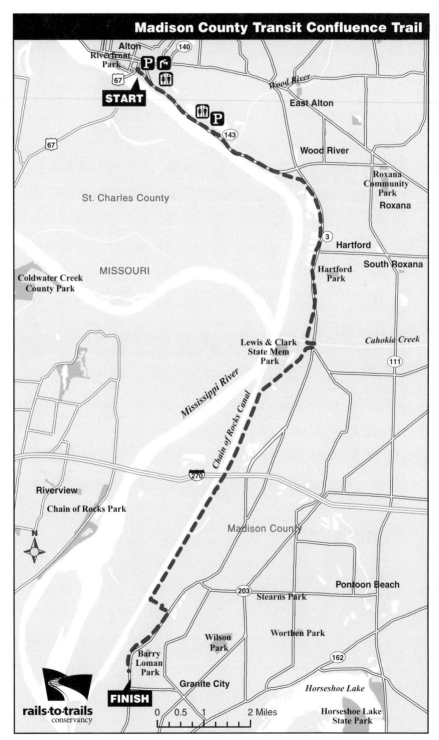

Madison County Transit Confluence Trail

Madison County Transit Confluence Trail

Bring your camera to the Madison County Transit Confluence Trail. Part of Illinois's Madison County Transit (MCT) bikeways network, this trail is a photographic patchwork of rivers, bridges, waterfront wildlife and industrial cityscape. The trail starts at Russell Commons Park in Alton and curves south, mostly along the Mississippi River levee to Granite City, offering spectacular views along the way. It is perfect for walking or biking, with a smooth trail surface that alternates between asphalt and chip-and-seal and some limestone sections.

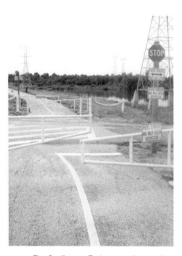

The Confluence Trail is one of several in the Madison County Transit system; this one takes you to the historic Chain of Rocks Bridge—exclusive to pedestrians and bicyclists.

Leaving the town of Alton, the trail maintains an elevated position so that you will be able to see the highway on your left and the river (and the state of Missouri beyond that) on the right. Heading south, after 1.5 miles, look for the Skinney Island facility, which has locks and a dam and offers great opportunities for taking photos. Soon after this, you arrive at the Amoco facility with its series of five gates that force cyclists to dismount and walk through them. There are also small hills associated with each of these gates. Be prepared to mount your bike and immediately pedal up the incline.

In the town of Hartford, the Lewis and Clark Confluence Tower appears along the left side of the trail, about 7.5 miles south of Alton and 0.75 mile from the Lewis and Clark Museum. The observation decks, historical displays and museum make for a great diversion.

Location
Madison County

Endpoints
Russell Commons Park in Alton to W. 20th Sreet in Granite City

Mileage
18.5

Roughness Index
2

Surface
Asphalt

In Granite City, the MCT on-road connector takes you along Highway 3 for 3 miles west to the historic Chain of Rocks Bridge. Today, the bridge is reserved exclusively for pedestrians, bicyclists and skaters. Historically, however, this bridge served as the Route 66 connection between Illinois and Missouri. The unique St. Louis skyline welcomes you on the far end of the 1-mile bridge.

Back on the trail heading away from the Lewis and Clark Interpretive Center, you come to the limestone-covered portion of the trail that parallels the Chain of Rocks Canal for 6.5 miles. Turn left on Bauer Road and continue for a quarter mile until the trail picks back up again.

For the next 1.75 miles, the trail becomes more urban and ends abruptly at the intersection of Illinois Route 3 and West 20th Street. There is no official trailhead or parking here.

This trail has many connections on its northern end, including a link to the 4-mile Alton Trail and a signed, mostly city street route to Piasa Park, where it meets the Vadalabene Bike Trail. Also from the northern section, you can cross the Clark Bridge in Alton. In Hartford, the trail meets New Poag Road, which offers a 5-mile connection east to the Bluff Trail.

DIRECTIONS

To access the start at Russell Commons Park in Alton, take State Route 140 west and turn left on Washington Avenue. After 1.3 miles, turn right on East Broadway Street and continue for 0.3 mile. Make a quick left onto the Broadway Connector and then travel for 0.25 mile to Landmarks Boulevard and turn right. After another 0.25 mile, turn left on Ridge Street and follow the curving road to the left. The trailhead is on the left in 0.3 mile.

To reach the East Alton trailhead on New Poag Road, take State Route 3 to East Alton and then travel east on New Poag Road/State Route 203. The trailhead is on the left.

Parking and trail access are also available at the Lewis and Clark Interpretive Center in Hartford and on both the Illinois and Missouri sides of the Chain of Rocks Bridge.

Contact: Madison County Trails
c/o Madison County Transit
One Transit Way
Granite City, IL 62040
(618) 874-7433
www.mcttrails.org

Madison County Transit Schoolhouse Trail

The Madison County Transit (MCT) Schoolhouse Trail is part of this county's premier, 85-mile system of urban and suburban trails—many of which are former railroad corridors and all of which are linked with public transit.

The trail begins at the southwest corner of Horseshoe Lake State Park at Harrison Street in Madison. The smooth asphalt path travels east over Route 203 via a trail bridge and then onto the old railroad corridor. For a few miles, the trail shares this route with a utility corridor and passes heavily industrial business areas. For this first part of the journey, Horseshoe Lake remains hidden from view to the southeast. But be patient. At mile 4, the lake bursts into view when the trail emerges from a pocket of trees. The lake offers excellent bird-watching. In late summer, the lake's southern portion is drained, drawing snowy egrets and great blue herons to feast on clams and snails. Just after the lake comes into

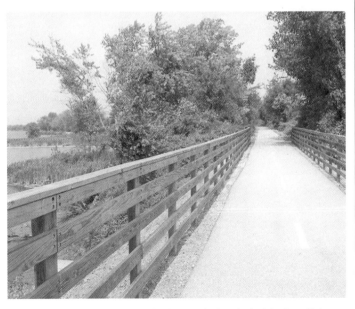

Broad lake views and dips into neighborhood woodlands make the Schoolhouse Trail a must-see of the Madison County Transit system.

Location
Madison County

Endpoints
Madison to Troy

Mileage
15.25

Roughness Index
1

Surface
Asphalt

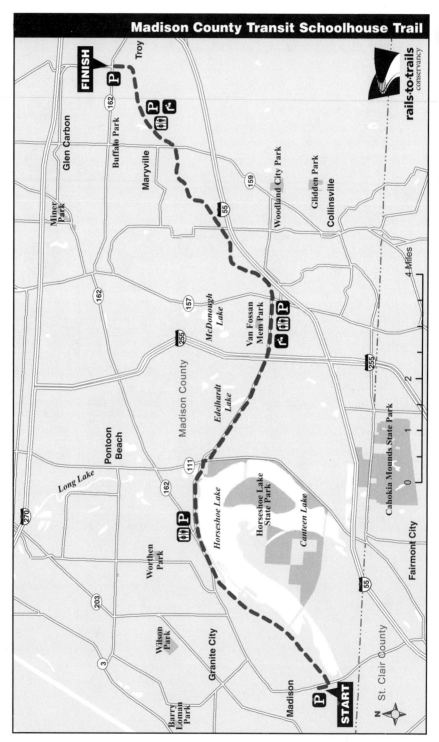

Madison County Transit Schoolhouse Trail

view, watch for a trail connection on the left. This is the MCT Nature Trail. Take this route if you wish to take an off-shoot trip 11 miles to the town of Edwardsville.

About 1 mile farther along, the trail leaves Horseshoe's shoreline and moves to a corridor parallel to Lake Drive. You soon cross Route 111 and the trail takes on a very rural feel, with vast farm fields on both sides. Interstate 55 looms ahead and crossing under it brings you to the outskirts of Collinsville. Just when it seems like a more urban environment will prevail, the trail plunges you into wonderful woodlands behind very tidy neighborhoods. It is very quiet through the hardwoods, disguising your proximity to a major interstate. The trees occasionally open to offer glimpses of the open fields that mark the landscape beyond the forest.

The town of Maryville almost sneaks by, but you will want to catch the respite offered by Drost Park on the trail's left. From here, you have just 1.6 more miles to the trailhead at Route 162. This trail's end marks the beginning of the MCT Goshen Trail, which offers 7 more miles of pavement into the town of Edwardsville.

DIRECTIONS

The Madison trailhead can be accessed from Interstate 55 by taking Route 203 north for 2.3 miles. Turn left onto Harrison Street; the trailhead is on the left.

For the trailhead in Troy, take Interstate 55 to Route 162 west. The trailhead is just over 1 mile ahead on the left, just past Kennedy Drive.

Contact: Madison County Trails
c/o Madison County Transit
One Transit Way
Granite City, IL 62040
(618) 874-7433
www.mcttrails.org

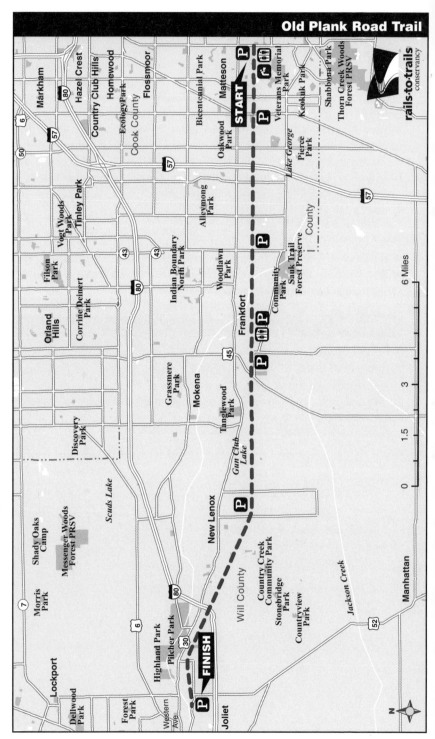

Old Plank Road Trail

The 21-mile Old Plank Road Trail travels over the original Michigan Central Rail Road (MCRR) line, a railroad started about 1850 that ran from Lake Station in East Gary to Joliet. Nicknamed the "Joliet Cut-Off" since it enabled trains to skip Chicago, the line was among the first to link to New York and Boston.

The trail starts in Park Forest and travels west, alternating between secluded, quiet sections and suburbs. The trail continues through Richton Park, Frankfort, New Lenox and finally ends on the western edge of Joliet. At mile 9.75, the trail reaches the award-winning Arrowhead suspension bridge, which takes you over Route 45.

You can almost feel the trail's history as you travel down the corridor. Originally a Native American transportation corridor, the route was used occasionally by traders, trappers and even missionaries. Later, European settlers used the pathway to find their own homesteads.

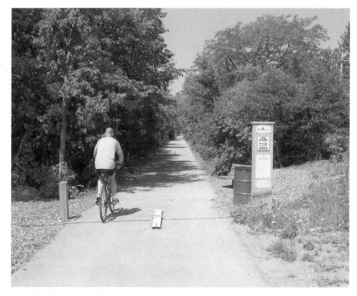

The Old Plank Road Trail has a long transportation history: from a Native American pathway and route for homesteaders, to a rail and finally a trail for bicyclists and walkers.

Location
Cook and Will counties

Endpoints
Western Avenue in Park Forest to S. Park Road in Joliet

Mileage
21

Roughness Index
1

Surface
Asphalt

Today, the oncoming traffic is more likely to be a pack of retired cyclists zipping by, or maybe a mom with a stroller.

Many areas along the trail have never been cultivated or developed. The Old Plank Road Trail, nearby nature preserve and other areas are as they were hundreds of years ago. The corridor remains one of the jewels of the area because of the ability and even sheer luck that allowed it to maintain its untouched characteristics.

DIRECTIONS

To reach the Western Avenue trailhead in Park Forest, take US Route 30 to the Western Avenue exit and follow Western Avenue south for about a half mile. The trailhead is on the right.

To reach the Joliet trailhead, take Interstate 80 to the east side of Joliet and exit at South Briggs Street. Follow South Briggs north to East Washington Street and travel east. Turn north on South Park Road. The trailhead is on the right, before the baseball diamonds.

Contact: Forest Preserve District of Will County
17540 West Laraway Road
Joliet, IL 60433
(815) 727-8700
www.oprt.org/index.html

Prairie Trail

The Prairie Trail—not to be confused with the Illinois Prairie Path—is a 28-mile route starting just 0.8 mile from the Wisconsin–Illinois border in Genoa City, Wisconsin, and ending in Algonquin, Illinois. The trail is a beautiful piece of nature tucked away in rural Illinois but still in the backyard of the greater Chicago area.

Before you head off, however, keep in mind that preparation is key for an excursion on this trail. Open spaces provide little shade and there are long stretches between water sources. Be sure to fill your water bottles and pack sunscreen if you're traveling in the warmer months. Throw in your camera, too, and capture this picturesque trail while enjoying a real outdoor adventure.

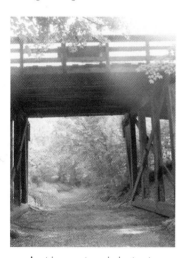

A quick escape to rural adventure is within easy reach on the Prairie Trail—not to be confused with the Illinois Prairie Path.

As the trail heads south from Genoa City, you'll enjoy serene travel on the crushed stone path. Several bridges and interpretive signs mark your journey. Nearly 8 miles in, the surface switches to smooth asphalt and the next 9 miles are enjoyably straightforward and relaxing.

Near mile 17, the trail becomes hilly—very hilly compared to the surrounding area. For the next 1.5 miles through Sterne's Woods, the trail leaves the rail corridor, undulating and twisting back and forth—a stretch that is likely to get your heart pumping if you're on a bike. The payoff is rich, however, because after the curvy, hilly challenge, you'll come to shining Crystal Lake, where there's a beach and swimming and picnic areas to spend a fun family day.

Location
Walworth (WI) and Algonquin (IL) counties

Endpoints
Genoa City, WI, to Algonquin, IL

Mileage
28

Roughness Index
2

Surface
Asphalt, dirt and crushed stone

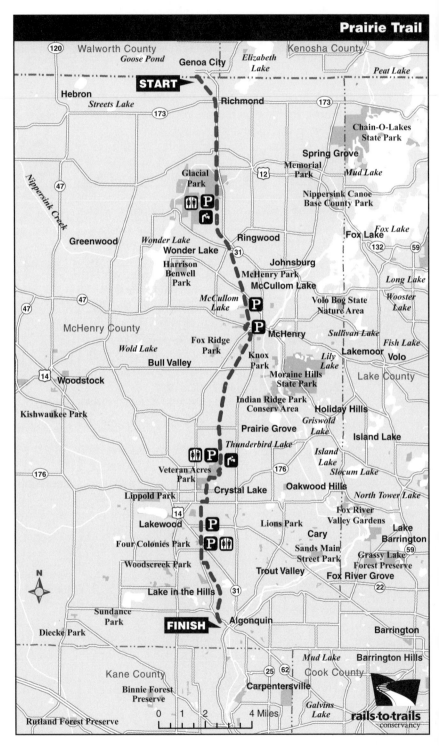

Prairie Trail

Walworth County · Kenosha County
(120)
Goose Pond · Genoa City · Elizabeth Lake · Peat Lake
START · Richmond · (173)
Hebron · Streets Lake · (173) · Chain-O-Lakes State Park
Spring Grove · Memorial Park · Mud Lake
Glacial Park · (12) · Nippersink Canoe Base County Park
(47) · Greenwood · Wonder Lake · Ringwood · Fox Lake
Nippersink Creek · Wonder Lake · (31) · Fox Lake · (132) · (59)
Harrison Benwell Park · Johnsburg · Long Lake
McHenry Park · Wooster Lake
(47) · McCullom Lake · McCullom Lake · Volo Bog State Nature Area
(47) · McHenry County · McHenry · Sullivan Lake · Fish Lake
Wold Lake · Fox Ridge Park · Lakemoor · Volo
Bull Valley · Knox Park · Lily Lake · Lake County
(14) · Woodstock · Moraine Hills State Park
Kishwaukee Park · Indian Ridge Park Conserv Area · Holiday Hills
Prairie Grove · Griswold Lake · Island Lake
Thunderbird Lake · Island Lake · Slocum Lake
Veteran Acres Park · (176)
(176) · Lippold Park · Crystal Lake · Oakwood Hills · North Tower Lake
Lakewood · Lions Park · Fox River Valley Gardens · Lake Barrington
Four Colonies Park · Cary · (59)
Woodscreek Park · Sands Main Street Park · Grassy Lake Forest Preserve
Trout Valley · Fox River Grove
Lake in the Hills · (31) · (22)
N · Sundance Park
Diecke Park · **FINISH** · Algonquin · Barrington
Kane County · Mud Lake · Barrington Hills
Binnie Forest Preserve · (25) (62) · Cook County
Carpentersville
Rutland Forest Preserve · 0 1 2 4 Miles · Galvins Lake · **rails·to·trails** conservancy

At this point, the trail begins to liven up. Count on consistently higher numbers of people using the trail and brace yourself for a few navigational changes. The farther south you get, the easier it is to get turned around if you're not familiar with the area.

DIRECTIONS

The Genoa City trailhead in Wisconsin is located on a city cul-de-sac and does not provide parking. To access the trail on this end, from US Route 12, take State Route H for a half mile to Grove Avenue and head south for a quarter mile. When you come to Southeastern Court, where the road curves left, follow it to a crushed stone path that leads through two yards and takes you to the trail. While it is an unconventional access point, there is a playground off the path and it is a short walk to the trail.

To reach the Algonquin trailhead from State Route 31, travel toward Algonquin and turn east on State Route 62. Head north on North Harrison Street and continue about a quarter mile to the parking lot at Riverfront Park.

Contact: McHenry County Conservation District
18410 US Highway 14
Woodstock, IL 60098
(815) 338-6223
www.mccdistrict.org/web/re-bicycling.htm

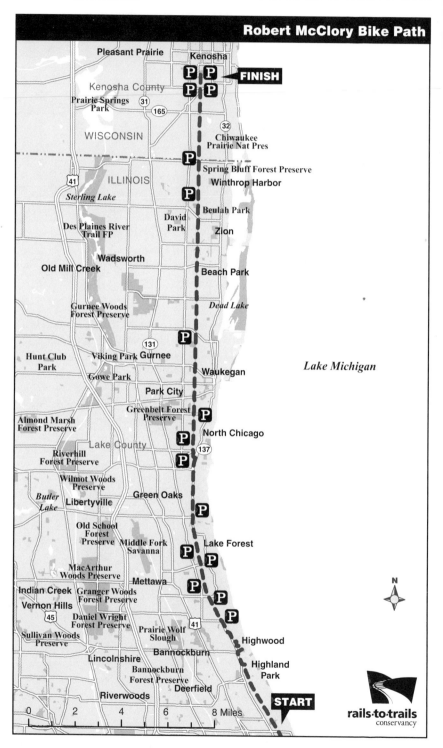

Robert McClory Bike Path

Pleasant Prairie

Kenosha

P P **FINISH**

P P

Kenosha County

Prairie Springs Park ③①

WISCONSIN ⑯⑤

③②

Chiwaukee Prairie Nat Pres

ILLINOIS ④①

P

Spring Bluff Forest Preserve

Winthrop Harbor

Sterling Lake

P

Des Plaines River Trail FP

David Park

Beulah Park

Zion

Wadsworth

Old Mill Creek

Beach Park

Gurnee Woods Forest Preserve

Dead Lake

P

⑬①

Hunt Club Park

Viking Park Gurnee

Gowe Park

Waukegan

Lake Michigan

Park City

Almond Marsh Forest Preserve

Greenbelt Forest Preserve

P

Riverhill Forest Preserve

Lake County

P

North Chicago

⑬⑦

P

Wilmot Woods Preserve

Butler Lake Libertyville

Green Oaks

P

Old School Forest Preserve

MacArthur Woods Preserve

Middle Fork Savanna

P

Lake Forest

P

Indian Creek Granger Woods Forest Preserve

Vernon Hills

Mettawa

P

④⑤

Daniel Wright Forest Preserve

Prairie Wolf Slough

④①

P

Sullivan Woods Preserve

Lincolnshire

Bannockburn

Highwood

Bannockburn Forest Preserve

Deerfield

Highland Park

Riverwoods

START

N

0 2 4 6 8 Miles

rails·to·trails
conservancy

Robert McClory Bike Path

The Robert McClory Bike Path (formerly the North Shore Bike Path) is notorious for its conglomeration of names over the years. At any given time—and depending on whom you ask—it has been called the Green Bay Trail, the North Shore Trail and the Robert McClory Trail. Its formal name, given in 1997, honors a bike-friendly government official.

The trail strings together the communities of Highland Park, Lake Forest, North Chicago and Waukegan and then seamlessly melds into the 3.5-mile Kenosha County Bike Trail at the Wisconsin state line.

Despite its modern-day identity crisis, the trail's past is clear. The majority of its 26.5-mile route follows a historic Chicago, North Shore and Milwaukee Railroad corridor. This railroad was an electric line and many of the old towers supporting the electric cables are visible along the trail. The trail surface alternates between asphalt and a finely screened limestone that offers a good, hard base for most trail uses.

Starting in the Chicago suburb of Highland Park, the smooth, paved trail travels through picturesque suburban communities (many of them among the most affluent in the Chicago area) that dominate most of the trail's first half. At Highwood, at the 1.25-mile mark, you must

Location
Kenosha County (WI) and Lake County (IL)

Endpoints
Laurel Avenue and St. Johns Avenue in Highland Park, IL, to 30th Street and 89th Avenue in Kenosha, WI

Mileage
26.5

Roughness Index
2

Surface
Asphalt and crushed stone

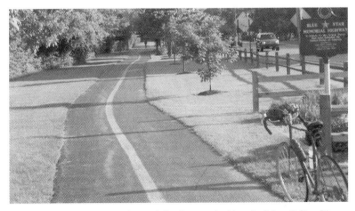

Stringing communities together much like the original rail line, the Robert McClory Bike Path is a neighborhood recreation and commuting amenity.

leave the trail and follow back streets. The road detour is very well marked, but you will want to stay alert.

Leaving Highwood and back on the rail-trail, you parallel active railroad tracks for most of the next 7 miles to just south of North Chicago. The trail and the tracks are separated by about 20 to 30 feet of thin forest most of this time.

Entering Lake Forest, at mile 6, the trail again detours onto streets, as well as through large parking lots that service the Metra commuter rail station. Again, this route is well marked and easy to follow.

The section between Lake Bluff and North Chicago still parallels the Metra tracks, on the left, but this stretch also opens up and quiets down, with expanses of woodlands and a golf course. North Chicago's section of the trail is very wide, housing the trail, utility lines and the old electric towers from the railroad days. Another unique feature along this section is mile after mile of community gardens. A lot of the trail's open space has been tilled and gardens sprout up everywhere, adding a charming country touch to the urban atmosphere.

As you head north, the subdivisions increasingly give way to fields. The Robert McClory Bike Path meets the Kenosha County Bike Trail on the bridge crossing Russell Road; this is the state line. The remaining 3.5 miles of trail take you through Wisconsin and this stretch is distinctly more rural, with a beautiful, tree-lined finish to the Kenosha trailhead.

DIRECTIONS

To access the Highland Park trailhead, take US Highway 41 (Skokie Hwy.) to Central Avenue and head east for just over 1 mile. Turn right onto St. Johns Avenue and park in any lot on the right. The trail starts along the west side of St. Johns Avenue, where it meets Laurel Avenue.

To reach the Kenosha trailhead from I-94, take 104th Street east for 4.25 miles. Turn left onto Springbrook Road and go just over a half mile. Turn left onto 39th Avenue and continue for 1.1 miles. Turn right onto 89th Avenue. The trailhead is a half mile ahead on the right, at the intersection of 89th Avenue and 30th Street.

Contact: Lake County Division of Transportation
600 West Winchester Road
Libertyville, IL 60048
(847) 362-3950
www.trailresources.com/trail-illinois-robert-mcclory-bike-path.html

Rock Island Trail State Park

The 29-mile Rock Island State Trail runs from Alta, in Peoria County, to Toulon, in Stark County, connecting the towns of Alta, Dunlap, Princeville, Wyoming and Toulon. This trail paints a great picture of Illinois, from its origin near the urban environment of Peoria, through numerous small towns and villages and unlimited expanses of classic Midwest farm and woodland in between. The trail owes its name to the Peoria and Rock Island Railroad Company trains that ran passengers and freight on this line until the 1950s.

Heading north from the Peoria Heights trailhead in Alta, have your camera ready to capture the views from the first overlook that comes up quickly. The farm and woodland setting of much of this trail is definitely picture-worthy.

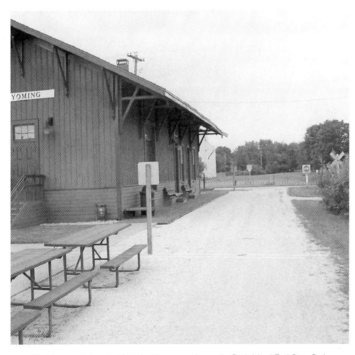

Ideal for an uninterrupted bicycle ride or smooth run, the Rock Island Trail State Park is an unwavering pathway through picturesque Illinois countryside.

Location
Peoria and Stark counties

Endpoints
Peoria Heights in Alta to Toulon

Mileage
29

Roughness Index
2

Surface
Crushed stone

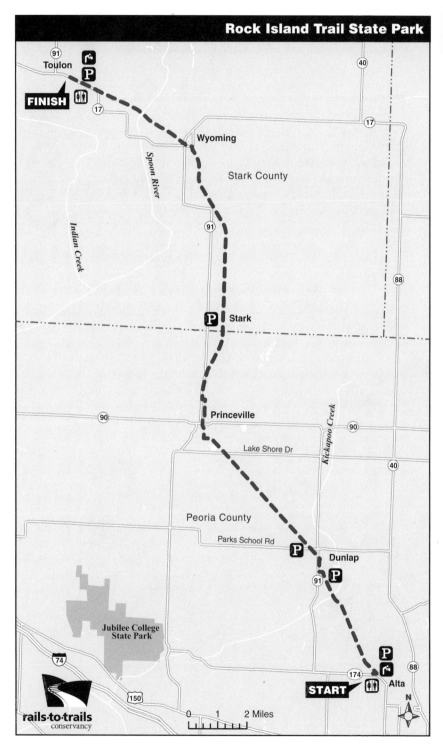

Rock Island Trail State Park

As the Rock Island Trail approaches the town of Dunlap, fields on one side and the emerging town on the other, the trail empties out onto 1st Street. This stretch requires some road riding, but traffic is light. Take 1st Street north three blocks, then turn left onto Walnut Street. Turn right onto 2nd Street, following its curve to the west. Just before 3rd Street, turn right onto a drive—the pick-up for the trail is visible from the road.

The corridor continues its straight-as-an-arrow path through farm fields as far as the eye can see. The trees lining the trail offer respite from the sun and also harbor a wide variety of bird life.

About 6 miles north of the county line trailhead, the fields start giving way to the outskirts of the small town of Wyoming. Upon entering Wyoming proper, look for the trail headquarters on the left. The restored Chicago Burlington & Quincy Depot, a bright, barn-red building, is absolutely beautiful, complete with the restored wooden cantilevers on the roofline. The depot also houses a visitor center and railroad museum.

In Wyoming, as you travel on quiet streets, look for the trail's green bike route signs to easily navigate the half mile street back to the trail. The scenery becomes more heavily wooded as you leave Wyoming and enter the Spoon River area.

The Spoon River, at mile 26, is a great spot to stop for a rest and to admire the trestle bridge that spans the creek. The bridge has observation "bump-outs" that offers a convenient rest stop with the wooded creek valley for a backdrop.

After a short mile, you leave the tree cover behind and the scenery switches back to farm fields for the remainder of your journey. The appearance of Route 17 indicates your imminent arrival at the town of Toulon. The endpoint trailhead is just 3 miles beyond the bridge.

DIRECTIONS

To access the trailhead in Alta, take Interstate 74 to Route 6 and then head north for 5.5 miles. Turn onto Route 174, which becomes Alta Lane. The trailhead is on the right in just under a mile.

To reach the midway point trailhead from Interstate 74, take Route 6 north for 2.5 miles to US Highway 150. Turn right at the exit and travel west on 150 for nearly a half mile. Take State Route 91 north through the towns of Dunlap and Princeville, for about 19 miles and then turn right on County Line Road. The trailhead is on the right in a half mile.

To access the Toulon trailhead from Interstate 74, take State Route 78 (South Randolph Street) north for 17 miles. Turn right on State Route 17 and follow it through the town of Toulon for just over 4 miles. The trailhead is on the left just south of town.

Contact: Illinois Department of Natural Resources
211 East Williams Road
P.O. Box 64
Wyoming, IL 61491
(309) 695-2228
www.dnr.state.il.us/lands/landmgt/parks/r1/
rockisle.htm

Sam Vadalabene Great River Road Bike Trail

Big bluffs, mighty rivers, the largest Illinois state park and one giant bird—you'll find them all along the Sam Vadalabene Great River Road Bike Trail. This unique rail-trail starts in the 8,050-acre Pere Marquette State Park (named for the first European to step on Illinois soil) and follows the Illinois River to its confluence with the Mississippi River. The enormous state park (the largest in Illinois) has a rich history and limitless sights, from Native American burial mounds to educational displays to lookouts with sweeping river views. It is best known, however, for its vivid fall foliage and a winter population of the majestic bald eagle.

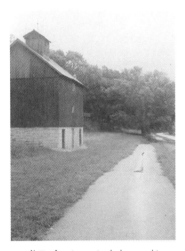

Native American petroglyphs carved in limestone bluffs, stunning river views, and historical sites like the above building are highlights on the Sam Vadalabene Great River Road Bike Trail.

Shortly after the park, the trail travels over a series of short but fairly steep hills and gullies. Around mile 5, you enter the town of Grafton, where the trail crosses the road and starts its run right along the riverbank at the confluence of the Mississippi and Illinois rivers. Across the river sits the state of Missouri. This is a beautiful, half-mile stretch with turtles, herons and a plethora of waterfowl. Soon, the trail veers off the rail corridor and passes through the quiet streets of Grafton.

The trail merges with the Great Rivers National Scenic Byway, otherwise known as Highway 100, outside of Grafton, traveling along a 3- to 4-foot painted bike lane that parallels the river, offering excellent water views. Traffic moves fast on this stretch, but the bike lane is wide enough for comfortable travel. Just south of

Location
Jersey and
Madison counties

Endpoints
Pere Marquette
State Park in
Grafton to Piasa
Park (on Hwy. 100)
in Alton

Mileage
20.4

**Roughness
Index**
1

Surface
Asphalt

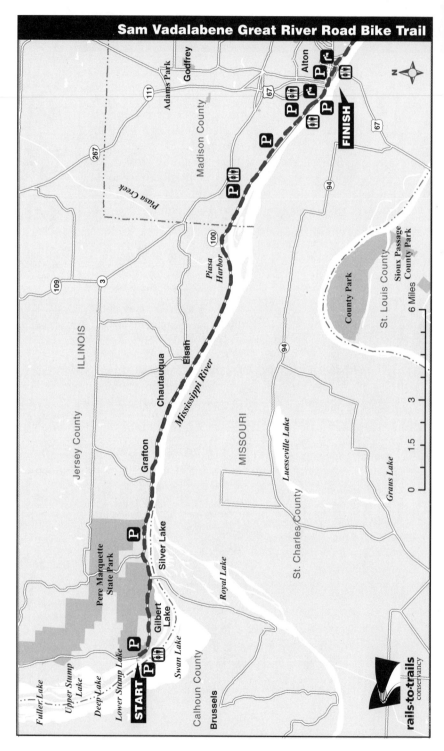

Sam Vadalabene Great River Road Bike Trail

Grafton is a visitors center with knowledgeable staff and a wide array of informative publications.

Four miles from Grafton, make a pleasant detour into the town of Elsah. Turn off the Scenic Byway at Mill Street to take a spin through the hamlet. Stone and brick houses line the narrow streets, lending Elsah a step-back-in-time quality that earned it a spot on the National Register of Historic Places in 1973.

Continuing on the Scenic Byway, in stark contrast to the wide river on your right, sheer limestone cliffs tower over the far side of the road for most of the 8 miles traveled along the roadway from Grafton to Piasa (PIE-a-saw) Harbor.

After passing the commercial harbor developments at Piasa Harbor, the bike lane crosses the road and resumes as trail. The final 6 miles roll along between the highway and the dramatic bluffs looming above. As you approach the southern trailhead at Piasa Park, look up at the huge limestone bluff to see a 48-by-22-foot Native American petroglyph of the fierce, warrior-killing Piasa Bird.

From Piasa Park, you can follow green bike-route signs to continue your journey on the 4-mile Alton Trail (mostly along city streets), which connects to the Madison County Transit Confluence Trail (page 47).

DIRECTIONS

To access the northern trailhead in Pere Marquette State Park, take Interstate 270 to Highway 3 and follow Highway 3 north for 6.6 miles. Turn left on Great River Road/Berm Highway and continue for 5 miles. Merge onto Great River Road/McAdams Parkway and head north for 20 miles. Turn right into the driveway to the Pere Marquette Lodge; the trailhead is on the right and parking is on the left.

To access the southern trailhead in Piasa Park, take Interstate 270 to Highway 3 and go north on Highway 3 for 6.6 miles. Turn left on Great River Road/Berm Highway and go 5 miles. Merge onto Great River Road/McAdams Parkway and head north for 0.8 mile. Piasa Park is on the right, just past Alton.

Contact: Illinois Department of Transportation
1102 Eastport Plaza Drive
Collinsville, IL 62234
(618) 346-3100
www.greatriverroad.com/vadalabene.htm

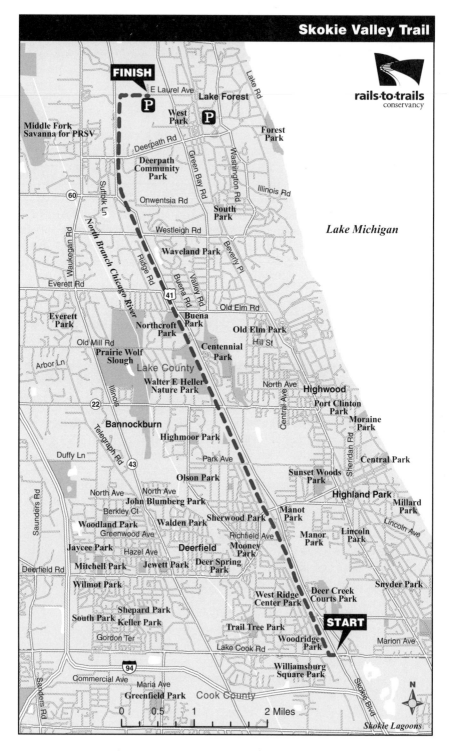

Skokie Valley Trail

rails·to·trails
conservancy

FINISH

E Laurel Ave

Lake Forest

West Park

Middle Fork Savanna for PRSV

Deerpath Rd

Deerpath Community Park

Lake Rd

Forest Park

Washington Rd

Illinois Rd

60

Suffolk Ln

Onwentsia Rd

Green Bay Rd

South Park

Waukegan Rd

North Branch Chicago River

Westleigh Rd

Waveland Park

Beverly Pl

Lake Michigan

Everett Rd

Ridge Rd

Buena Rd

Valley Rd

41

Old Elm Rd

Everett Park

Old Mill Rd

Northcroft Park

Buena Park

Old Elm Park

Hill St

Arbor Ln

Prairie Wolf Slough

Lake County

Centennial Park

Walter E Heller Nature Park

North Ave

Highwood

Illinois

22

Bannockburn

Highmoor Park

Port Clinton Park

Moraine Park

Duffy Ln

Telegraph Rd

43

Park Ave

Sheridan Rd

Central Park

Saunders Rd

Olson Park

Sunset Woods Park

Highland Park

North Ave

North Ave

John Blumberg Park

Berkley Ct

Woodland Park

Greenwood Ave

Walden Park

Sherwood Park

Manot Park

Millard Park

Lincoln Ave

Jaycee Park

Hazel Ave

Deerfield

Richfield Ave

Mooney Park

Manor Park

Lincoln Park

Deerfield Rd

Mitchell Park

Jewett Park

Deer Spring Park

Wilmot Park

Snyder Park

Shepard Park

South Park

Keller Park

West Ridge Center Park

Deer Creek Courts Park

Gordon Ter

Trail Tree Park

START

94

Woodridge Park

Marion Ave

Commercial Ave

Maria Ave

Greenfield Park

Cook County

Williamsburg Square Park

Sanders Rd

N

0   0.5   1   2 Miles

Skokie Lagoons

Skokie Valley Trail

An excellent example of land use in greater Chicago, the entire Skokie Valley Trail corridor is a rail-with-trail, paralleled by double tracks that sit about 40 feet to the left of the trail surface. The well-maintained, paved asphalt path offers a nice, smooth experience for a multitude of uses. (And indeed, this corridor serves a variety of different users. The trail shares right-of-way with a major residential electricity service company and you will see high-voltage electrical wires overhead.)

The trail connects Highland Park in the south to the northern trailhead in Lake Forest. Although there is no parking or proper trailhead in Highland Park, you can park less than a quarter mile to the south at the Village Square at Northbrook, a large shopping mall off of Skokie Boulevard.

Once you're underway, it's amazing to see how nature can flourish in such an urban environment. Even as

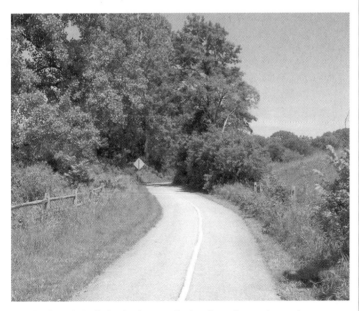

The Skokie Valley Trail multitasks as a rail-with-trail as well as a utility corridor.

Location
Lake County

Endpoints
Highland
Park to Lake
Forest

Mileage
8.3

**Roughness
Index**
1

Surface
Asphalt

69

you pass suburban Chicago life along each side of the corridor, it's not uncommon to come across rabbits, deer, blackbirds, hawks, robins and a plethora of tree and low-brush species. The trail is sandwiched between US Highway 41 and the train tracks for most of its course, and there are several major road crossings. While these are well marked and include crosswalks, use caution when crossing.

The 200-plus-foot trail bridge over Highway 22 signals the mid-point of the trip. The remainder of the trail passes through mainly commercial and light industrial developments and, as you approach Lake Forest, some residential subdivisions. After you make a dramatic 90-degree turn east around the edge of a golf course, the northern trailhead appears out of the trees. If you wish to continue, it is a 0.75-mile shot to meet up with the 26.5-mile Robert McClory Bike Path (page 59). To get there, go straight along Laurel Avenue for 0.7 mile, turn right on Western Avenue. Take the first left on East Woodland Road, which goes under the railroad tracks and then under the trail bridge. Take a left and this trail will take you all the way to Wisconsin. Or turn right to loop back toward Chicago on the bike path.

DIRECTIONS

To access the trail in Highland Park (remember, there is no parking here), take Interstate 94 to Skokie Valley Road (US Route 41) north. After just under a mile, turn left on County Line Road. The trail is accessed from the gas station parking lot on the right, just past Skokie Valley Road. To park, take County Line Road to Skokie Road and turn left, traveling just a tenth of a mile south to a large shopping mall on the left.

To reach the Lake Forest trailhead from Interstate 94, take West Kennedy Road (County Road 60) east 1.5 miles. Turn left onto North Waukegan Road (County Road 43), go 0.5 mile and then turn right on West Deerpath Road. After 1.4 miles, turn left on North Green Bay Road (County Road 131) and travel for 0.70 mile. Turn left on East Laurel Avenue. The trailhead (with parking), is just under a half mile away, at the dead end of Laurel Avenue.

Contact: Lake County Division of Transportation
600 West Winchester Road
Libertyville, IL 60048
(847) 362-3950

Tunnel Hill State Trail

Southern Illinois's Tunnel Hill State Trail is a gem of a route, with 23 trestle bridges (including one that is 450 feet long), several ghost towns, a beautiful park, a comfortable trailhead in Vienna Station and, of course, its namesake tunnel, an impressive corridor that once measured 800 feet long until a collapse in 1929 shortened it by some 300 feet. The first railroad tracks laid on this corridor caused such a stir that in 1870, local farmers, anticipating shipment-ready crops, planted orchards even before the line's tunnel was complete. In 1991, the corridor was donated to the state and just 10 years later, the entire 47.5 miles was opened to the public as a multiuse trail.

The trail begins at the Barkhausen Wetlands Center and serves up instant trailside gratification within the

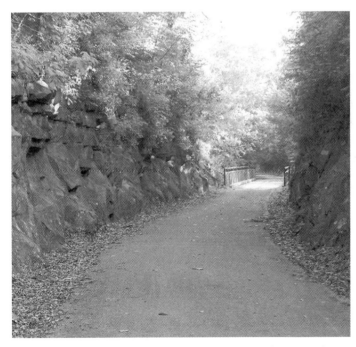

A cavernous, 543-foot-long tunnel marks both the literal (in terms of elevation) and figurative highlight of the Tunnel Hill State Trail.

Location
Johnson, Pulaski, Saline and Williamson counties

Endpoints
Barkhausen Wetlands Center in Cypress to Harrisburg

Mileage
47.5

Roughness Index
2

Surface
Crushed stone

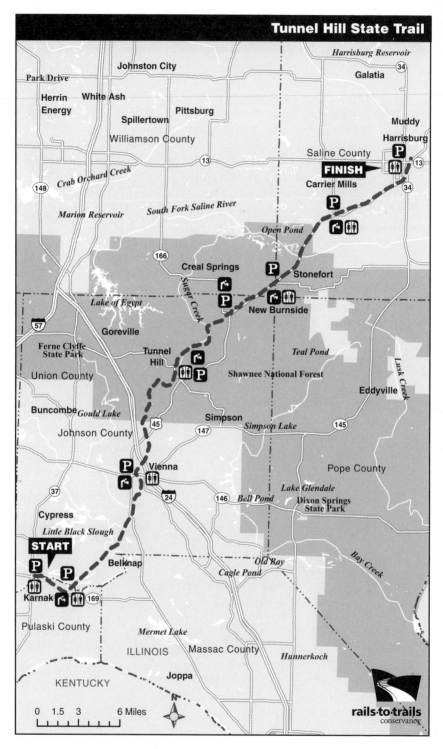

Tunnel Hill State Trail

first 2.5 miles, showcasing a bridge and scenic overlook even before reaching the town of Karnak. Karnak offers restrooms, a water fountain and ample parking. A few miles farther in, you will come to the polar opposite, the ghost town of Forman (to your left) that hints at a scary movie set from a Hollywood backlot.

The scenic trail passes more bridges as you make your way to the town of Vienna Station. A nice park here makes for an ideal rest and picnic spot, especially if you have children along.

Leaving Vienna Station, you head toward Tunnel Hill and the trail's midpoint. In the 9 miles bewteen Vienna Station and Tunnel Hill, there are four more bridges before the landmark tunnel. It's handy to use a flashlight as you travel through the cavernous, 543-foot trail namesake. If you're cycling, you may want to dismount and walk your bicycle through the tunnel. Be especially careful of other trail users coming in the opposite direction through the tunnel.

After Tunnel Hill—the highest point on the trail—there is a gentle 2 percent grade downhill for the remaining 25 miles. Soon after leaving the Tunnel Hill trailhead, the trail travels through the Shawnee National Forest, a stunning landscape with a high tree canopy that shades a trickling brook off to the right. You're more likely to hear the birds here than you are to see them, but the local rabbit population is everywhere. The journey here is amazingly quiet and rural.

After 6 miles, you arrive in the town of New Burnside, which takes its name from Civil War General Ambrose Burnside, a founder of the original railroad. The terrain here is marked by looming bluffs, providing a dramatic contrast to the forest you traveled through earlier.

Another 4.4 miles of travel takes you out of the forest and into a very flat section along US Highway 40 to Stonefort, whose trailhead includes a well-restored railroad depot. The next 6.7-mile stretch of trail remains within sight of US Highway 40 most of the way to Carrier Mills. Keep an eye out for turtles and snakes, which also like to use this trail.

After Carrier Mills, the last 7.5 miles of trail into Harrisburg meander past farm fields and neighborhoods. The route for the final 2.5 miles in Harrisburg is a mix of trail and sidewalk, ending at the trailhead on the north side of town.

DIRECTIONS

To access the Barkhausen Wetlands Center in Cypress, take Interstate 57 to State Route 146 and proceed east for about 9.5 miles. Turn right on State Route 37 and continue for 9 miles. Pass through the town of Cypress and look for the wetlands center on the left.

To reach the trailhead at Tunnel Hill (the midpoint), take Interstate 24 to US Highway 45 and head north. Turn left on Tunnel Hill Rd. and look for the trailhead on the right, just before Possum Road.

To reach the Harrisburg trailhead from Interstate 57, take State Route 13 east approximately 24 miles. Turn left on US Highway 45 and head north for just 0.15 mile. Turn left on Walnut Street, and then turn right on Industrial Drive. The trailhead is on the right.

Contact: Tunnel Hill State Trail
P.O. Box 671
Vienna, IL 62995
(618) 658-2168
www.dnr.state.il.us/lands/Landmgt/PARKS/R5/
tunnel.htm

Virgil Gilman Trail

The smooth, asphalt Virgil Gilman Trail travels through forest and prairie land from a quiet, rural community college campus all the way into suburban Chicago. The trail's namesake, Virgil Gilman, served as director of the Fox Valley Park District for 30 years and successfully championed public access to the river—indeed, access grew from 66 feet in 1946 to more than 30 miles today.

Beginning at Waubonsee Community College, the trail heads into open native prairie land for the first mile. (Don't be alarmed if you hear gunshots for the first few miles, as the Aurora Sportsman's Club shooting range is nearby.) After traveling through the grasslands, you enter the Bliss Woods Forest Preserve, marked by beautiful, large white and black oak trees. The preserve is also home to many other tree species, including sycamore, white poplar and cottonwood. Keep your eyes open for birds. It's not uncommon to encounter red-winged

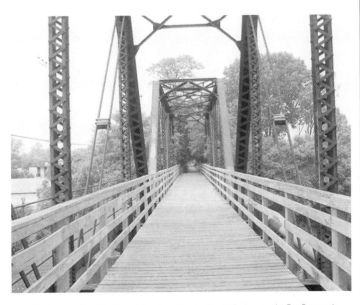

The former railroad trestle and its adjacent pedestrian bridge across the Fox River make for good picture-taking time on the Virgil Gilman Trail.

Location
Kane and Kendall counties

Endpoints
Waubonsee Community College in Sugar Grove to Route 30 (Hill Road) in Montgomery

Mileage
11.5

Roughness Index
1

Surface
Asphalt

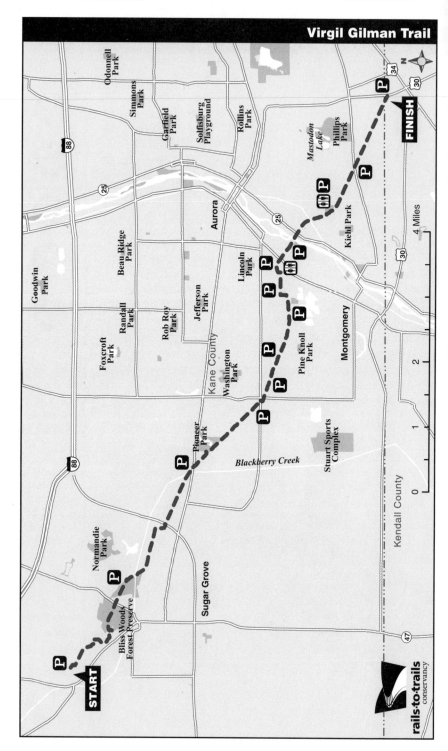

Virgil Gilman Trail

blackbirds, downy woodpeckers, cardinals and blue jays along the trail.

From Bliss Woods, the trail travels alongside a rolling brook until it crosses Route 56 on an overpass. Now the landscape becomes large farm fields as you slowly begin to enter a more developed area with subdivisions of single-family homes.

After crossing another bridge over Orchard Road, the route becomes a 1.75-mile rail-with-trail stretch and you may hear the active tracks through the thick vegetation that acts as a natural buffer between the two corridors. Emerging onto Terry Avenue the trail briefly continues on quiet side streets that are very easy to navigate. Take a left on Terry Avenue followed quickly by a right on Rathbone Avenue. Follow Rathbone a short distance until you cross the active rail line. The trail begins immediately after this crossing, at Copley Park, a nice rest stop.

Shortly after leaving the park, the trail crosses the Fox River via an original trestle bridge. Off to one side of the bridge, you can see the old pedestrian walkway—a testament to days gone by. Once across the river, follow the smooth path for 2.75 miles, through the suburban developments of Montgomery, to the trailhead on Route 30—the eastern terminus of the Virgil Gilman Trail.

DIRECTIONS

To access the start at Waubonsee Community College, take Interstate 88 to Highway 56 south and continue 3.8 miles. Turn right on Highway 47 and after a little more than 2 miles, turn right on Waubonsee Drive. Continue to the community college and look for the trailhead at the far end of the parking lot.

To reach the Montgomery trailhead from Interstate 88, take North Farnsworth Avenue south for 4.5 miles. Turn right on Montgomery Road and travel a quarter mile to US 30 and turn left. The trailhead is a half mile ahead, on the right.

Contact: Fox Valley Park District
712 South River Street
Aurora, IL 60506
(630) 897-0516
www.foxvalleyparkdistrict.org/index.php?q=node/50

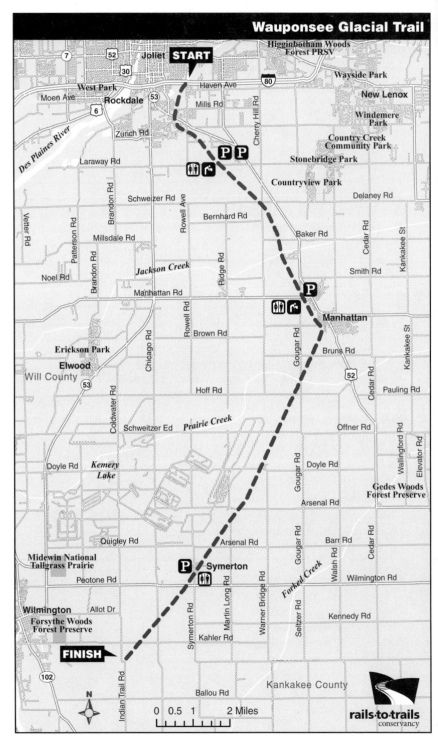

Wauponsee Glacial Trail

Wauponsee Glacial Trail

Traveling along the Wauponsee Glacial Trail, you'll be surprised just how quickly you can move from an urban environment into the rolling fields of the Midwest. Starting in Joliet, within shouting distance of Interstate 80 overhead ramps, you might think you're in for a busy urban trail experience. But after just 1.5 miles, the trail takes you through a sparse forest with only an occasional train passing by on the active tracks a few hundred yards away.

A few large warehouses signal the end of the forest as you enter a subdivision and travel along the backyards of nearby homes. Over the next 1.5 miles, you make multiple small stream crossings, where there are excellent birding opportunities.

The Sugar Creek Administrative Center of the Will County Forest Preserve serves as this trail's northern trailhead. If you are driving to the trail, this is where you will park and start your trip. (The Joliet access point does not have parking.) The preserve building offers information on its trails, permits for picnicking, camping,

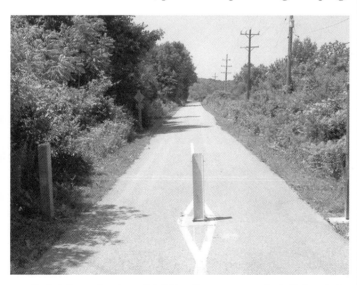

Thanks to its smooth surface and straight corridor, you can move at a decidedly unglacial pace on the Wauponsee Glacial Trail.

Location
Will County

Endpoints
S. Rowell Ave. under I-80 in Joliet to S. Old Indian Rd. between Symerton and Lakewood Shores

Mileage
18.5

Roughness Index
2

Surface
Asphalt and crushed stone

programs and dog parks, as well as workshops on gardening and green building techniques.

As you head south from the Sugar Creek Administrative Center, the trail surface changes from asphalt to crushed stone. You may begin to feel very small along this stretch, as vast farm fields stretch out farther than the eye can see. The farmland gives way for a short time as you enter the town of Manhattan, where there is a trailhead with restrooms and drinking water.

Leaving Manhattan, the trail parallels another very short section of railroad tracks that dead-ends at a maintenance facility. South of Manhattan, you'll see some of the largest cornfields around. To the west, you'll see 19,000-acre Midewin National Tallgrass Prairie, which was federally designated as tallgrass prairie in 1996—the only such area to receive that status. (For information about visiting the prairie, which is only partially open to the public due to restoration activities, see www.fs.fed.us/mntp.)

The southernmost trailhead—but not the end of the trail—is near mile 15, in the quaint town of Symerton. The trail currently extends about 3.5 miles past Symerton, to just beyond South Old Indian Trail Road.

DIRECTIONS

To reach the endpoint in Joliet (remember, no parking available) take Interstate 80 to Richards Street Exit North. Take a right onto Richards Street, go one block and take a right onto 4th Avenue. After 0.6 mile, take a right onto Rowell Avenue. The trail endpoint is on the right just 0.3 mile from 4th Avenue and just past the I-80 overpass.

To reach the Sugar Creek Administrative Center from Interstate 80, take South Briggs Street south for 2.7 miles and turn right onto East Laraway Road After 0.7 mile, look for the center on the right, before the Chicagoland Speedway.

To reach the Symerton trailhead from Interstate 57, take West Wilmington Road west 12.25 miles and turn right onto South Symerton Road. After a half mile, turn right on West Commercial Street and continue for just over a tenth of a mile. The trailhead facilities are on the left.

Contact: Forest Preserve District of Will County
17540 West Laraway Road
Joliet, IL 60433
(815) 727-8700
www.fpdwc.org/regional.cfm

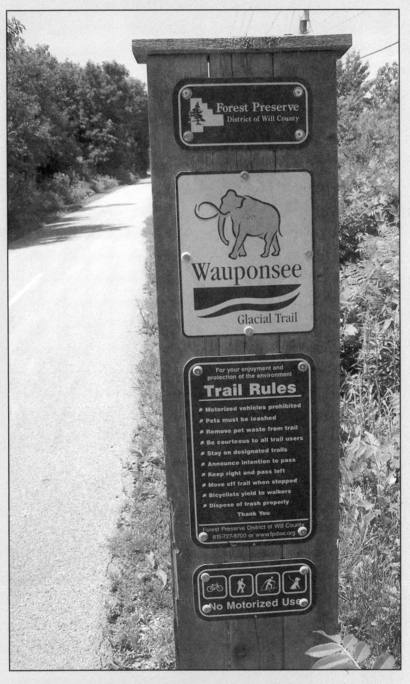

In Illinois the 18.5-mile Wauponsee Glacial Trail offers surprising diversity of landscape—from urban centers to farmland and from quaint neighborhoods to a forest preserve.

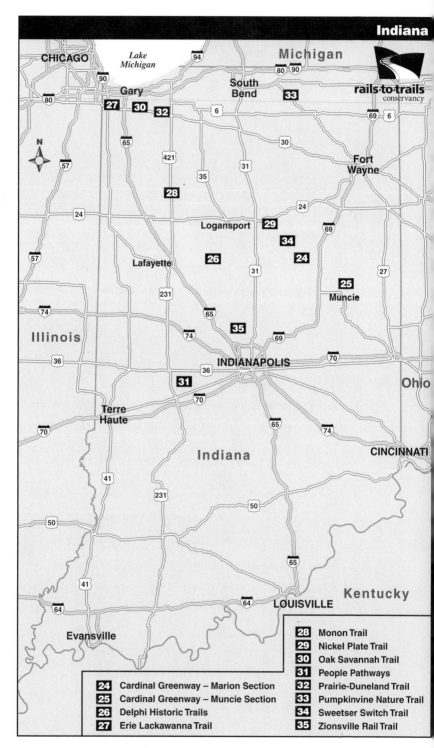

Indiana

rails·to·trails
conservancy

CHICAGO
Lake Michigan
94
Michigan
80 90
90
Gary
South Bend
33
Fort Wayne
69 6
80
27 30 32
6
65
30
421
28
35
31
57
24
29
Logansport
34
69
57
Lafayette
26
24
27
231
25
Muncie
74
65
35
31
69
Illinois
36
74
INDIANAPOLIS
70
36
Ohio
31
70
Terre Haute
65
74
CINCINNATI
70
Indiana
41
231
50
65
50
Kentucky
41
64
LOUISVILLE
64
Evansville

24	Cardinal Greenway – Marion Section
25	Cardinal Greenway – Muncie Section
26	Delphi Historic Trails
27	Erie Lackawanna Trail

28	Monon Trail
29	Nickel Plate Trail
30	Oak Savannah Trail
31	People Pathways
32	Prairie-Duneland Trail
33	Pumpkinvine Nature Trail
34	Sweetser Switch Trail
35	Zionsville Rail Trail

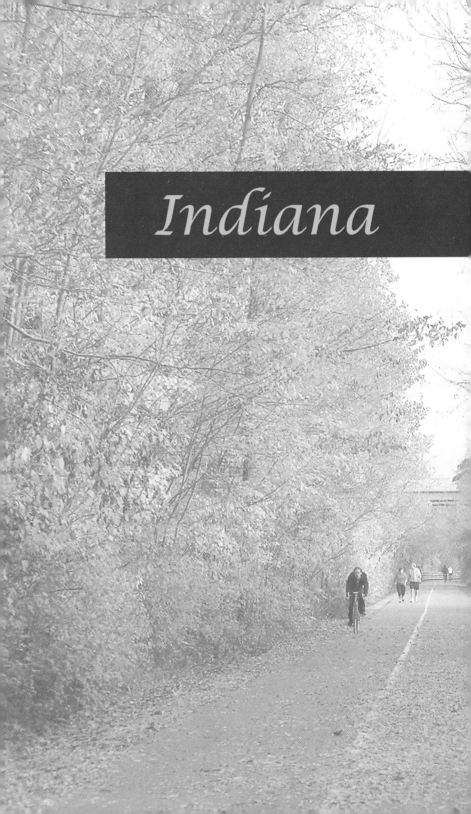

Indiana

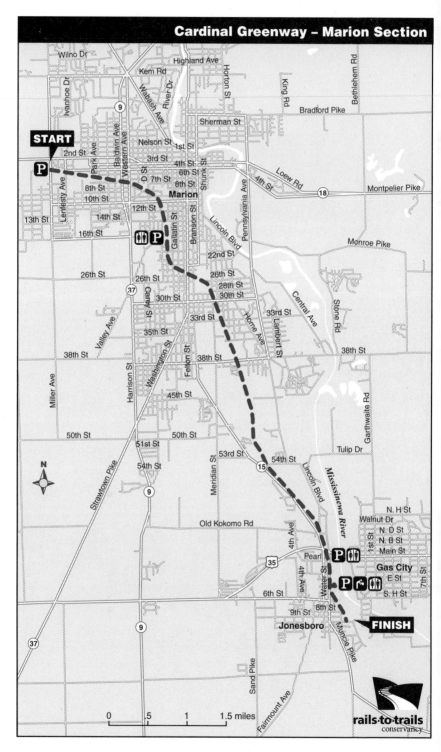

Cardinal Greenway – Marion Section

Cardinal Greenway – Marion Section

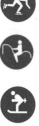

The Cardinal Greenway in Marion is the northern section of a larger planned trail system that will eventually connect Marion, Muncie and Richmond, Indiana. One of this pleasant trail's best attributes is that it links many neighborhoods and provides a non-motorized transportation corridor through the town.

Another attribute of this trail is its starting point in Marion, a town that takes great pride in its "coolness"—and for good reason. Marion was the birthplace of James Dean, who starred in film classics such as *East of Eden* and *Rebel Without a Cause* before his death at age 24. Depending on your definition of cool, another famous Marionite—Jim Davis, the creator of Garfield, the lasagna-loving comic strip cat—still remains local, with a studio in Muncie. (If this cat is up your alley, be sure to head to the 3-mile Sweetser Switch Trail, page 115, just north of Marion. At that trailhead, next to a retired

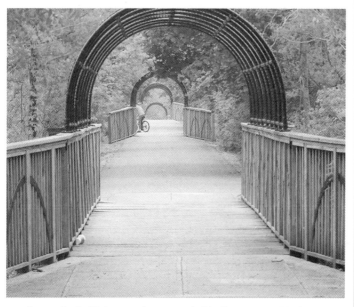

A string of arched bridges are a distinctive mark of the Marion section of the Cardinal Greenway.

Location
Grant County

Endpoints
Miller Road in Marion to E. 10th Street in Jonesboro

Mileage
7.25

Roughness Index
1

Surface
Asphalt and dirt

train car, a 4-foot Garfield statue makes for a perfect photo-op to commemorate your trail trip.)

From the trailhead in Marion, where there is an information kiosk and ample parking, you continue to another trailhead at Hogin Park, on the far side of a small tunnel. That trailhead features parking, picnic tables, covered shelters and basketball courts.

After Hogin Park, you cross the first of nine bridges, all of which add a unique flavor to this trail. Once the trail winds its way into Jonesboro, at approximately 6.5 miles, you cross US Route 35. The trailhead is on the left. A slight uphill takes you to a bridge that serves as an overlook over the Mississinewa River; students who attend school on the far side of the bridge often use this bridge. After the school, it is a mere half mile to the trail's end at East 10th Street.

DIRECTIONS

To access the Marion trailhead, take State Route 18 (West 2nd Street) in Marion and turn south on South Miller Avenue. The trailhead is located on the left after about a quarter mile, just beyond the railroad crossing.

To reach the Jonesboro trailhead from US Route 35, turn south on South Lincoln Boulevard and look for the trailhead immediately on the right.

Contact: Cardinal Greenway Inc.
700 East Wysor Street
Muncie, IN 47305
(765) 287-0399
www.cardinalgreenways.org

Cardinal Greenway – Muncie Section

The Cardinal Greenway in Muncie stretches through Indiana countryside that may well have inspired the lyrics to "America the Beautiful": Spacious skies, fruited plains and amber waves of grain provide the backdrop to the rural parts of this trail.

The rail-trail travels through the city of Muncie, but each end offers rich rural landscapes. Beginning in Gaston, population 1010, the trail is flanked by wildflowers. Early risers will be rewarded with the sight of hundreds of spiderwebs thick with morning dew and glistening in the new day's sun.

As you reach the 400 North trailhead, the urban fingers of Muncie start to reach out. An influx of runners, walkers and inline skaters—many of them students at nearby Ball State University—hit the trail. The McColloch Boulevard trailhead introduces you to the true Cardinal Greenway experience. First is the connector at mile 10 to the White River Greenway, which follows

Location
Delaware County

Endpoints
Gaston to
Losantville

Mileage
27.5

Roughness Index
1

Surface
Asphalt and dirt

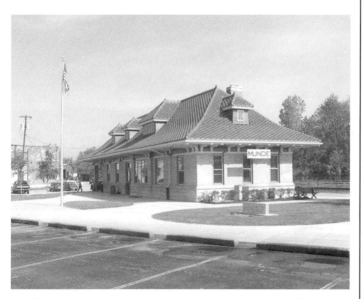

Restored railroad depots and train bridges are just part of the magic of the Muncie section of the Cardinal Greenway.

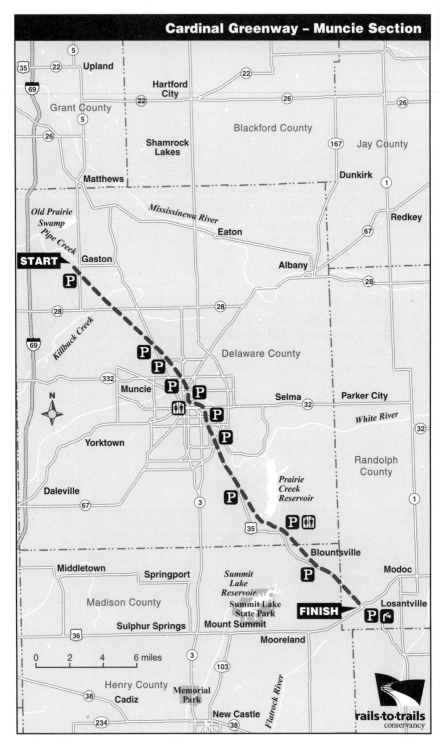

Cardinal Greenway – Muncie Section

(naturally) the White River. Second, you are faced with two bridges—to the right a historic trestle bridge and to the left the bicycle and pedestrian bridge that takes you across the White River. Another third of a mile along is the beautifully restored Wysor Street Depot and the office of Cardinal Greenway, Inc. The historic depot is a perfect place to stop for a picture, get a souvenir, or look at the model train. You also can pick up a free loaner bike at the depot; simply leave a valid picture ID and borrow a bike to cruise the trail.

Heading south from the depot, you will find yourself in the neighborhoods of Muncie. Passing under Route 35 you reenter the sun-drenched Indiana countryside. Note that the rocks marking the mileage here show it decreasing; these numbers signify the mileage to Cincinnati, the original destination of the railroad.

The trail ends just beyond the tiny town of Losantville, population 280. When you arrive at the trail end, you'll see that the corridor continues on to the horizon. Soon, the trail will continue to Richmond, extending this beautiful American experience by almost another 20 miles.

DIRECTIONS

To access the Gaston trailhead, from Interstate 69 take Route 35 east to North 600 West, which becomes South Sycamore Street in the town of Gaston. Follow South Sycamore Street to West Elm Street, turn left on West Elm Street and left again on Broad Street. At the end of Broad Street you dead-end into the parking area for the trail.

To get to the Muncie depot, follow Interstate 70 to Route 35 north. Follow Route 35 to Muncie and exit at Route 32. Follow Route 32 west until it turns into East Main Street. Stay on East Main Street, then turn north onto Vine Street. Follow North Vine Street across East Wysor Street and into the depot parking lot.

Contact: Cardinal Greenway, Inc.
700 East Wysor Street
Muncie, IN 47305
(765) 287-0399
www.cardinalgreenways.org

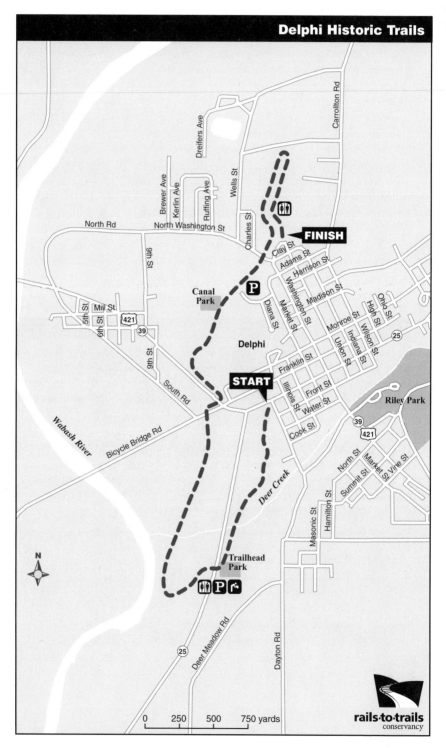

Delphi Historic Trails

Delphi Historic Trails

Tucked into rural north-central Indiana, the Delphi Historic Trails should not be overlooked by outdoors enthusiasts or history buffs. While access is convenient from Trailhead Park, printing out the map of the trail system (see website in "Contact" information) is a good idea. The route described below is composed of seven different named trails. These trails blend together fairly seamlessly, but without a map can be confusing. The entire system runs along a crushed stone surface suitable for walking and off-road bicycles (road bikes are not recommended).

Upon leaving Trailhead Park, you cross Deer Creek on a stunning suspension bridge that provides an excellent view of the crystal-clear water below, as well as the healthy fish population that inhabits it.

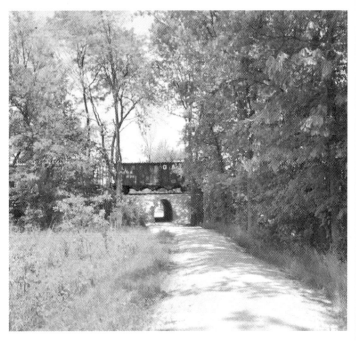

Delphi Historic Trails meanders along canals and rivers, through tunnels and over bridges for a rustic tour of the city and its outskirts.

Location
Carroll County

Endpoints
Near corner of State Route 25 and State Route 39 to N. Union Street and E. Packet Avenue in Delphi

Mileage
4

Roughness Index
2

Surface
Crushed stone

Across the bridge, you reach a junction: To the right is the Robbins Trail, which travels along Deer Creek past some wonderful swimming and fishing holes. The Robbins Trail connects with the Happy Jacks Loop just beyond Highway 25, and from there it is only 1 mile to the end of this section of the trail.

Instead of taking the Robbins Trail, however, you should turn left after the bridge to access the Van Scoy Towpath Trail. At this intersection, you are rewarded with an amazing view of the Wabash River as well as the Wabash and Erie Canal.

Turn right onto the Van Scoy Towpath and be sure to stop to read the interpretive panels along this stretch that provide interesting historical information about the canal. This section of trail also crosses a historic stone arch bridge and then tunnels under Highway 39, where it becomes the Underhill Towpath Trail.

Shortly after that, the trail goes through another tunnel under the active rail line that still services the town. From this point on, the trail follows the restored section of the canal. At 468 miles, this was once the longest canal in the northern hemisphere and second longest in the world. This trail section—just over a mile in length—is reminiscent of how the canal looked in its heyday in the 1850s. As you go by, keep a lookout for the occasional "explosions" in the clear water—many large carp call this stretch home. Anglers may want to cast a line for the bluegill, bass and catfish that also live in the canal.

Other highlights of this stretch include the town of Delphi, which has an excellent interpretive center located right along the trail. A restored canal boat moored here offers canal rides on the weekends during the summer.

After 1 mile on the Underhill Towpath Trail, you pass another historic stone bridge at Washington Street, built in 1901. At this point, you begin the Founders Towpath Trail. Although it's only a half mile long, this portion of the trail takes you past the beautifully restored Paint Creek Bridge, an old iron highway bridge built in 1873. This section ends at Founder's Point, where you can see the water intake that feeds the restored section of the canal. The local limestone quarry pumps in more than 3 million gallons of water a day to keep the canal filled to capacity.

From Founder's Point, your path becomes the North End Trail, which passes between the canal and Canal Park Annex, a park setting with restrooms and picnic areas. A half mile from Founder's Point, the trail ends. Cross the stone arch bridge at Washington Street and then return to the starting point.

DIRECTIONS

To access the starting point at Trailhead Park, take Interstate 65 to State Route 25 and head north for 12 miles. Trailhead Park is on the left just a mile before the town of Delphi. This is the preferred access point as it offers public parking.

Contact: Wabash and Erie Canal Park
1030 North Washington Street
Delphi, IN 46923
(765) 564-2870
www.wabashanderiecanal.org/subpage/
parktrails/trails.html

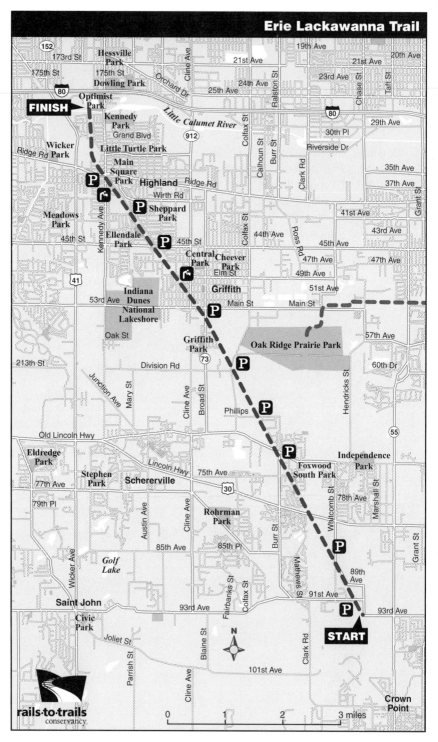

Erie Lackawanna Trail

FINISH

START

rails·to·trails
conservancy

Crown
Point

0   1   2   3 miles

Erie Lackawanna Trail

R unning from Crown Point to Highland, the Erie Lackawanna Trail passes through wetlands and open space on an unusually wide, paved corridor. The northern section is a popular thoroughfare that lends green space to an urban landscape on this neighborhood rail-trail.

From Crown Point, head north and very shortly you come upon the first of many street crossings and convenient trailheads. You also will see one of the many makeshift community access points. The first is for the Pine Island neighborhood and provides residents convenient backyard access to the trail.

Near mile 2, a tunnel takes you under US Route 30, where the trail traffic increases. Here, notice one of the most interesting characteristics of the trail—spectacular inlaid tile markers and overhead signs bearing the Erie

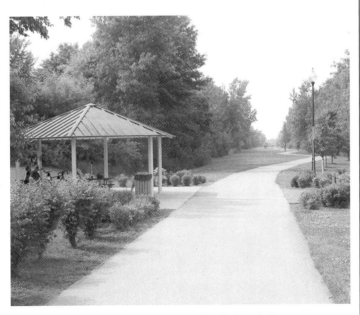

Access along the Erie Lackawanna Trail is plentiful in this "green" urban environment.

Location
Lake County

Endpoints
Main St. in Crown Point to the Little Calumet River in Highland

Mileage
9.9

Roughness Index
1

Surface
Asphalt

Lackawanna name. In a lovely combination of function and form, these elements double as fun and functional trail art.

At South Broad Street, the route briefly departs from the old railroad corridor. For about 0.8 mile, you follow a well-marked independent bike lane on city streets across seven active rail lines. Just before this detour, take a break at the convenient trailside shelter, which features picnic tables, restrooms and a tremendous Erie Lackawanna sign. The trail sign alone makes the visit worthwhile. Like an old railroad sign, this trail marker is elevated above the rail-trail.

There are big plans for this little trail. One day soon, it will connect with Hammond, 2 miles to the northeast and to other area trails. Longer-range plans include linking this trail to other trail systems in the greater Chicago area. Until then, this trail comes to a quiet and peaceful close in a nondescript Highland neighborhood.

DIRECTIONS

To access the Crown Point trailhead from State Route 55, take West 93rd Avenue west. In about a half mile, when the road turns 90 degrees to the right, continue straight (do not turn right) to access trailhead parking. This is the preferred trail access point as it has public parking.

Contact: Hammond Parks Department
5825 Sohl Avenue
Hammond, IN 46320
(219) 853-6378
www.indianatrails.org/Erie_Lackawanna_Trail_
Hammond.htm

Monon Trail

The Monon Trail is a colossus in the world of Midwest rail-trails. The 15-mile trail is attractive and well designed, also functioning as an urban transportation corridor. The trail stitches together neighborhoods, recreational facilities, cultural centers and schools between Indianapolis and the northern suburb of Carmel.

Beginning in Indianapolis, at the trail's south end, the Monon is undeniably an urban trail. You will travel beneath the ramps that comprise the intersection of Interstates 70 and 65, passing a mixture of residential areas and light industrial zones. After 2.7 miles, you come upon the first of this trail's bridges; the fire-engine red, transformed railroad trestle is a true marvel. After crossing a bridge and a couple overpasses, you arrive at the Indiana State Fairgrounds, an enormous complex with a popular annual fair that many people bike to via the Monon Trail.

Beyond the fairgrounds, the trail travels along the backyards of suburban Indianapolis through a corridor

Location
Hamilton and
Marion counties

Endpoints
10th Street, Indianapolis to
146th Street in
Carmel

Mileage
15.7

**Roughness
Index**
1

Surface
Asphalt

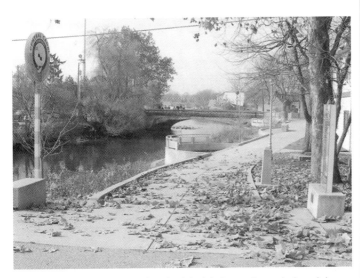

The Monon Trail is a wildly popular rail-trail that links homes, shops, schools, workplaces and fun destinations.

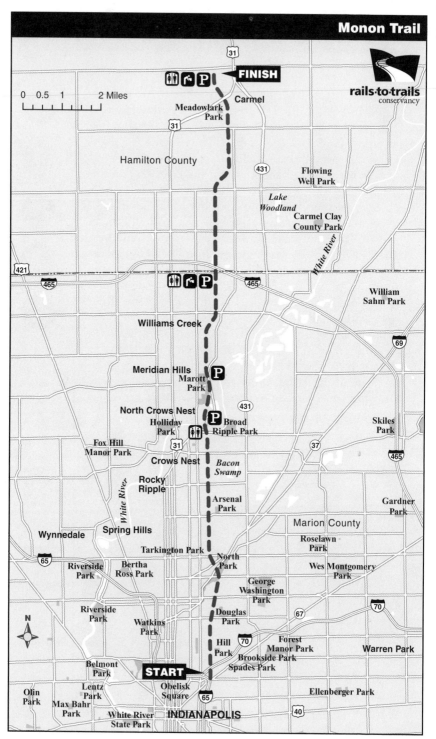

Monon Trail

rails-to-trails
conservancy

0   0.5   1   2 Miles

FINISH

Carmel

Meadowlark
Park

Hamilton County

Flowing
Well Park

Lake
Woodland

Carmel Clay
County Park

White River

William
Sahm Park

Williams Creek

Meridian Hills

Marott
Park

North Crows Nest

Holliday
Park

Broad
Ripple Park

Skiles
Park

Fox Hill
Manor Park

Crows Nest

Bacon
Swamp

Rocky
Ripple

White River

Arsenal
Park

Gardner
Park

Wynnedale

Spring Hills

Tarkington Park

Marion County

Roselawn
Park

Wes Montgomery
Park

Riverside
Park

Bertha
Ross Park

North
Park

George
Washington
Park

Riverside
Park

Watkins
Park

Douglas
Park

Belmont
Park

START

Hill
Park

Forest
Manor Park

Brookside Park
Spades Park

Warren Park

Olin
Park

Lentz
Park

Max Bahr
Park

Obelisk
Square

White River
State Park

INDIANAPOLIS

Ellenberger Park

lined with a ribbon of trees and green space. Local artwork placed randomly along this stretch adds a unique flavor to this trail, with pieces ranging from bright community murals to a network of pipes painted on the sides of a utility storage building.

At 63rd Street (mile 11), you reach the gateway to Broad Ripple, a beautiful village with a bright red bridge. This town practically vibrates with culture, offering many eateries, galleries, breweries and shops—a must-stop destination on your Monon trip.

After crossing two more impressive red bridges, the trail meanders through quiet neighborhoods for another 2.5 miles before crossing busy 86th Street. From here, it is just 1 mile to the trailhead at 96th Street, which marks the beginning of the trail's Carmel section. Interstate 465 looms overhead just beyond the trailhead, but soon you again travel past lovely backyards. Some wonderful trailside displays and rest areas—sponsored by local residents and community associations—provide nice spots for respite along the trail.

At 111th Street, you reach the Monon Center, a new development with a water park, fitness center, skate park and meeting facilities. The trail then cuts through downtown Carmel, where you may want to detour to shop along bustling Main Street. From here, the Monon Trail's end at 146th Street is just 1.5 miles away.

DIRECTIONS

The best access points for the Monon are the Broad Ripple and 96th Street trailheads.

To reach the Broad Ripple trailhead from Interstate 70, take Keystone Way north for 5 miles. Turn left on Broad Ripple Avenue and travel for 1 mile to Winthrop Avenue and turn right. After a quarter mile, turn left onto 64th Street and then take an immediate right on Cornell Avenue. Parking is available all along the right side of the trail.

To access the 96th Street trailhead in Carmel, take Interstate 465 to US Route 31 (North Meridian Street) and drive south for a quarter mile. Turn left onto East 96th Street and continue for 1.25 miles to the trailhead, on the left.

Contact: Greenways Foundation
The Depot
900 East 64th Street
Indianapolis, IN 46220
(317) 327-7431
www.indygreenways.org/monon/monon.htm

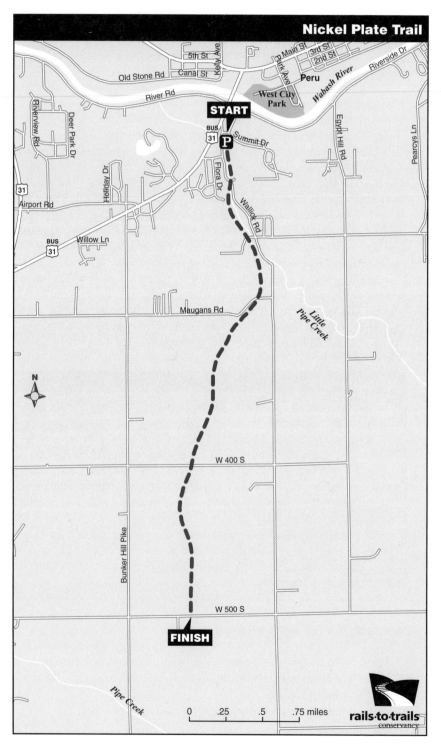

Nickel Plate Trail

Nickel Plate Trail

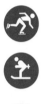

Although the Nickel Plate Trail is currently only 3.4 miles long, it represents the first step toward a nearly 40-mile rail-trail through north-central Indiana. Don't let its length deter you—this little trail promises a bounty of dense forests, water views and wildlife.

The path starts a quarter mile south of the mighty Wabash River and follows the gentle babbling waters of Little Pipe Creek south for its first mile. Around mile 1, a bridge spanning the water gives you an excellent view of the rock formations that make up the bed of Little Pipe Creek. You soon find yourself in a forest thick with willows and maple trees. Summer foliage creates a canopy over the trail that in many sections shields you from the withering sun. If you're cross-country skiing here in winter, this trail is nothing short of a snowy wonderland.

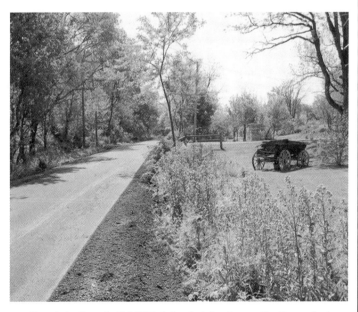

For a short pathway, the Nickel Plate Trail packs in the pleasure with willow woodlands, creek views and trailside rural homesteads.

Location
Miami County

Endpoints
Ellis Road and State Route 125 West to County Road 500 South in Peru

Mileage
3.4

Roughness Index
1

Surface
Asphalt, gravel and dirt

It may seem quiet here in the forest, but you are not alone—deer, rabbits, squirrels and chipmunks are likely to cross your path. A wide variety of bird species make their homes in these trees.

The view on the east side of the trail opens up about 1.5 miles into your trip. Near here, look for an old concrete dam that sits low in the creekbed; it has a lookout platform along the edge of the creek. The dam was originally built to supply water for the steam boilers on the locomotives pulling trains along the tracks. In spring and summer, a lovely flower bed next to the viewing platform flaunts cheerful blooms. The final 2 miles continue through the forest canopy with classic small farms and rural homesteads before the trail ends at County Road 500 South.

Future plans for the Nickel Plate Trail include extending it almost 10 miles south from County Road 500 and close to 24 miles north from the trailhead in Peru. One day, it will be a part of the 6,800-mile, cross-country American Discovery Trail.

DIRECTIONS

To access the northern trailhead, take US Route 31 north to US Route 31 Business and follow this for 1.5 miles. Turn right on Ellis Road and drive about 800 feet. Turn left on State Route 125 west (Wallick Road). Look for the trailhead, with parking, on the right after about 800 feet. This is the preferred access point as it has public parking.

Contact: Nickel Plate Trail Inc.
P.O. Box 875
Peru, IN 46970
(765) 473-9363
www.indianatrails.org/Nickel_Plate_Trail.htm

Oak Savannah Trail

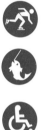

T he Oak Savannah Trail takes its name from the unique ecosystem that it runs through. Once pervasive throughout northern Indiana, the oak savannah is a transitional zone between forest and prairie, with grassland marked by a smattering of oak trees. Unfortunately, development, drought and the suppression of natural fire cycles (which allows other species to dominate) have all contributed to the massive decline of the oak savannah ecosystem. The fact that this prairie environment is now endangered makes this an important trail to visit.

Built in 1893, this corridor served the Elgin, Joliet and Eastern Railroad, whose track made a semicircle around Chicago to avoid the congestion of the city's rail yards. Because of this shape, it became known as the "J" line. In its prime, the trains carried grain, meat, fruit, vegetables and coal.

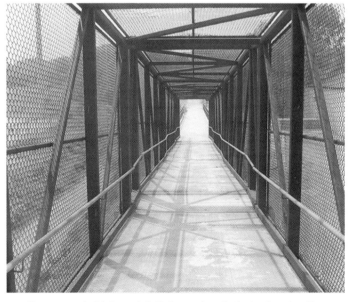

The arrow-straight Oak Savannah Trail links several neighborhood parks and neighborhoods on this once bustling former rail line.

Location
Lake and Porter counties

Endpoints
Wisconsin Street in Hobart to Oak Ridge Prairie Park in Griffith

Mileage
6.25

Roughness Index
1

Surface
Asphalt

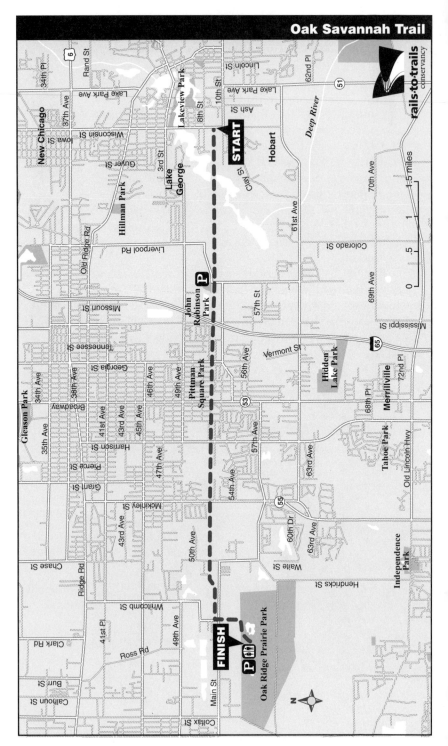

Beginning in Hobart, the well-maintained, asphalt trail very quickly takes you to the edge of Lake George—an excellent spot to fish for bass, crappie and other species; the lake is also home to a permanent population of geese, ducks and ring-billed gulls. From the trail bridge, you can walk onto platforms overlooking the lily-pad-covered neck of the lake between the lake's larger main bodies.

The next few miles of trail beyond the lake travel west through excellent representations of an oak savannah ecosystem. Shortly, you emerge along another lake at John Robinson Park (parking), where you may want to take a rest in the small field of grass along the lakefront.

At the tunnel beneath Interstate 65, the trail enters a more urban setting with a variety of road crossings, the most significant of which is at busy Broadway Street in Merrillville. Broadway is best negotiated by heading south one block and using the crosswalk at 53rd Avenue.

After crossing Broadway, you soon return to the quiet forest and prairie that dominates the trail. After passing a large private fishing club, you will see the end of the county airport runway, just west of the corridor. Here, just past mile 5.5, a very dense forest marks the entrance of Oak Ridge Prairie Park. A wonderful yet short stretch of the trail winds through the woods to the Griffith trailhead in the park's parking lot. If you want to linger, explore Oak Ridge Prairie Park, where a trout-stocked fishing lake, picnic areas and a large playground provide activities for all ages.

DIRECTIONS

To reach the Hobart trailhead, take Interstate 94 to Highway 51 (Ripley Street) and travel south for 2.3 miles. Turn right on US Route 6 (37th Avuene) and go 1.5 miles. Turn left on Wisconsin Street. The trailhead is on the right in 1.9 miles, between 8th and 10th streets. Parking is on-steet only.

To reach the Griffith trailhead in Oak Ridge Prairie Park, take I-94 to the Burr Street exit and head south for 1.5 miles. Turn right on US Route 6 (Ridge Road) and drive for 2.2 miles to the exit for Colfax Street. Look for the park's parking lot on the left.

Contact: Lake County Parks and Recreation
6400 Harrison Street
Merillville, IN 46410
(219) 945-1543
www.indianatrails.org/Oak_Savannah_Trail.htm

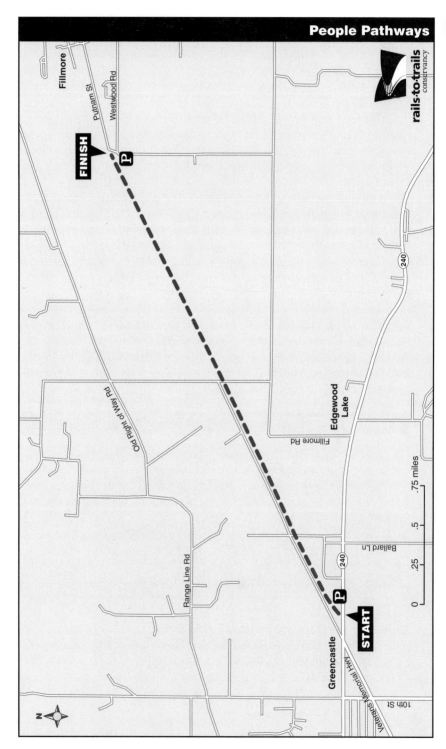

People Pathways

Its name might imply that this path is crowded with people, but in fact the People Pathways is a quiet trail through rural Midwest farmland. The rail-trail has a big past and a promising future: It follows the old Vandalia-Pennsy corridor that was the main rail line between St. Louis and Indianapolis and it is slated to be part of a 150-mile cross-state greenway known as the National Road Heritage Trail.

The trail is named for the local group that championed its development. The organization aims to establish an extensive trail system and they are well on their way—this relaxing stretch of trail was funded and constructed entirely by community volunteers.

From the gazebo and parking lot that serve as the trailhead in Greencastle, the path follows the paved shoulder of Veterans Memorial Highway, a quiet road with a wide shoulder for trail use. After a mile, the trail leaves the roadway on a crushed limestone surface and

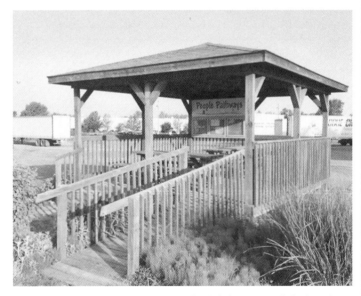

Simplicity suits the straight and unassuming People Pathways, especially for those who visit the trail to watch the local bluebird population.

Location
Putnam County

Endpoints
Calbert Way Park
in Greencastle to
County Road 475
East in Fillmore

Mileage
3.4

Roughness Index
2

Surface
Asphalt and
crushed stone

sets off into the countryside. Farm fields stretch out to the south and the old Vandalia corridor—a bed of ballast with the old train tracks—runs along to the north.

The fact that you are on one of Indiana's most rural rail-trails becomes evident rather quickly. The route is uninterrupted by road crossings, or even neighborhoods. This makes for some excellent birding opportunities. As locals know, the resident bluebird population frequents this corridor, so expect to see birders with binoculars in tow.

The trail ends in a simple gravel parking lot outside the town of Fillmore.

DIRECTIONS

To access the trailhead in Greencastle, take Interstate 70 to US Route 231 and continue north for just over 8.5 miles. Turn right on Washington Street, drive a half mile and turn left on Indianapolis Road. After 1.5 miles, turn left on Veterans Memorial Highway and look for the trailhead on the left.

To reach the Fillmore trailhead, take I-70 to US Route 231 and continue north for just over 8.5 miles. Turn right on Washington Street, drive a half mile and turn right on Indianapolis Road. After 2.7 miles, turn left on County Road 50 south (South Fillmore Street) and drive for 2.3 miles. Turn left onto South County Road 475 east. The trailhead is on the left after just over a mile, at the end of Country Road 475.

Contact: Greencastle/Putnam County Development Center
2 South Jackson Street
Greencastle, IN 46135
(765) 653-2474
www.pcfoundation.org/giving/PeoplePathways.htm

Prairie-Duneland Trail

As its name implies, a trip on the beautiful Prairie-Duneland Trail offers snapshots of the flora and fauna—from hardwood forest to remnant prairie grasslands—that once dominated this region. In spite of the rapid development of the south Chicago suburbs spilling into northwest Indiana, this trail ensures the preservation of these invaluable pockets of land. The trail also offers a classic rail-trail experience, with a long, level grade and a 10-foot-wide asphalt surface that is suitable for bicycles and inline skates (and cross-country skis in winter) and is ADA accessible.

Starting in Chesterton, the trail makes its way toward Portage and on west to Hobart, passing well-manicured subdivisions. The sights and signs of town life begin to fade away a mile and a half into the ride as you enter a lightly forested area with farm fields interspersed along the way. In between and in some cases

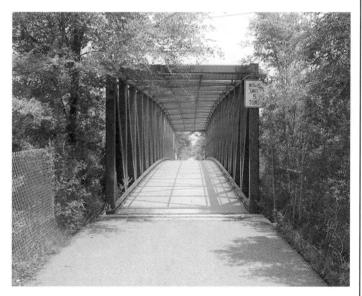

The Prairie-Duneland Trail is a mini-escape from town life and alternates between open farm fields and wooded canopy.

Location
Lake and Porter counties

Endpoints
S. Jackson Avenue in Chesterson to South Hobart Road in Hobart

Mileage
10.3

Roughness Index
1

Surface
Asphalt

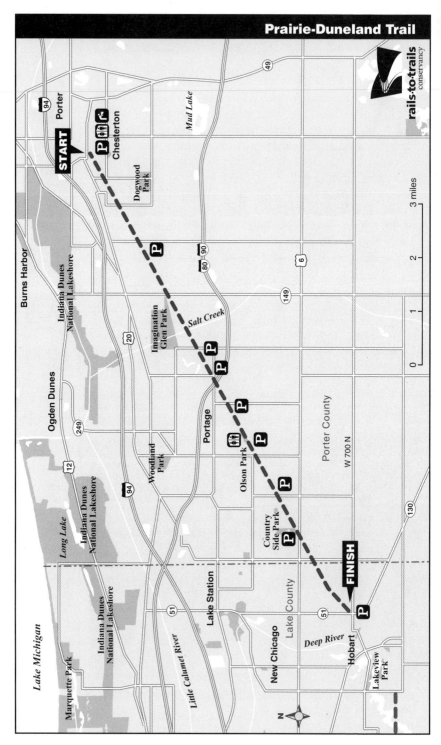

intermingled with these areas, you will encounter remnants of tall-grass prairie environments.

In several sections, a veritable tunnel of vegetation envelops the trail, with the dense forest canopy creating a lush passageway. Coming out of one such section at just past 3 miles, you encounter a 130-plus-footbridge that travels over Route 149 and takes you into the section of trail through Portage. The next stretch—approximately 2 miles—takes you through an area crossing a small creek drainage, as well as a couple streets.

Near mile 5, backyards and residential subdivisions begin to dominate the landscape. After the trail passes beneath Interstate 80, it travels through another pocket of forest. The remaining 5-mile stretch to the trail's end at Highway 51 in Hobart is bordered mostly by neatly kept backyards.

In the future, the Prairie-Duneland Trail will link with other trails, including the Oak Savannah Trail (page 103), to form the Lake Michigan Heritage Greenway and connect communities all along the south shore of Lake Michigan. This system will cross three counties and stretch over 40 miles from Hammond, Indiana, to Michigan City, Indiana.

DIRECTIONS

To access the eastern trailhead on South Jackson Avenue in Chesterton, take Interstate 94 to Highway 49 and head south for 1.25 miles. Turn right on Porter Avenue and go 1.5 miles. Turn right onto South 15th Street and turn left on West Morgan Avenue after 0.2 mile. After 0.1 mile, turn right on South Jackson and look for the trailhead on the right.

To reach the trailhead in Hobart, take I-94 to Highway 51 (Ripley Street/Adam Benjamin Highway) and head south for 3.25 miles. (Highway 51 changes names twice in this short distance—first Randolph Street, then Hobart Road). The trailhead is on the left of Hobart Road, just prior to the intersection of Hobart Road and Cleveland Avenue.

Contact: City of Portage Parks and Recreation
2100 Willowcreek Road
Portage, IN 46368
(219) 762-1675
www.indianatrails.org/
Prairie_Duneland_Trail_Portage.htm

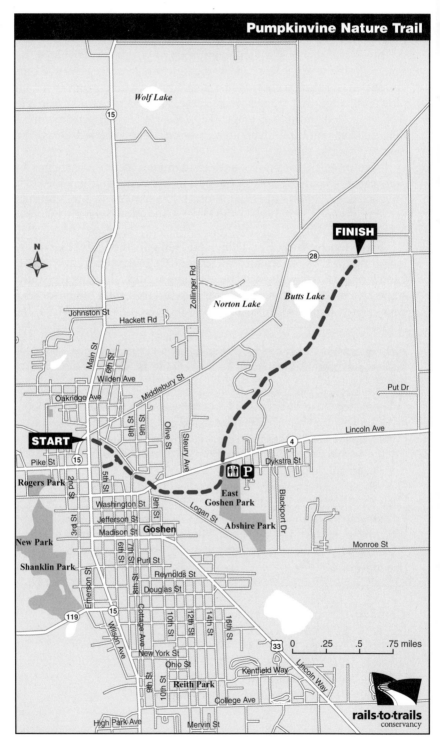

Pumpkinvine Nature Trail

The railroad line between Goshen and Middlebury was a popular passenger route at the turn of the century and its numerous curves and turns led to its being nicknamed after the rambling pumpkin vine. Today, the trail that shares this famed line's route is only 2.8 miles long, but it will one day extend for 16 miles.

The trail starts as a smooth, paved path near an active rail line in the bustling downtown of Goshen, a small Midwestern town. In the first quarter mile, keep your eyes open for the interpretive signs explaining the railroading history of this area. A restored railroad viaduct carries you across a small creek and into a quaint neighborhood. A second bridge, equally well preserved with vibrant blue paint, is a short distance ahead. After the trail crosses State Route 4 at a crosswalk, it immediately enters a wooded area en route to Abshire Park, the trail's approximate halfway point. Here you'll find a playground and restroom facilities, as well as an outdoor

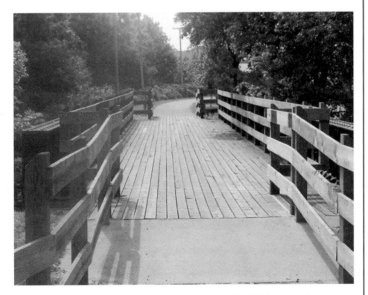

The Pumpkinvine Nature Trail and its brightly painted bridges link the surrounding communities to fun, year-round recreation destinations.

Location
Elkhart and Lagrange counties

Endpoints
5th Street and Pike Street to County Road 28 in Goshen

Mileage
2.8

Roughness Index
1

Surface
Asphalt and crushed stone

skating rink, sledding hill and warming hut, providing ample activities for every season.

When the trail crosses Route 4 again, the surface changes from asphalt to hard-packed, crushed stone. The remaining 1.5 miles travel through a thick, beautiful forest of maple and oak trees. Emerging from the trees, the trail hits County Road 28, the eastern terminus of the current trail. The undeveloped corridor lies in wait across the road, providing a tantalizing look at the future of this delightful, winding route.

DIRECTIONS

To access the starting point at 5th Street in Goshen, take US Highway 15 south, then turn left on Oakridge Avenue. Go one block then turn right on 5th Street. The trailhead is not quite a half mile ahead on the left, just before the active railroad tracks. (If you're coming from US Route 33 heading north, turn right onto 5th Street and follow the directions above.)

To reach the Abshire Park trailhead, head south on 5th Street and turn left on East Lincoln Avenue. The trailhead is on the right.

Contact: Goshen Parks and Recreation
607 West Plymouth Avenue
Goshen, IN 46526
(219) 534-2901
www.pumpkinvine.org

Sweetser Switch Trail

It may be only 3 miles long, but the Sweetser Switch Trail is nearly bursting with unique features and small-town charm. Like many things in Sweetser, the main trailhead is located right in the middle of downtown and the route is often packed with users beyond what one would expect from a local population over just 900 people. Perhaps one of the draws is the larger-than-life statue of Garfield, the comic strip cat—a nod to Garfield creator and area native Jim Davis. The trailhead also has two restored railcars that provide a wonderful backdrop for pre-trip pictures. There are restrooms, water and parking available at the trailhead.

The trail's midpoint is the town of Sweetser itself and, because of its parking and amenities, it also serves as the best starting point for your trip. Heading west out of town, wildflowers and evenly distributed solar lights line the trail. And pull that camera back out, because at the trail's western and remote endpoint, you'll find a

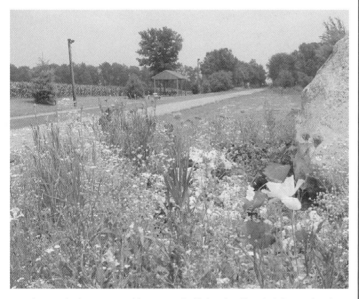

Attractive landscaping, annual festivities and added touches like solar lights speak to the local appreciation of the Sweetser Switch Trail.

Location
Grant County

Endpoints
County Road 400W to County Road 700W in Sweetser

Mileage
3

Roughness Index
1

Surface
Asphalt

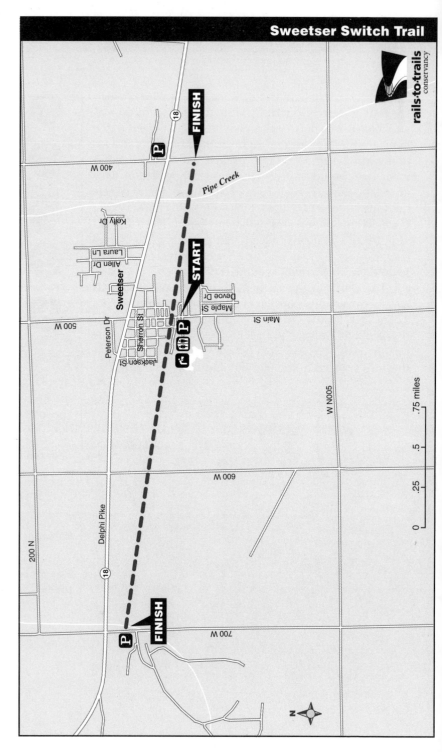

covered bridge. Pack a picnic to enjoy at the tables provided here for just such an outing.

The eastward journey from the trail's midpoint toward the town of Marion follows a similar pattern—wildflowers and solar lights, but also bird boxes so ornithologists may enjoy a sighting or two. The trail ends just outside of Sweetser. It will eventually be extended east to meet the Cardinal Greenway in Marion (page 85) and an extension northwest could bring it to the developing Nickel Plate Trail (page 101). For now, though, this robust 3-mile stretch of the Sweetser Switch is just plenty. And while the trail is popular nearly all year long, consider visiting around Halloween. The annual pumpkin walk, with a parade of jack-o'-lanterns lighting the rail-trail, is a popular event for all ages.

DIRECTIONS

To access the start point at the Garfield statue in Sweetser, follow Interstate 69 to County Route 18 and travel west for 12 miles through the town of Marion to Sweetser. Turn left (south) on N. Main Street and drive a quarter mile. The trailhead is before the railroad tracks. Look for the Garfield statue on the left by the retired rail cars.

To access the County Road 700 West from downtown Sweetser, take Main Street north to State Road 18. Turn left and follow State Road 18 west for 2 miles. Turn left onto County Road 700. The trailhead is on the left just before the railroad tracks. To access the County Road 400 West from downtown Sweetser, take Main Street north to State Road 18. Turn right and follow State Road 18 east for 1 mile. Turn right onto County Road 400. The trailhead is on the right just before the railroad tracks.

Contact: Greenways Foundation
P.O. Box 80091
Indianapolis, IN 46280
(317) 848-7855
www.indianatrails.org/Sweetser_Switch_Trail.htm

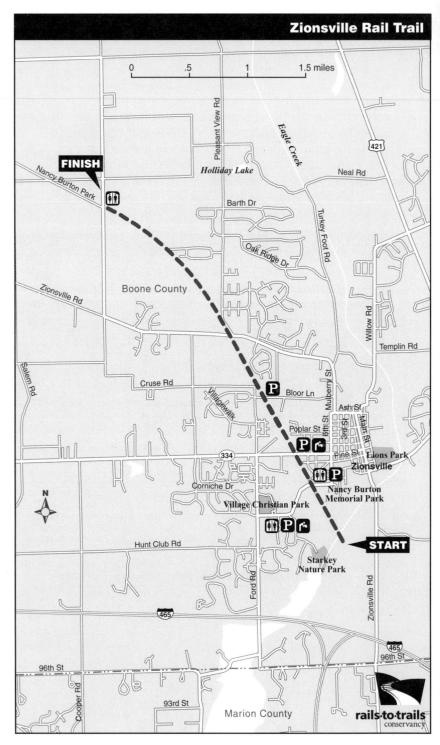

Zionsville Rail Trail

Zionsville Rail Trail

W hen greenways are done well, they deftly weave into the fabric of a town and become a material part of people's lives. Indianapolis suburb Zionsville's rail-trail system masterfully exhibits great greenway design: It threads through neighborhoods, tying together schools, churches and shops. Children use the corridor to travel safely to school and across town, while employees of local business use it for leisurely lunch-hour walks.

The trail's south end in Nancy Burton Memorial Park starts with a dramatic view of Eagle Creek from a bridge over the water 60 feet below. A descent down a mammoth boardwalk brings you to Starkey Nature Park and an extensive system of walking trails in the Eagle Creek flood plain. This system is not a part of the rail-trail, but it makes a nice side trip. This southern mile of the trail, built atop a massive embankment, travels northwest deep into old-growth woods. The hard-packed limestone surface makes for easy walking and biking and there are plenty of pleasant picnic spots, including on the bridge over Eagle Creek. In the winter, cross-country skiers flock to this corridor.

Leaving the park and the tree cover that has dominated the landscape, the trail goes through a tunnel underneath State Route 334 and the surface changes to asphalt for the remaining 2.5 miles. As it continues north and west, the trail progresses from a rural setting into a small town, passing under bridges, beneath roadways and curving past churches and the town hall. For a short stretch, just past the tunnel, you briefly depart from the old rail corridor, but the trail picks up the rail corridor again. At this point it is below street level, almost tunneling through the surrounding neighborhoods. Connecting trails drop down from the streets above.

A mere half mile east of the Route 334 tunnel is the brick-street downtown area of Zionsville with its immaculately preserved 19th-century village. Enjoy exploring the town after your trip down the rail-trail.

Location
Boone County

Endpoints
Nancy Burton
Memorial Park to
downtown
Zionsville

Mileage
3.5

**Roughness
Index**
2

Surface
Asphalt and
crushed stone

DIRECTIONS

To get to the south trailhead from Interstate 65, take Russell/State Route 334 east for 4.6 miles. Turn right on 6th Street and after a quarter mile, turn right again on Starkey Road. In 0.2 mile, you go under the trail bridge; after just 130 feet, turn right into the trail parking lot.

To get to the trailhead in downtown Zionsville from I-65, take Russell/East SR 334 for 4 miles to Zionsville Town Hall, at 1100 West Oak Street. Park in the lot in back of building, where you will also find the trail.

Contact: Zionsville Parks
1075 Parkway Drive
Zionsville, IN 46077
(317) 733-2273
www.zionsville-in.gov/parks

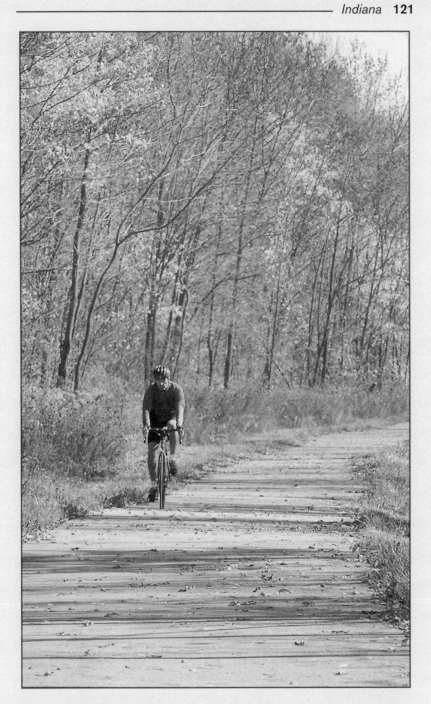

Tree-lined and limestone surfaces for much of its route, the Zionville Rail Trail is a well-used bicycling route in the summer and a popular cross-country skiing destination in the winter.

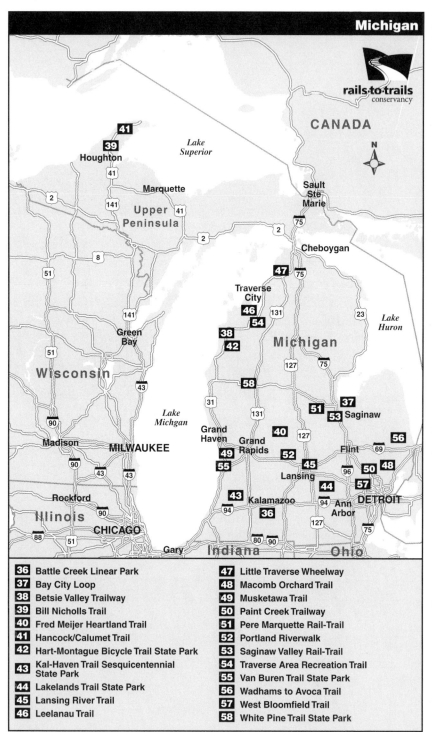

Michigan

rails·to·trails
conservancy

36	Battle Creek Linear Park	47	Little Traverse Wheelway
37	Bay City Loop	48	Macomb Orchard Trail
38	Betsie Valley Trailway	49	Musketawa Trail
39	Bill Nicholls Trail	50	Paint Creek Trailway
40	Fred Meijer Heartland Trail	51	Pere Marquette Rail-Trail
41	Hancock/Calumet Trail	52	Portland Riverwalk
42	Hart-Montague Bicycle Trail State Park	53	Saginaw Valley Rail-Trail
43	Kal-Haven Trail Sesquicentennial State Park	54	Traverse Area Recreation Trail
44	Lakelands Trail State Park	55	Van Buren Trail State Park
45	Lansing River Trail	56	Wadhams to Avoca Trail
46	Leelanau Trail	57	West Bloomfield Trail
		58	White Pine Trail State Park

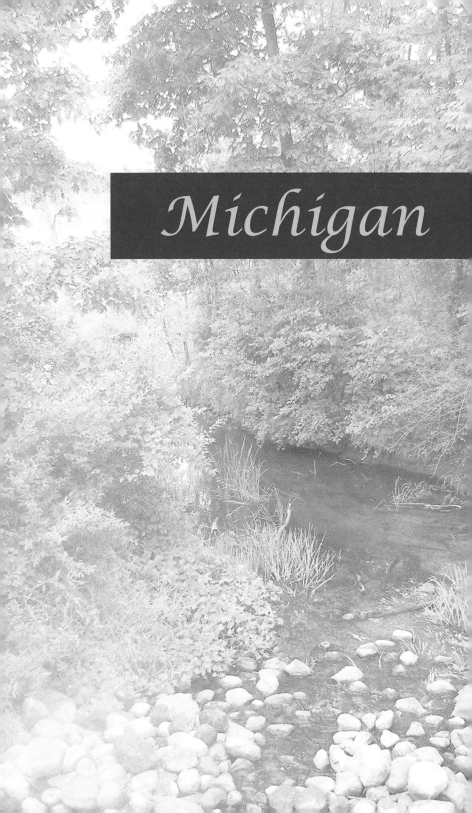

Michigan

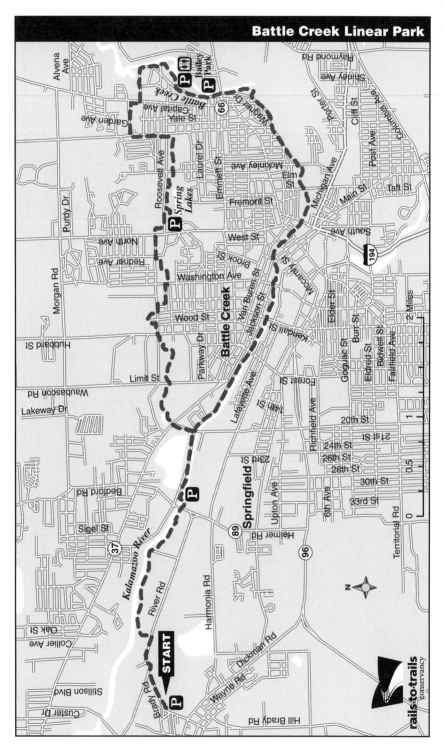

Battle Creek Linear Park

A former railroad line is the spine of this system, hugging the banks of the Kalamazoo and Battle Creek rivers, and several pathways departing and rejoining the main corridor form distinct trail loops. The Battle Creek Linear Park covers 22 miles of interconnected paved path in and around the city of Battle Creek, which is situated at the confluence of the Kalamazoo and Battle Creek rivers. Despite its urban setting, the trail takes you over winding waterways and past woodlands before heading straight through the heart of downtown Battle Creek. The trail provides education as well as recreation: Dozens of signs describe the surrounding animal and plant life, as well as the area's history and culture.

To experience this trail system fully, start at the westernmost point, off Dickman and Brady roads. Here, the trail passes through a country setting as it winds east through neighborhoods and parks and past schools and

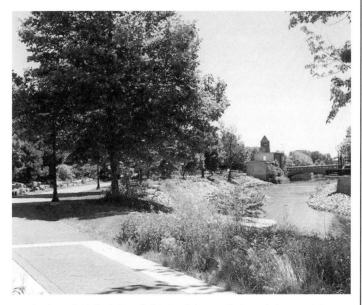

Locals use Battle Creek Linear Park to tour their namesake town, picnic, commute to school and enjoy their green space.

Location
Calhoun County

Endpoints
Dickman and Brady roads to Bailey Park in Battle Creek

Mileage
22

Roughness Index
1

Surface
Asphalt

museums. Just a mile from the start, the trail begins to travel along the banks of the Kalamazoo River.

Before you cover too much ground, pick up a trail map and brochure from one of the boxes along the path. These brochures detail the four distinct loops (color-coded on the map) that the system is divided into, which will help you plan a self-guided tour. When you reach downtown Battle Creek, there are numerous points of interest, such as a bronze statue paying tribute to the Underground Railroad and the W. K. Kellogg House, the former home of the founder of the cereal company that still dominates this city. Bailey Park, at the trail system's northeast corner, offers picnic areas, a ballpark, playgrounds and restroom facilities. From here, you can follow the winding trail back to your starting point at Dickman and Brady roads.

DIRECTIONS

To reach the trailhead at Dickman and Brady roads, take Interstate 94 to Exit 92 and follow Battle Creek Road north to Dr. Martin Luther King Drive and turn left. Turn right on Dickman Road and follow it to the corner of Brady Road. The trail will be on your right.

To access the trail in Bailey Park, take I-94 to Exit 98 and drive north to downtown Battle Creek. The trail runs throughout downtown Battle Creek and you can park almost any place to access the trail.

Contact: Battle Creek Parks and Recreation Department
35 Hamblin Avenue
Battle Creek, MI 49017
(269) 966-3431
www.bcparks.org/jsps/linear_park.jsp

The Bay County Riverwalk/Railtrail System's Bay City Loop shows community at its best, offering plenty of sights, sounds and activities along its route through Bay City and its parks and through the residential and agricultural areas of Portsmouth, Hampton and Bangor townships. There are dozens of places to access and jump off the trail and each one offers convenient parking and facilities, as well as clear signs to help you navigate the route. In the future, this trail system will extend south along the Saginaw River to link with additional communities.

The trail's striking scenery is as diverse as the type of path you will follow: As scenery changes from woodlands and marshes to riverfront views and ball fields, the trail surface changes from asphalt to sidewalk alongside major roads, to boardwalk along the waterfront and back to asphalt through the residential neighborhoods and rural township lands.

The trail is shaped like a noose, with access points all along it. One starting point is on the northern end at the Bay City State Park (parking fee) where you are treated to a sweeping vista of Saginaw Bay and the adjacent Tobico Marsh. In the first mile, the path connects with hiking trails on your right and an overlook platform with views of the marsh and the bay. Keep your eyes out for the interpretive signs along the trail and stop to visit the nature center with its exhibits on the area's unique topography.

After 2.5 miles, you leave the recreation area and travel through fields of wildflowers along an asphalt utility corridor to downtown Bay City.

At mile 7, follow the wide sidewalk connectors to and through Bay City's commercial and entertainment district, where you can access ball fields, a skate park and playgrounds at Defoe Park. A half mile later, you arrive at Liberty Bridge, marking the start of the 9.5-mile Bay City Loop part of the system, which travels through downtown Bay City and the surrounding agricultural lands. A half mile into this loop, you reach the heart of

Location
Bay County

Endpoints
Bay City to Hampton Township

Mileage
17.5

Roughness Index
1

Surface
Asphalt, concrete and boardwalk

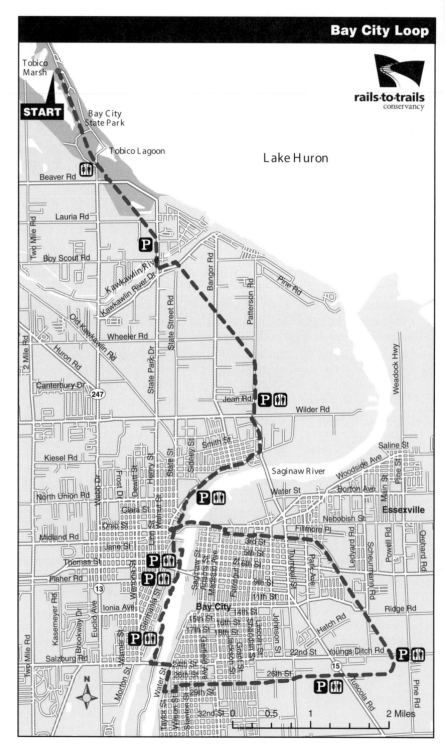

Bay City Loop

rails·to·trails
conservancy

Tobico
Marsh

START

Bay City
State Park

Tobico Lagoon

Beaver Rd

Lake Huron

Lauria Rd

Two Mile Rd

Boy Scout Rd

Kawkawlin River

Kawkawlin River Dr

Old Kawkawlin Rd

State Street Rd

Bangor Rd

Patterson Rd

Pine Rd

Wheeler Rd

State Park Dr

2 Mile Rd

Huron Rd

Canterbury Dr

247

Jean Rd

Wilder Rd

Weadock Hwy

Kiesel Rd

Frost Dr

DeWitt

Henry St

State St

Sidney St

Smith St

Saginaw River

Saline St

Woodside Ave

North Union Rd

Webb Dr

Cleata St

3rd St

Water St

Borton Ave

Main St

Pine St

Essexville

Ohio St

Elm St

Walnut St

Nebobish St

Midland Rd

Jane St

Fillmore Pl

Powell Rd

Orchard Rd

Thomas St

Isabella St

3rd St
5th St
6th St
7th St
9th St

Saginaw St

Adams St

Madison Ave

Grant St

Trumbull St

Park Ave

Ledyard Rd

Scheurmann Rd

Fisher Rd

13

Washington Ave

11th St

Ionia Ave

Kasemeyer Rd

Brookway Dr

Euclid Ave

Germania St

Bay City

15th St
16th St
17th St

Lincoln St

Sheridan Ave

Johnson St

Hatch Rd

Ridge Rd

22nd St

Youngs Ditch Rd

Warner St

Van Buren St

Jackson St

Grant St

15

Salzburg Rd

Morton St

Water St

26th St

Tuscola Rd

Pine Rd

Two Mile Rd

Taylor St

Wilson St

Stanton St

29th St

32nd St

N

0   0.5   1   2 Miles

downtown, where eateries will tempt you with a variety of ethnic cuisines.

From downtown, the trail continues to a bustling marina and the popular waterfront Veteran's Memorial Park, featuring beautiful gardens, riverside benches and memorials of shipbuilding days gone by. The waterfront section features several ball fields, picnic areas and playgrounds.

At mile 9, bird-watchers will enjoy the stretch of trail that follows a boardwalk for a few blocks over the Saginaw River. A mile later, the trail courses through a distinctly residential district, where private gardens are resplendent with delightfully bright blooms.

After Youngs Ditch Road near mile 13 and about halfway through the loop, the corridor opens up for a smooth pass through agricultural lands and countryside that will appeal to nature lovers.

Be sure to print a copy of the rail-trail map at www.bayfound ation.org before you go. The map consists of two pages and covers the loop as well as the newer extension to the Bay State Recreation Area.

DIRECTIONS

The easiest access point for the trail is in Bay City at Veterans Memorial Park. Coming from the north or south, take Interstate 75 to Bay City and take Exit 162. Go east (toward Bay City) on Business I-75/State Highway 25 for 2.5 miles. This becomes Thomas Street in town. When you reach John F. Kennedy Drive, you can turn left or right to either of the park's entrances.

To reach Bay City State Park from Interstate 75, exit east in North Williams onto East Beaver Road. East Beaver Road crosses North Euclid Road to become State Park Road, and just past North Euclid Road you cross the trail. Parking is another quarter mile ahead on the right.

Contact: Bay City Convention and Visitor's Bureau
901 Saginaw Street
Bay City, MI 48708
(989) 893-1222
www.tourbaycitymi.org/parks-and-camping-12/416/416/

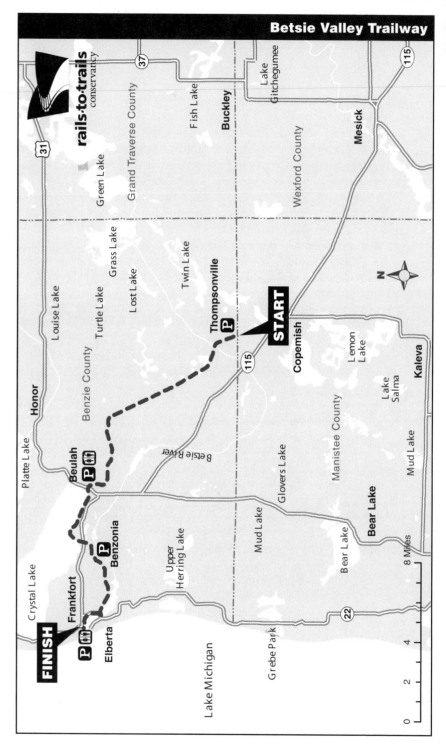

Betsie Valley Trailway

Northern Michigan's natural splendor is on display during a trip along the 23-mile Betsie Valley Trail. Stretching north and west from Thompsonville to Frankfort, the crushed limestone and asphalt trail travels through Pere Marquette State Forest and along the waters of Crystal Lake, the Betsie River and Betsie Lake. Some parts of the limestone sections of the trail are quite soft and road bikers should follow signs indicating an alternate route for the section from the town of Beulah to Mollineaux Road.

Thompsonville's Crystal Mountain Resort Area, which offers lodging, dining and bike rentals, serves as the starting point for this journey. (If you choose to start from the trail's southern terminus, there is parking at the ball field just north of Lindy Road.)

In the 13-mile section from Thompsonville to Beulah, you travel the former Ann Arbor Railroad corridor through forest and fields; 6 miles of this portion passes

Location
Benzie County

Endpoints
Thompsonville to Frankfort

Mileage
23

Roughness Index
2

Surface
Asphalt, crushed stone and ballast

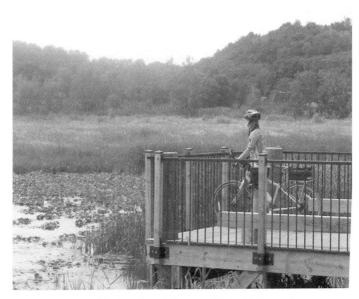

Make a vacation of the Betsie Valley Trailway and all its local features such as water sports on Lake Michigan and Crystal Lake, resorts, culinary delights and a restored

through the naturally beautiful Pere Marquette State Forest. Also along the way are several historical remnants, including the old turbine from the dam that was once the sole source of electricity in this area and the ghost town of Homestead, where railroad maintenance workers lived in boarding houses at the turn of the 19th century. While the limestone surface may be soft in spots, the trail offers a nice, gradual descent along the 5.3-mile stretch between Aylsworth Road and Beulah.

Once you arrive in Beulah, stop by the historic rail depot for visitor information, bathrooms and historic memorabilia. (There is also ample parking if you choose to start or end your journey here.) Shops, bicycle and kayak rentals, a public beach and a playground are also located here.

Just west of Beulah, the trail meets the south shore of Crystal Lake. Here, the trail winds through a row of beachside cottages and the lake lives up to its name, with hues of deep sapphire and turquoise shimmering in the sunlight. Be sure to abide by signs warning trail users that dogs are not allowed within this segment. Trail users must stay within the 10-foot trail easement and adhere to a speed limit of 10 miles per hour for the short segment to Railroad Point Natural Area.

This beautiful 67-acre Railroad Point Natural Area offers a 1-mile stretch of county-preserved beach along Crystal Lake. Here, the waves lap up against shady stands of birch, aspen, pine and hardwood maple. Take a swim, enjoy a picnic and, above all, take time to enjoy this slice of lakeside splendor.

At Mollineaux Road, near mile 15, the trail surface becomes asphalt and the route veers into the woods and soon begins following the Betsie River. At an overlook jutting out above the river, peer down for a bird's-eye view of the fish jumping in the waters below.

More wildlife viewing awaits in the village of Elberta. The Audubon Society built a wooden viewing platform overlooking the marsh and wetlands at the mouth of the Betsie River and lucky visitors will spot herons and all sorts of migrating waterfowl and marsh birds, including ducks, geese, snipes and rails. Cross State Highway M-115 and in seconds you reach another observation deck overlooking Betsie Lake, which is the access waterway to Lake Michigan. From here, the trail travels along the shore to the public marina, which offers a safe haven for Great Lakes boaters.

The small town of Frankfort, at trail's end, serves up culinary delights and overnight lodging if you're ready for a meal and a bed. There is also a bike-rental shop in Frankfort, if you plan to start your journey there.

DIRECTIONS

To reach the Thompsonville trailhead, take State Highway M-115 to Thompsonville and then follow Thompsonville Road north to Beecher Road. The parking area is on left side of Thompsonville Road.

To reach the Frankfort trailhead, take State Highway M-115 to 9th Street in Frankfort and turn left to access the trailhead.

Contact: Friends of the Betsie Valley Trail
P.O. Box 474
Beulah, MI 49617
(231) 775-9727 ext. 6045
www.betsievalleytrail.org

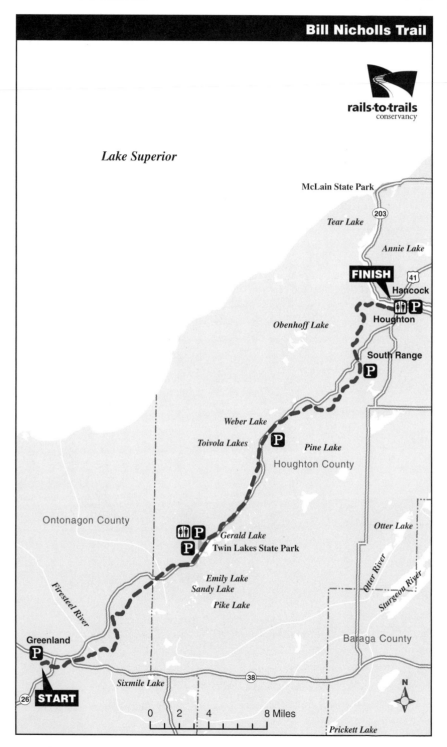

Bill Nicholls Trail

Both scenic and challenging, the Bill Nicholls Trail (a portion of designated Snowmobile Trail #3) covers 41.5 miles of sometimes steep, sometimes sandy and sometimes soaring terrain. The trail takes you over the west and east branches of the Firesteel River on three successive steel bridges that total nearly 1300 feet in length, with a maximum clearance over the water of 85 feet, providing a breathtaking experience.

Nearly 40 miles of the trail follows the route of the Copper Range Railroad, built between 1899 and 1901. When the state acquired the line in 1974, it was among the first inactive railroad corridors in Michigan to be converted to a public trail. The beginning of the trail at the Ontonagon County Fairgrounds outside of Greenland is not a rail-trail at all. This 1.9-mile section of the Bill Nicholls Trail, called the "Adventure Trail" in memory of local trail advocate Peter H. Wolfe, is quite challenging in parts. A rock escarpment, steep grades and mine tailings

Location
Houghton and
Ontonagon
counties

Endpoints
Greenland to
Houghton

Mileage
41.5

**Roughness
Index**
3

Surface
Gravel, ballast, dirt
and sand

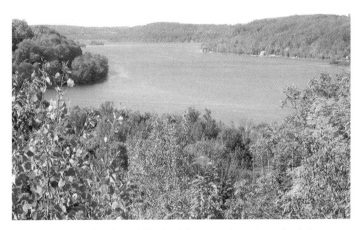

The Bill Nicholls Trail offers a 41.5-mile, challenging—and rewarding—rail-trail adventure.

135

placed on the trail to prevent erosion force you to watch your step or walk your bicycle. Heading east, you soon pass the Adventure Mine, where copper was excavated from 1850 to the 1920s. The mine now offers tours and is part of the Keweenaw National Historical Park, a collection of heritage sites celebrating the region's rich copper mining history.

After less than 2 miles, the trail heads northeast and merges with the former railroad line and its level cinder surface. There is plenty more adventure to come and not just because the trail surface keeps changing between cinder, dirt, sand and rocks.

After crossing State Highway M-38, you enter the trail's most scenic section, which stretches for nearly 11 miles. Highlights include the three Firesteel River bridges, near mile 4.2. This area is remote—there are no major road crossings until you cross State Highway M-26—so plan accordingly.

The trail attracts motorized users in all seasons and is in parts heavily impacted by ATV use. The most noticeable wear and tear is found near the few communities along the trail and at the Twin Lakes State Park, near mile 16.4. As you approach the state park, the trail parallels State Highway 26. This allows easy access to the park and to nearby businesses that cater to park users. The park offers a day-use area and camping.

From the state park to the small community of Toivola, the trail passes several small lakes, traverses scenic woodlands and is periodically lined with wild blackberry and thimbleberry bushes. With a tower as your beacon, you arrive at Toivola, which offers a restaurant and a small grocery store near mile 25.2.

A bridge is currently out near mile 31.4 at Painesdale. As you make the steep descent, you enter an area heavily impacted by mining activities and pass old ruins and mine-tailing piles. After crossing State Highway M26 into South Range, you can visit the Copper Range Historical Museum. Read the sign over the trail that describes the many offerings at the surrounding community near mile 34.4.

The last 4 miles into Houghton are all downhill. Be careful because unexpected surface changes make for a challenging descent. About 1.5 miles from the trail's end is a scenic overlook onto the Portage Lake Ship Canal, which played a big role in the copper mining industry. The final leg of the trail parallels the canal. With about 1 mile to the finish, you pass another large bridge that has been removed. A stone surface leads you down to the road and back up to the trail on the other side. The slope is steep and the stone is loose, so be careful. The trail comes to an end at the City RV Park in Houghton, near the Raymond C. Kestner Waterfront Park, where picnic facilities, restrooms, a beach and a playground will restore your energy for the return trip.

DIRECTIONS

To access the Greenland trailhead, follow State Highway M-26 and turn left on State Highway M-38. Veer left onto Plank Road, the turn left on Depot Street. There is parking on the right.

To access the trailhead in Houghton, follow State Highway M-26 north to Houghton. Turn left onto Canal Drive just before the river. Parking is available at the Raymond C. Kestner Waterfront Park.

Contact: Michigan Department of Natural Resources
Forest Management Division
427 US 41 North
Baraga, MI 49908
(906) 353-6651
www.exploringthenorth.com/keweenaw/billnichols.html

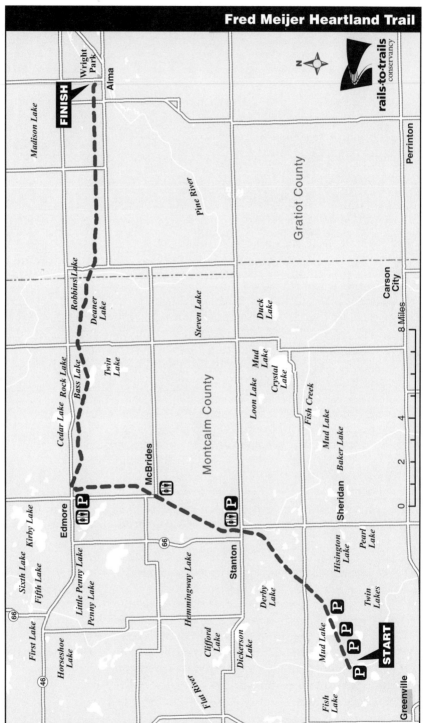

Fred Meijer Heartland Trail

Fred Meijer Heartland Trail

The story of the 41-mile Fred Meijer Heartland Trail is one of generosity, dedication and can-do attitudes. Fred and Lena Meijer helped purchase the unused corridor in 1994, Rails-to-Trails Conservancy held it for safekeeping and a very active citizens group took over the trail's operation and development in 2000. Since then the corridor has blossomed into a scenic asphalt trail from the northern edge of Greenville to Edmore. The remaining 20 miles, from Edmore to Alma, are open but awaiting pavement.

From Lake Road in Greenville to the Village of Edmore, you will find a peaceful 22-mile stretch of paved trail through prime agricultural lands, woods, meadows, wetlands and small historic towns. Just 1.5 miles down the trail, you reach the first attraction: a connecting trail to the Heritage Village at Montcalm Community College, a cluster of 20 historical buildings with artifacts depicting life in Michigan at the turn of the 20th century. While the grounds are open year-round, visitors to the annual Heritage Festival in August and other special events throughout the year can enter many of these buildings, including a one-room schoolhouse, a blacksmith shop and a town jail. Costumed reenactments make history come alive at those times. A historic 1887 trestle bridge (former road bridge) gets you over Fish Creek at mile 6, halfway between Sidney and Stanton.

Just 2 miles from Stanton at mile 5.5 the trail passes through the first of two wildlife areas along this trail, the Stanton State Game Area. In the warm months, the trail is abloom with many native wildflowers, all of which are documented and on display at the herbarium exhibit at Montcalm Community College. Another trailside attraction paying tribute to the past is the Railroad Worker Memorial in Stanton at mile 7.5. Stanton, the county seat for Montcalm County, offers a variety of eateries, from fast food to home cooking and a few local shops that carry clothing and other supplies. Back on the trail, you run right up to the Mid-Michigan Motorplex Dragstrip at mile 9.5, where you may be able to catch a glimpse of

Location
Gratiot and Montcalm counties

Endpoints
Greenville (Lake Road) to Alma

Mileage
41

Roughness Index
2

Surface
Asphalt, gravel and ballast

the dragsters being put through their paces in the warmer months. The historic town of Edmore is next at mile 14.5, with memorabilia at the Old Fence Rider Museum and in the local antique shops. It is here that the trail sharply changes direction from north to east as you make your way toward Vestaburg.

Halfway there the trail travels through the Vestaburg State Game Area. This area, so rich with the natural beauty of woods and waters, became even better environs for wildlife when the water washed out the rail corridor in the mid-1980s and beaver and other wetland species took up residence.

The beauty of this section of trail is that it goes for 2.5 miles without a single road crossing. Many white-tailed deer, fox, muskrat and other animals can be spotted traversing this open space along the way. A short trail link at mile 25 to Cedar Lake Academy, a Seventh Day Adventist school, presents a most unique historic artifact—a two-story outhouse. The story has it that the local hotel owner had seven daughters living with him on the hotel's second floor. He did not want them to interact with the railroad workers and lumberjacks who frequented the first floor and so he provided them with their own outhouse.

The town of Riverdale at mile 33 boasts the Riverdale Museum where you can visit a restored one-room schoolhouse and cross the Pine River trestle bridge. The town of Elwell 2 miles farther has limited services for trail users, but your journey ends 4 miles later in the largest town along the trail: Alma, the home of Alma College and many grocery stores, a bike shop and several other businesses.

DIRECTIONS

The Lake Road entrance to the trail holds a couple cars, but is not an official trailhead. You may find parking at many of the cross streets and at a sizeable shared use parking lot at Sidney, but the official trailheads are in Stanton, McBride and Edmore.

To start the trail in Greenville, follow Lafayette Street north out of Greenville to County Farm Road. Turn right on Lake Road. Turn left and continue a half mile to the trailhead.

To start in Edmore, take State Highway M-46 in downtown Edmore to 3rd Street. Turn south on 3rd Street to reach the trailhead.

Contact: Friends of the Fred Meijer Heartland Trail
6125 North Douglas Road
Riverdale, MI 48877
(989) 235-6170
www.montcalm.org/trail

Hancock/Calumet Trail

Take a trip through the heart of "Copper Country" on the Hancock/Calumet Trail. When more than three-quarters of the nation's copper came from this region of the Keweenaw Peninsula, Mineral Range Railroad cars hauled hard-rock copper along this route. Today the rolling corridor is home to 13.4 miles of trail that also goes by the names "Jack Stevens Calumet-Hancock Rail Trail" and "Snowmobile Trail #17."

The Portage Lift Bridge, the heaviest and widest double-decked vertical lift bridge in the world, serves as the backdrop for the southern end of the trail, but it is more convenient to park and start your journey from just west of the bridge at Hancock's Porvoo Park. Faced with starting a climb cold from the park, you might want to warm up your legs by heading first over to the lift bridge to visit Turtle Garden and Labyrinth Park. Check out the sights, then hit the trail.

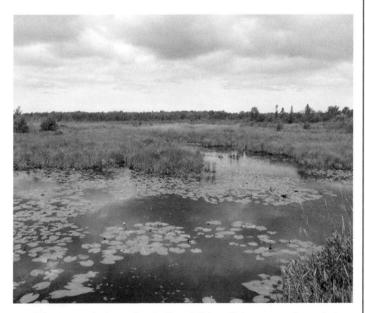

Lakes are a regular feature along the Hancock/Calumet Trail, as are some hearty climbs that reward bicyclists especially with easy downhill coasting.

Location
Houghton County

Endpoints
Hancock to Calumet

Mileage
13.4

Roughness Index
2

Surface
Asphalt, gravel, ballast and dirt

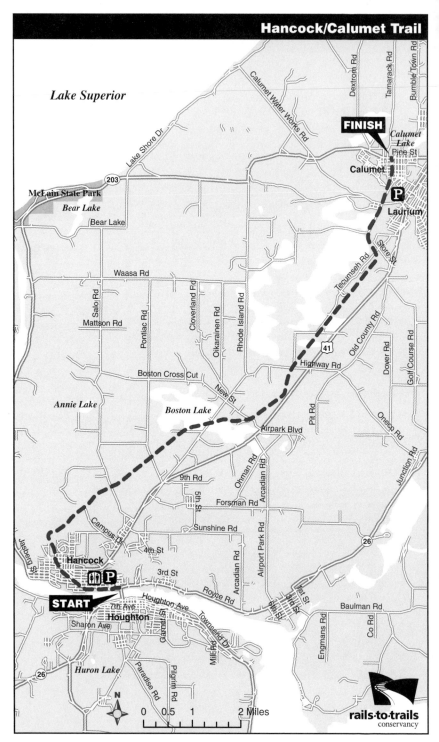

Hancock/Calumet Trail

The first few miles of the trail within the city of Hancock from Porvoo Park are paved—a rarity for Upper Peninsula rail-trails—and steep. As you huff and puff up the incline, you can appreciate the energy required to move trains up this hill. Coasting downhill on your return will soon put a smile on your face and so will this: The trail levels off near mile 4. After leaving the asphalt surface in Hancock, the trail alternates between crushed stone and dirt and you sail past numerous ponds, wetlands, fishing spots, mine tailing piles (piles of rock brought to the surface during mining) and other relics of the copper mining era.

As you approach the Calumet area the trail skirts the Swedetown Recreation Area and Swedetown Trails. Formerly just for cross-country skiers, these trails now welcome mountain bikers too. Closer to downtown Calumet an old railroad bridge frames the boarded-up Mineral Range depot. This idle bridge now stands as a gateway to Calumet for trail users as they pass beneath it. The depot serves as a logical ending point for the trail.

Calumet is the headquarters for the Keweenaw National Historical Park that preserves and celebrates the mining history of Michigan's Keweenaw Peninsula. If you're interested in learning about this area when copper was king, pick up a brochure and take a walking tour of the historical downtown. Summer visitors have greater opportunities for enjoyment, when the seasonally operated heritage center and the Coppertown Mining Museum are open.

DIRECTIONS

To start at the southern end in Hancock, take US Highway 41 or State Highway M-26 north to cross the Portage Lake Lift Bridge, exit right (east) along the ramp for State Highway M-26 and turn right at the first access road to loop under the Lift Bridge to the trailhead, or continue west along Navy Street to park at Porvoo Park at the end of Tezcuco Street.

To start at the northern end in Calumet, take US Highway 41 north and turn left on 6th Street. Turn left on Elm Street to reach the trailhead by the old depot.

Contact: Upper Peninsula Mountain Biking
(906) 353-6651
www.traillink.com

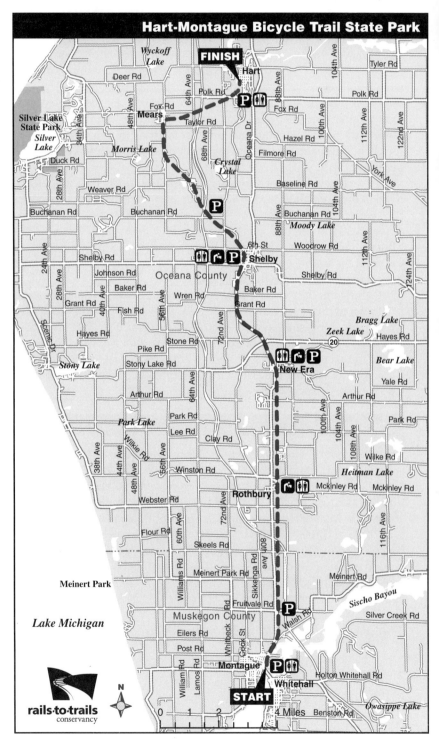

Hart-Montague Bicycle Trail State Park

Hart-Montague Bicycle Trail State Park

The paved 22-mile Hart-Montague Trail State Park is one of Michigan's great rural rail-trails. The trail is located in Oceana County, the "asparagus capital of the world," and the town of Hart hosts an annual asparagus festival complete with a parade, floats and an Asparagus Queen. Agriculture may have a hold on this area today, but Montague, Mears and Hart all have museums showcasing the time when the railroad and lumber industry reigned.

The trail begins in Montague. From the trailhead in Montague, a connecting trail—the 4-mile White Lake Trailway—heads south, crosses the White Lake River and continues through the City of White Hall. For the Hart-Montague Trail, head north. Whichever way you go first, this is the spot to see the world's largest weathervane, a 48-foot structure depicting a Great Lakes schooner that went down in a 1901 storm.

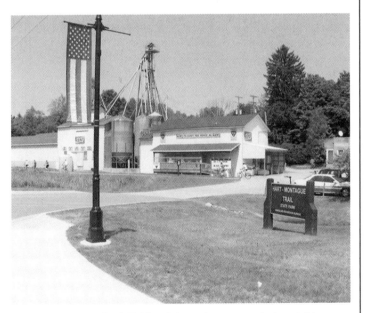

The Hart-Montague Bicycle Trail State Park is as American as apple pie—or in this case homemade ice cream and the annual crowning of the Asparagus Queen.

Location
Muskegon and Oceana counties

Endpoints
Hart to Montague

Mileage
22

Roughness Index
1

Surface
Asphalt

The southern segment of the trail is straight and flat. Christmas tree farms and orchards line the trail—look for cherries, peaches, apples, even apricots and plums. Be on the lookout for deer milling around in the fields and orchards, especially in the morning and evening. Springtime features a colorful and fragrant trip past the blossoming fruit trees, while autumn brings the crunch of leaves of spectacular reds, oranges and gold.

As the trail moves north through the small towns of Rothbury, New Era, Shelby and Mears, it becomes hilly and winding. Between Rothbury and Mears there are viewing platforms with picnic tables offering scenic views of the wooded areas. The Village of New Era is near the halfway point of the trail, and during the summer trail users can stop for homemade ice cream at the trailside dairy bar. In the town of Mears, which has plenty of places to stop for food and water, you can spot remnant prairie grasses along the trail. The gently rolling terrain offers nice country vistas, with plenty of places to stop for a rest.

The rail-trail winds down in Hart, but your adventure could be just heating up: Hart is the gateway to the beautiful beaches and giant sand dunes of Silver Lake and Lake Michigan.

DIRECTIONS

To reach the southern trailhead in Montague, take US Highway 31 north to Whitehall/Montague exit. Turn right on Bus. 31/Colby Street. Follow Business 31 past the stoplight in Montague and to trailhead parking on the right.

To reach the Hart area trailhead, follow US Highway 31 north and turn right onto Tyler Road/Main Street. Gurney Park and the trailhead is at the corner of Tyler and Oceans roads.

Contact: Michigan Department of Natural Resources
Mason Building, Third Floor
P.O. Box 30031
Lansing MI 48909
(517) 373-9900
www.michigandnr.com/parksandtrails/Details.
aspx?id=452&type=SPRK

Kal-Haven Trail
Sesquicentennial State Park

The nine towns that once stood between Kalamazoo and South Haven were connected by train from 1870 to 1970. Some of those towns have faded into the past, but the old railroad corridor linking Kalamazoo and South Haven still hums with activity as the 34.5-mile Kal-Haven rail-trail, itself a state park.

Begin at the eastern trailhead on 10th Street in Kalamazoo. A refurbished caboose serves as the trail office and information center. The beginning of the trail is paved—though the majority of the route is crushed slag and limestone—and slopes gently downward. Trees flanking the trail offer many miles of shade before you enter the open fields of Mentha. Almost nothing remains of the old Mentha Plantation that built this area's reputation for producing some of the world's finest peppermint oil.

Continuing west you pass the south edge of Kendall and Gobles. The restored Bloomingdale Depot stands as

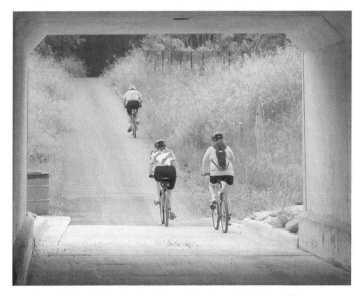

Restored railroad relics add authenticity and charm to popular Kal-Haven Trail Sesquicentennial State Park.

Location
Kalamazoo and Van Buren counties

Endpoints
Kalamazoo to South Haven

Mileage
34.5

Roughness Index
2

Surface
Crushed stone

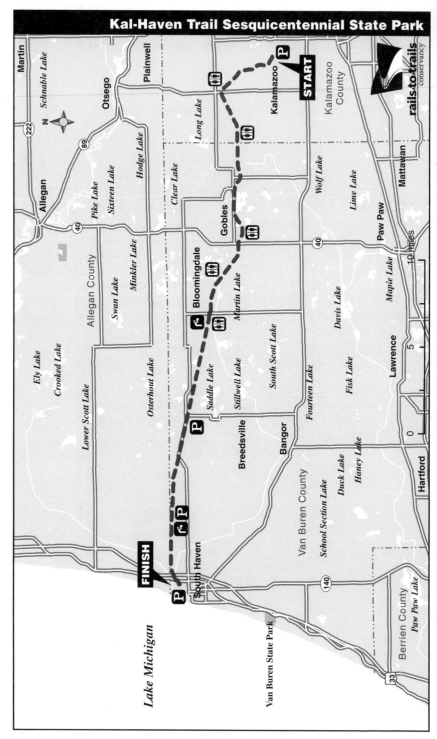

the halfway point of the trail and houses a museum filled with railroad and local history.

One mile east of Grand Junction, a bridle trail starts and follows the trail until 1 mile beyond the town of Kibbie. In Grand Junction a pedestrian walkway carries you over active train tracks. Just 2 miles past Grand Junction you cross the Camelback Bridge, named for its unique curved camelback style, over Barber Creek. In early spring the trail here is lined with a white carpet of wild trilliums.

The covered bridge over the Black River signals that you are nearing the end of the trail and you begin winding uphill to the South Haven staging area. Trail passes are required to use this trail (purchase daily or yearly tickets at trailheads), but you will be glad for the chance to explore this rambling corridor where trains once rolled.

DIRECTIONS

To reach the Kalamazoo trailhead, take Interstate 131 to Exit 38. Turn left on 10th Street and follow 10th Street for 2 miles. The trailhead is on your left.

To access the South Haven trailhead, take Interstate 196 to Exit 20. Take Phoenix Road west to Bailey Road. Turn right on Bailey Road and left onto Wells Sreet. The trailhead will be on your left.

Contact: Friends of the Kal-Haven Trail
P.O. Box 20062
Kalamazoo, MI 49019
(269) 674-8011
www.kalhaventrail.org

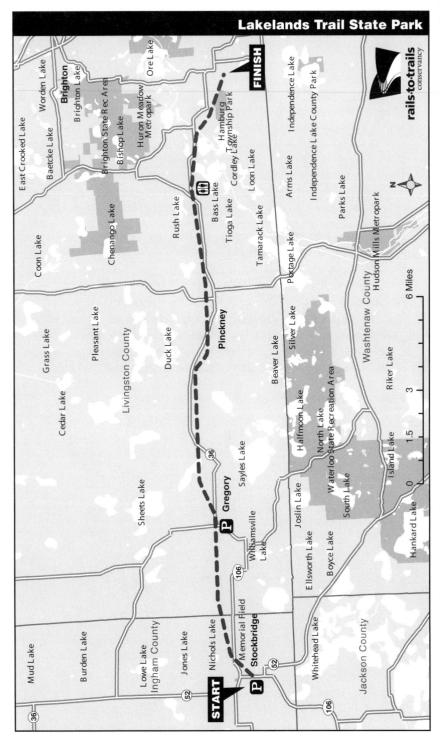

Lakelands Trail State Park

Lakelands Trail State Park

Stretching 26 miles through central Michigan, this rail-trail has two personalities: rural and suburban. Twenty miles of soft limestone surface from Stockbridge to Pinckney offer a pastoral backdrop, and 6 miles of smooth asphalt carry you through rapidly growing Hamburg Township. The trail is an easy drive from the major population centers of Detroit, Lansing, Jackson and Ann Arbor, which contributes to its popularity.

Heading east from the Stockbridge Trailhead amid working farms, wide-open fields and woods, you will understand why equestrians feel right at home on this trail. A diverse collection of wildflowers and butterflies flourish here. The small town of Gregory, followed by the equally quaint Pinckney, add charm to this quiet agricultural area and are good stopping points to enjoy lunch or ice cream or to stock up on supplies.

Mountain bikers and walkers have a seamless transition to the trail's recently paved 6-mile section, where

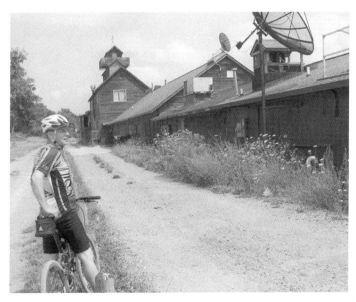

Horseback riders, mountain bikers and families pushing strollers will all find their home at some point on the diverse and pastoral Lakelands Trail State Park.

Location
Ingham and Livingston counties

Endpoints
Stockbridge to Hamburg Township

Mileage
26

Roughness Index
2

Surface
Asphalt, crushed stone and ballast

they join skinny tires and strollers to continue through the swiftly developing suburb of Hamburg Township. The woods grow thicker and frequently arch into a canopy as the trail meanders to Zukey Lake, a popular destination for swimming, boating and fishing.

Trail traffic increases as you head east, but the corridor remains a peaceful getaway. Just before reaching Pettysville Road at mile 15.5, there is a tunnel under State Route 36, transporting you safely under the road. At that point there is a large trailhead. A little farther along, the trail skirts along behind shops, restaurants and snack stops in Hamburg Township.

Locals are looking to expansion plans that would take the Lakelands Trail another 16 miles to Jackson, where it would link to Jackson's urban pathway system and provide a journey from sweeping rural vistas to urban conveniences.

DIRECTIONS

To access the Stockbridge trailhead, take State Route M-106/M-52 south through Stockbridge, crossing Main Street in downtown Stockbridge. After crossing Main, the trail is approximately 0.5 mile ahead on the left.

To access the Hamburg Township trailhead, take Interstate 23 to Exit 54. Head west on State Route M-36/Nine Mile Road. Turn left to head south on Merrill Road. The trailhead at Manly W. Bennett Memorial Park is on the left.

Contact: Lakelands Trail State Park
10405 Merrill Road
Hamburg, MI 48139
(810) 231-4295
www.hamburg.mi.us/lakelands_trail_state_park

Lansing River Trail

Michigan's state capital boasts a rail-trail, coursing along scenic riverbanks for 8 miles from the campus of Michigan State University to Old Town Lansing. The Lansing River Trail follows the Red Cedar River west to its junction with the Grand River and then follows the Grand River north. Despite the urban setting you will experience wetlands and woodlands and probably catch sight of the trail's resident ducks, squirrels and butterflies. The paved path has sections of wooden boardwalk passing under highways and skirting out over the water, avoiding almost all contact with motorized traffic.

From the Clippert Street trailhead at the trail's southeast end you travel 1 mile before coming to the Aurelius Road trailhead and another half mile to Potter Park. The park is beautifully landscaped and its location—right on the Red Cedar River—offers a soothing atmosphere to

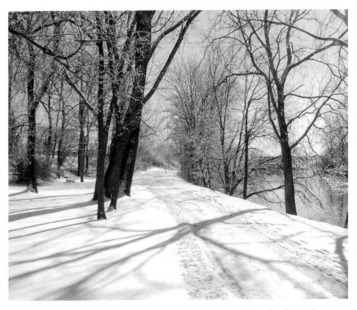

Used year-round, the Lansing River Trail is a green escape in the midst of a bustling city.

Location
Ingham County

Endpoints
Michigan State University campus (Lansing) to Old Town Lansing

Mileage
8

Roughness Index
1

Surface
Asphalt

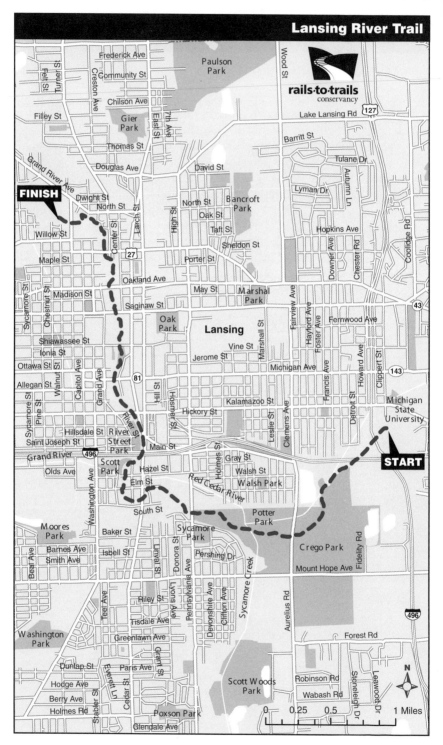

Lansing River Trail

rails·to·trails
conservancy

feed ducks or simply take a break. It is also home to the Potter Park Zoo and is a popular stop for post–zoo picnics.

Next the trail crosses Pennsylvania Avenue via a wooden pedestrian bridge. An active railroad bridge parallels the trail at this point, and if your timing is right you may find yourself racing a train. Where the Red Cedar and Grand rivers join, you head due north along the Grand River toward downtown Lansing. A collection of historical and cultural locations speckle the route from here, starting with the Impression 5 Science Center and its planet walk. Next door is the River Walk Theater and the R. E. Olds Transportation Museum.

Continuing north, beside the trail at mile 4 is the Lansing City Market. The market—in operation since 1909—is the place to stop for fresh local produce and handmade crafts. Shaded benches and tables in Adado Riverfront Park, adjacent to the market, make a great picnic spot.

Old Town Lansing—and the northern end of the rail-trail—provide some beautiful scenery. Simply stick to the path and you will see the peaceful Burchard Dam and the architecturally striking Brenke Fish Ladder, which allows fish to bypass the dam by scaling spiral steps. To wander through an art gallery or find a charming cafe, hop off the trail at mile 5 and visit downtown Old Town. The Turner-Dodge House is located at the trail's endpoint. This magnificent brick mansion, one of Lansing's most recognized landmarks, has been restored to reflect life in the 1800s. Arrange for a tour, drink tea on the porch, or at the very least stop to admire the beautifully manicured lawns and gardens before returning along this urban oasis of a trail.

DIRECTIONS

To access the East Lansing trailhead, take Interstate 127 north to Exit 8 onto Kalamazoo Street. Turn right on East Kalamazoo Street, then turn right onto South Clippert Street. Turn right to reach the trailhead.

To access the Turner Dodge Park trailhead, take Interstate 496 through Lansing. Take Exit 6 north on Martin Luther King Boulevard for 3 miles, then turn right on North Grand River Avenue. The trailhead in Dodge Park is 0.5 mile on the right.

Contact: City of Lansing
124 West Michigan Avenue
Lansing, MI 48933
(517) 483-4277
www.re-news.net/update/year2/maps/
rivertrail.htm

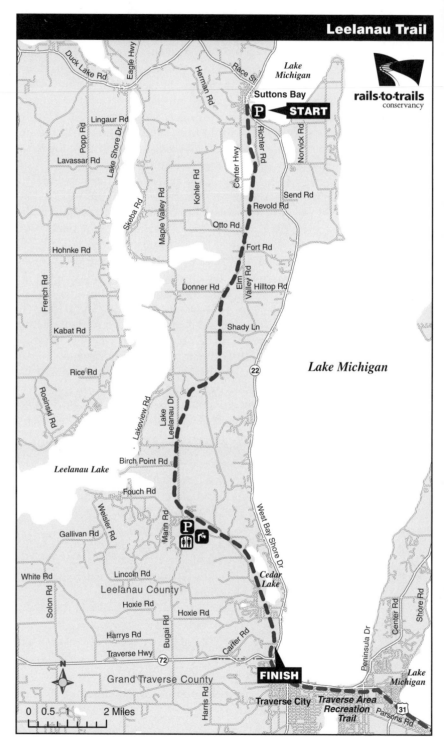

Leelanau Trail

rails·to·trails
conservancy

Leelanau Trail

The 15-mile Leelanau Trail, half paved and half sandy and rocky gravel, presents two distinct adventures along the former Leelanau Scenic Railroad line. Farm fields are followed by lush woods and smooth cruising finishes off country rambling as the trail stretches south from Suttons Bay to Traverse City.

You can pick up the trail in the village of Suttons Bay at 1st Street and Cedar Street, though the first trailhead is a short distance ahead at 4th Street. The first 2.5-mile section is paved. The experience is pure country: wide-open vistas, rolling hills, picturesque fruit orchards, working farms and peaceful meadows. Just be sure that you are wearing your walking shoes or have fat tires with a lot of tread on your bicycle to navigate the sandy and rocky gravel terrain.

The 7.5-mile paved portion begins at the junction with Lakeview Road, the midpoint of the trail. The trailhead at Fouch Road is approximately 2.5 miles into the

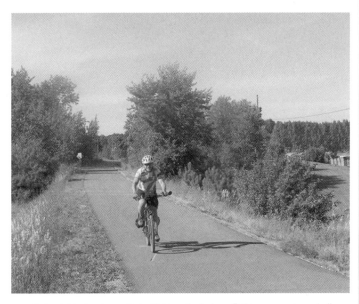
Bookended by the shores of Lake Michigan, the Leelanau Trail is pure country, and offers connections to even more rail-trail miles at its southern endpoint.

Location
Grand Traverse and Leelanau counties

Endpoints
Traverse City to Suttons Bay

Mileage
15.3

Roughness Index
2

Surface
Asphalt, gravel, ballast and dirt

paved segment and conveniently connects to hiking trails on 145 acres of farmland owned by Leelanau Conservancy. Drinking water, a parking lot and restroom facilities are available for hikers.

Continuing toward Traverse City, lush forest canopies arch over the paved rail-trail, and you can feast your eyes on gorgeous greenery and an aquatic medley of streams, lakes and ponds. The trailhead at Cherry Bend Road just before you reach Traverse City is the trail's official endpoint, marked by an historic caboose from the Leelanau Scenic Railroad.

The end, however, is only the beginning if you follow the connecting Traverse Area Recreation Trail (page 181) 11 miles through Traverse City and along Traverse Bay.

DIRECTIONS

To start at Traverse City Cherry Bend Park, from Traverse City take State Highway 22 north to East Cherry Bend Road. The trailhead is at Cherry Bend Community Park.

To start at Suttons Bay, follow State Highway 22 north to Suttons Bay. Just before you get to the town, turn left on 4th Street and go a couple of blocks. The trailhead will be on your left.

Contact: TART Trails, Inc.
232 East Front Street, Suite 11
Traverse City, MI 49685
(231) 941-4300
www.traversetrails.org/trails/leelanau

Little Traverse Wheelway

The 26-mile Little Traverse Wheelway provides exciting changes of scenery—including many views over sparkling Lake Michigan—as it winds from Charlevoix to the northern outskirts of Petoskey and eventually to Harbor Springs. Most of the route is paved, with several sections on boardwalk, sidewalks and area roads.

If you park at the trailhead at Charlevoix Township Hall, your journey begins with a half mile on Waller Road with light traffic. Once you reach the trail, you begin a 7-mile breezy ride sandwiched between Lake Michigan and US Route 31. A lightly wooded buffer helps to shield you from the fast-moving traffic along the highway and the trail is entirely paved except for a 0.6-mile wooden boardwalk across a quiet wetland between the Charlevoix Country Club and Big Rock Road.

A magnificent view of the lake awaits you at the Adams Rest Area, offering a chance to lunch at one of many picnic tables. Following that is Nine Mile Point, a particularly lovely strip of land along Little Traverse Bay. The shop- and restaurant-studded village of Bay Harbor lies 2 miles ahead, followed later by a 1.2-mile temporary

Location
Charlevoix and Emmet counties

Endpoints
Charlevoix to Harbor Springs

Mileage
26

Roughness Index
1

Surface
Asphalt

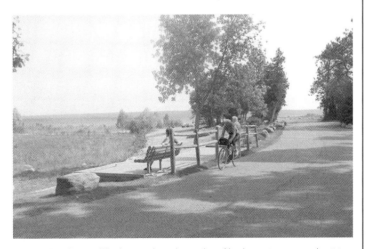

The Little Traverse Wheelway is a leisurely marathon of local attractions, seasonal activities, architectural sightseeing and brilliant Lake Michigan vistas.

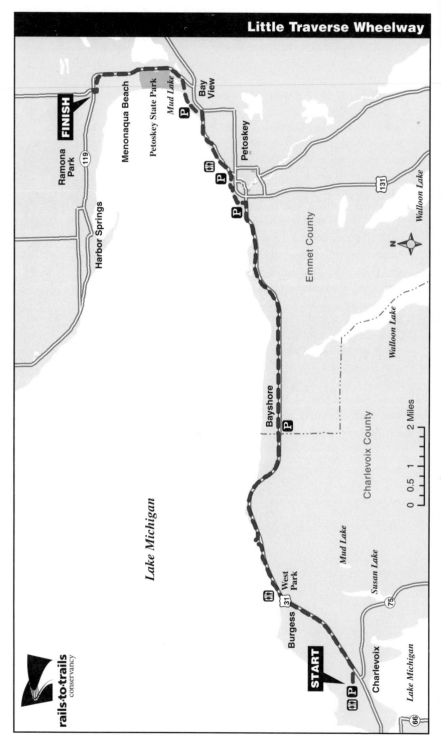

detour that takes you along the shoulder of US Route 31. This section is rather precarious and noisy and is not recommended for families with children. Fortunately the main trail is expected to reopen once paving and landscaping are completed (expected summer 2008, but check the website for updates). Back on the trail, you soon curve through woods and descend into Magnus Park on the lakeshore. You are now in Petoskey and the city-owned public campground offers rustic tent sites as well as RV hookups.

Just after Magnus is Bayfront Park, where history comes alive. This portion of the Little Traverse Wheelway dates from the late 1880s when it was a bikeway. This purpose actually predates the railroad, which was completed in 1892. Three arches (also called gates), which say NO TEAMING OR DRIVING, are replicas of a gate that once stood where the third arch stands now; they refer to the time when trail users were prohibited from bringing horses or horse-drawn carriages on the trail. Bicycles were the recreation rage for a couple decades prior to 1900 and they also served as inexpensive transportation. This bicycle history is commemorated in the Little Traverse History Museum, located on Depot Court, just off Lake Street near City Hall and is symbolized by a sculpture of an antique "boneshaker" bicycle within Bayfront Park.

Other Bayfront Park destinations include the Midway and Lime Kiln Pond. The Midway was once the shopping area on lower Lake Street that ran from today's business district down to the dockside area at the waterfront. It was Petoskey's cosmopolitan shopping center and included three "Persian Bazaars" run by Armenian families dealing in rugs, spices and other Oriental products popular in late Victorian America. On summer nights residents and visitors could listen to concerts performed by brass bands on shore or the many large boats docked in the harbor. As a growing commercial and tourist center, Petoskey was kind of an "emporium of the upper lakes." The Midway has since been bisected by the relocation of US Highway 31; the park is now accessible through an underpass near the foot of Bay Street.

Lime Kiln Pond was the heart of Petoskey pioneer Hiram Rose's quarry operation that dated from 1874 and greatly altered the appearance of the waterfront. The kilns "cooked" the limestone as the first step of the process of making lime. At one time it was one of Petoskey's most important industries, employing 30 to 40 workers, and sent lime used in fertilizer, cement and a variety of other industrial applications throughout the Great Lakes region. Today the pond, created by the quarry operation, is stocked with panfish and is a popular spot for parents to teach their children how to fish. The pond maintains a water level several feet above that of Little Traverse Bay only a few steps away. The exposed cobble on the bay is a good place to look for

Petoskey stones, organic matter from the ancient past fossilized in the limestone.

Upon leaving the park, salmon-colored sidewalks signal your entry into the historic Bay View neighborhood. This elite community, dominated by charming Victorian homes, has long been a summer getaway for prominent Michiganians. At the east end of Bay View is the Fettis-McCue Overlook, a covered wooden gazebo with benches offering a particularly pleasant view of the bay and a mural on the back of a grocery store depicting a historical timeline of transportation along the corridor. Soon after that, you arrive in Petoskey State Park with its sweeping sand dunes and fine swimming beach.

After the park the trail continues 2.5 miles on an off-road path along busy State Route M-119 before cutting away to follow the northeast edge of the Harbor Springs Airport. The trail currently ends at Pleasant View Lane, just 4 miles short of Harbor Springs. Future plans are to connect the trail to this quaint resort settlement in 2009, but your best bet for now is to backtrack toward the main entrance of the state park and turn off on Beach Road for a 4-mile trip into the heart of downtown Harbor Springs. Use caution on Beach Road, as sight lines on this twisting and densely forested road are limited. Turn right on Bay Street and follow it into town.

DIRECTIONS

To reach the Charlevoix trailhead, go north from the town of Charlevoix, on US Highway 31 for about 3 miles to Waller Road. Turn left and proceed for a half mile to Charlevoix Township Park on your right.

The next trailhead is at Resort Township's West Park, just several hundred yards north of the trail and US Highway 31 on Townline Road, offering parking and restrooms; however, there is an additional parking area located right next to the trail.

To reach the northernmost trailhead at the Harbor Springs Airport, go north from the city of Petoskey on US Highway 31 to State Route M-119. Turn left on State Route M-119 and follow it until you see the Harbor Springs Airport on your left and State Hwy. 81. Just beyond the airport on your left is the trail parking lot, near the trail's end at Pleasant View Lane.

Contact: Top of Michigan Trails Council
445 East Mitchell
Petoskey, MI 49770
(231) 348-8280
www.trailscouncil.org

Macomb Orchard Trail

Named for the rich assortment of fruit trees in southeast Michigan, this trail cuts a 23.5-mile arc across the northern portion of Macomb County. Regardless of where you begin, the entire route is relatively flat. Running east to west, the trail starts out as urban trail and then turns into rural countryside as it passes through townships and connects the villages of Romeo and Armada. You will find lots of fruit orchards, crop fields and dairy farms before ending in the city of Richmond.

The western end is perhaps the most attractive portion of the trail. Within the first few miles you cross the Clinton River Bridge with large turnout platforms on each side on which you can stop and view the pastureland and the Clinton River or try your hand at catching some trout. The trail is paved for the 10 miles between Dequindre Road and 32 Mile Road in Romeo. After leaving Romeo, the trail crosses busy State Highway 53. A

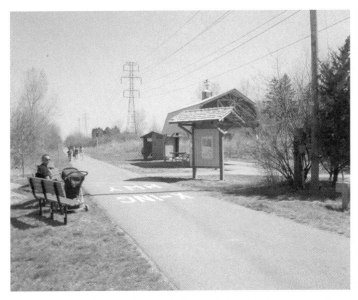

True to its name, fruit orchards pepper the Macomb Orchard Trail, which connects with other trails including the Paint Creek Trailway.

Location
Macomb County

Endpoints
Shelby Township
to Washington
Township

Mileage
23.5

**Roughness
Index**
1

Surface
Asphalt

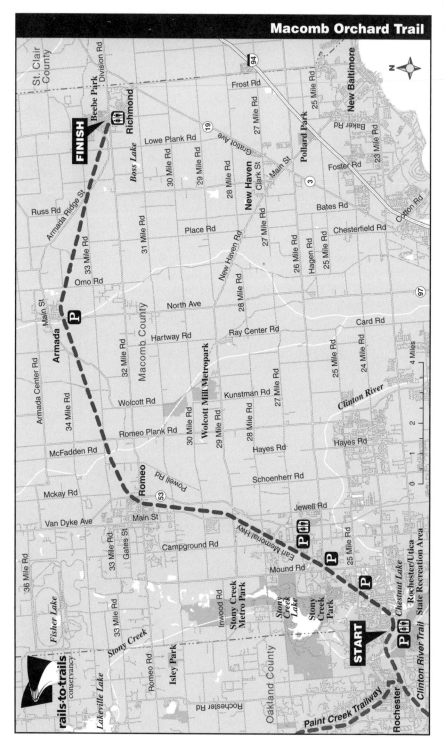

bridge is scheduled to be completed over the highway soon. The next 6.5 miles is sandy gravel and it is paved from 6 miles before you reach Richmond until the trail's end.

The trail ends in the heart of Richmond at a trailhead park, with a gazebo, restrooms, picnic tables, benches and a path to the municipal parking lot. A 10-mile section for an equestrian trail from Romeo Plank Road to Lowe Plank Road is being developed.

At its west end the Macomb Orchard Trail connects to two other trails, the 16-mile Clinton River Trail and the 8.5-mile Paint Creek Trailway (page 169) via the Rochester City River Walk.

DIRECTIONS

To reach the access point in Richmond, take Interstate 94 and exit west onto Fred W. Moore Highway/Division Road. Turn right onto State Route M-19/Main Street. Turn left onto Water Street. The trailhead is at the intersection of Water and Parker streets.

To reach the access point in Washington, take State Route M-53 toward Washington. Exit at 26 Mile Road, then turn right on Van Dyke Road. Turn left onto West Road. The trailhead is 0.4 mile ahead on the right.

Contact: Macomb Orchard Trail Commission
Freedom Hill County Park
1500 Metropolitan Parkway
Sterling Heights, MI 48312
(586) 979-7010
www.macomborchardtrail.com

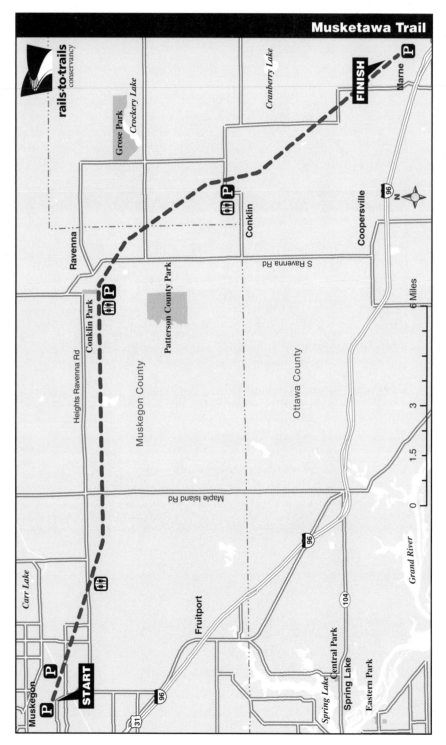

Musketawa Trail

Musketawa Trail

The 25-mile Musketawa Trail provides a patchwork of scenery from Muskegon to Marne, neatly divided by its four trailheads. From west to east the trailheads are in Muskegon at Broadway and in Ravenna, Conklin and Marne. Grand Rapids is only 4 miles east of the Marne trailhead, making it the most heavily used of these facilities.

Leaving Muskegon on the paved trail you pass through light industrial and residential areas and skirt the county prison and the fairgrounds. Then sprawling hay fields and crops of blueberries, corn and cucumbers dominate the rest of the way to Ravenna. Ravenna, at mile 13, is considered the midpoint of the trail. Look closely at the old railroad water tower along the trail; the base was recently repaired and restored, and a replica wooden tank was installed to mirror its appearance when the Grand Rapids and Indiana Railroad ran this line. The Ravenna business district, located about a half

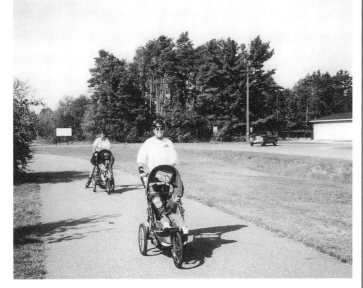

The Musketawa Trail offers a distinctly rural oasis from nearby Grand Rapids, making it a popular destination trail for locals.

Location
Muskegon and Ottawa counties

Endpoints
Muskegon to Marne

Mileage
25

Roughness Index
2

Surface
Asphalt and gravel

mile north of the water tower and trailhead, is a good place to stop for a rest or to eat or stock up on snacks. The Crockery Creek trestle, just ahead, rises 45 feet above Crockery Creek.

The eastern portion of the trail is more heavily shaded, passing through long stretches of open farmland and wooded landscapes of pines and maples. At the small village of Conklin, about halfway between Ravenna and Marne, there is another trailhead with no amenities.

Despite its proximity to Grand Rapids, the Marne trailhead is in a rural area. Nevertheless, it is a hopping spot in every season. Bicyclists, runners, walkers, inline skaters and even horseback riders head here in warmer months, while snowshoers, cross-country skiers and snowmobilers take to the trail when the snow flies. The Musketawa Trail will only get busier, as long-term plans call for extending it east to connect with Grand Rapids trails and west from Muskegon to meet the Hart-Montague Bicycle Trail State Park (page 145).

DIRECTIONS

To access the Muskegon trailhead, take US Highway 31 to Exit 72B. Take Sherman Avenue east for 1 mile. Turn left onto Broadway Avenue and travel for 1 mile. The trailhead will be on your left.

To access the Marne trailhead, take westbound Interstate 96 to Exit 25. Take 8th Avenue (turn right at the bottom of the ramp and then left at the T-intersection) and follow it north for approximately 1.5 miles. The trailhead will be on your left just past Garfield Road.

Contact: Friends of the Musketawa Trail
3734 Center Street
Ravenna, MI 49451
(616) 738-4810
www.musketawatrail.com

Paint Creek Trailway

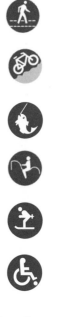

It is Michigan's oldest rail-trail, but the charms of the Paint Creek Trailway add up to more than its 1974 birth date. This 8.5-mile trail has wildlife, historical sites, picnic tables and a lovely creek filled with jumping trout. To help keep tabs on your trip and connect with other area trails, the six trailheads provide large billboard maps and folding trail guides to take with you. Mile markers, left over from the days when this path was a railway, are additionally helpful.

Following Paint Creek from Lake Orion south to the city of Rochester, the trail slopes gently downhill. Its crushed limestone surface is a draw for mountain bikers, walkers and joggers. Equestrian riders share the path until just outside the Rochester city limits. Just 2 miles from Lake Orion, a prominent historical marker notes the site of the water-powered Carpenter Rudd Mill that stood here until 1926. This is also where you can connect to the Bald Mountain Recreation Area for fishing, swimming and mountain biking. Take special care as you leave the trail and cross Adams Road, as there is a high volume of traffic and no crossing signal.

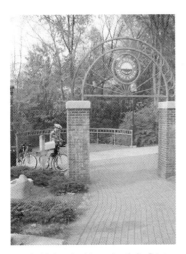

As Michigan's oldest rail-trail, the Paint Creek Trailway has retained a sense of its own history with historical markers along its former railroading path.

Continuing on the trail you find an abundance of wildlife, including deer, turtles, frogs and many species of birds, as well as wildflowers. There are lots of opportunities to fish along the trail as Paint Creek meanders alongside and crosses the trail.

In Oakland Township, Goodison area, there are two trailheads. At mile 5 there is parking only at the

Location
Oakland County

Endpoints
Lake Orion to Rochester

Mileage
8.5

Roughness Index
2

Surface
Crushed stone, ballast and dirt

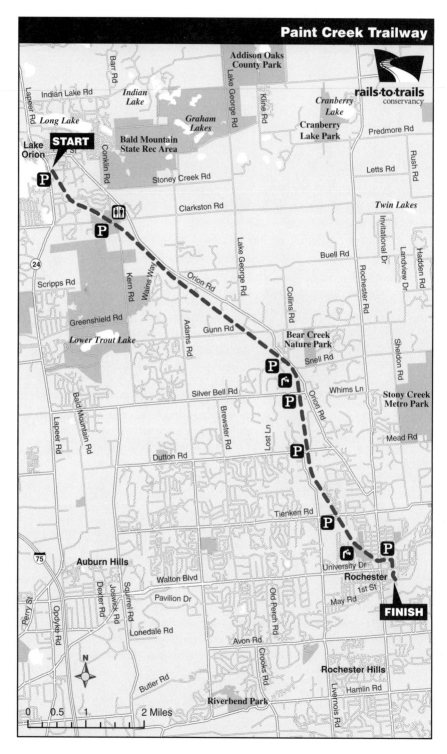

Paint Creek Trailway

Gallagher Road trailhead, and parking is available at the Silver Bell Road trailhead at mile 6. At Tienken there is parking and picnic tables. At mile 8.5, Dinosaur Hill Nature Preserve offers hiking trails through 16 acres of all-season beauty. A short way beyond the nature preserve, Rochester Municipal Park on your right provides parking, restrooms and drinking water. Just past the local police department and outside the park are bicycle shops, restaurants, a bank and shops.

The rail-trail ends along Rochester Municipal Park, where the Rochester River Walk begins. Follow the walkway south along Paint Creek, through the city of Rochester and behind the Rochester Hills Public Library. When the walkway forks at a gazebo, bear to your left to reach the 16-mile Clinton River Trail. At this point you can go west on the Clinton River Trail or turn east for 2 miles and connect to the Macomb Orchard Trail (page 163).

DIRECTIONS

To reach the Lake Orion trailhead, follow State Route M-24 (Lapeer Road) to Atwater Road. Parking and two trailheads are behind the strip mall on the southeast corner.

To reach the Clarkston Road trailhead, follow State Route M-24 (Lapeer Road). Turn east onto Clarkson, traveling 1 mile before turning right onto Kern Road. Parking is on the left.

Contact: Paint Creek Trailways Commission
4393 Collins Road
Rochester, MI 48306
(248) 651-9260
www.paintcreektrail.org

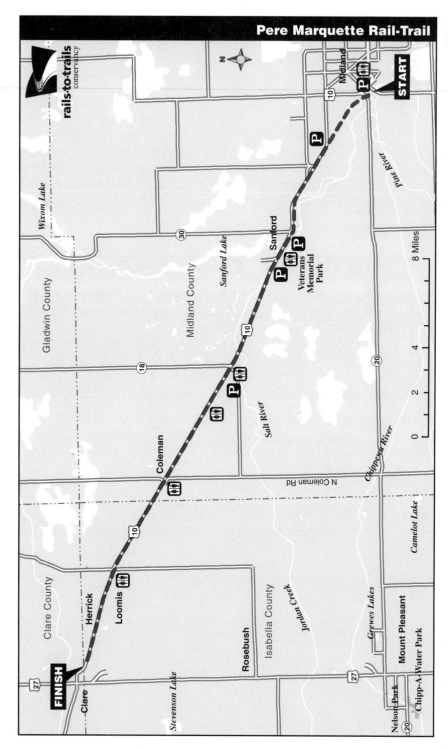

Pere Marquette Rail-Trail

If a trip on the Pere Marquette Rail-Trail leaves you in love with this 32-mile greenway, you are not alone. The Pere Marquette is one of the most heavily used trails in Michigan, according to a 2002 Michigan State University study. The serene, paved corridor welcomes all nonmotorized users, including equestrians on an adjacent path for approximately 5 miles between State Route 18 and Coleman Road. There are numerous access points along the trail, as well as benches on which trail users can rest and take in the beautiful scenery of maple and pine trees.

Kick off your trip in downtown Midland at the Tridge, a unique three-way bridge located at the confluence of the Tittabawassee and Chippewa Rivers. Stay straight to follow the rail-trail all the way to Clare. One section leads to the Chippewassee Park.

The trail is a haven for deer, chipmunks and an assortment of bird species. There are cultural attractions

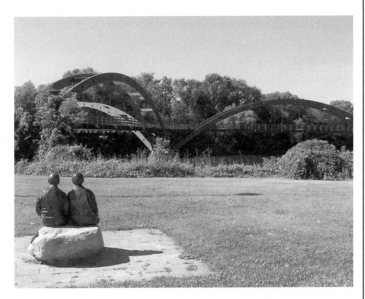

The Pere Marquette Rail-Trail is a backyard playground—or resting spot as the statues above suggest—to all Michiganders as well as a draw for trail-lovers around the country.

Location
Midland County

Endpoints
Midland to Clare

Mileage
32

Roughness Index
1

Surface
Asphalt

to be had from the very start. Just off the trail in Midland is the Dow Historical Museum, where you can find information and displays concerning the pioneering chemical experiments of Herbert H. Dow. Another interesting cultural attraction, located just off the trail, is the Bradley House. This restored 1874 home offers visitors a glimpse into the everyday life of an early Midland family.

The town of Sanford at mile 8.4 is a good spot for a lunch break. It has shops and restaurants as well as Sanford Village Park, where you can dip a fishing line or a canoe into the Tittabawassee River. If you are up for a quarter-mile side trip, head north and cross Saginaw Road to reach Sanford Lake County Park, which has a beach, pavilions, boat launch and playground.

Just ahead at mile 9.3 is Veterans Memorial Park, which features 180-year-old red and white pines. The Pine Haven Recreation Area, located at 8 Mile Road, has 8 miles of trails for hiking, mountain biking and cross-country skiing.

In Coleman the trail has been made the focal point for the city. Exit the trail at the Coleman Staging Area if you want to stop, shop or grab a bite to eat. A bike shop is also located adjacent to the trail. Continuing north, you may decide to stop at the general store in Loomis for a snack.

Although the Pere Marquette Rail-Trail ends in Clare, the rail-trail system continues to Baldwin, Michigan.

DIRECTIONS

To start in Midland, from the intersection of State Route M-20 and Business Route M-10 go east on Buttles Street/State Route M-20 for 3 blocks to Ashman Street. Turn right and follow the street right to the trailhead, which has plenty of parking and restroom facilities.

To reach the trailhead in Clare, from US Highway 127, exit onto McEwan and follow it to 5th Street. Go east for 1 mile. The trailhead will be on your right by the freeway underpass.

Contact: Friends of the Pere Marquette Rail-Trail
P.O. Box 505
Midland, MI 48640
(989) 832-3703
www.lmb.org/pmrt

Portland Riverwalk

Portland, Michigan, is known as the City of Two Rivers and the 8-mile Portland Riverwalk could well be called the Trail of Two Rivers. The paved rail-trail serves as a spine for a series of connecting trails, loops and city paths that circle Portland for approximately 15 miles.

The trail is suburban by location, but quiet enough to let you think you are in the country. Built and maintained by the Portland Parks and Recreation Department, the path connects schools and five parks and follows the Grand and Looking Glass rivers. Be sure to bring your camera, because there are four historic bridges, one railroad trestle bridge and three steel truss bridges over the rivers and through the woods along the rivers.

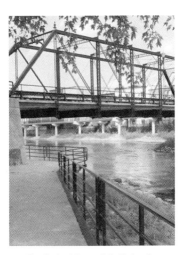

The Portland Riverwalk highlights the town's main waterways, the Looking Glass and Grand rivers.

A good place to start is at Portland High School, where a slight downhill carries trail users through a canopy of maples and pines. After only three-quarters of a mile you can choose to turn onto a spur trail that enters the Bogue Flats Recreation Area of soccer and baseball fields and follows the Grand River for a short distance with many scenic turnouts overlooking the river. Stop, sit on a bench and listen to all that nature has to say.

Returning to the main trail, a half mile farther along than where you left it, a lovely old railroad bridge takes you over the Grand River. This is the first of three bridges, all of which allow fishing; you will likely see anglers casting for smallmouth bass, perch or trout from the structures. On the far side of the bridge another spur

Location
Ionia County

Endpoints
Portland

Mileage
15

Roughness Index
1

Surface
Asphalt

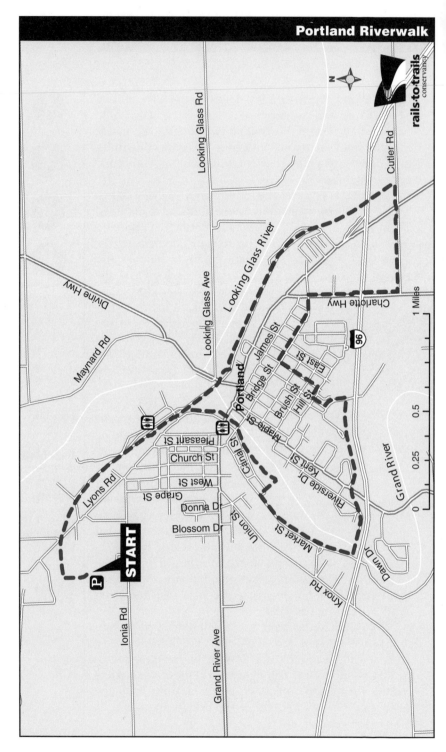

Portland Riverwalk

loops through a residential area and back to the trail; a spur from that loop heads into the historic part of town for shopping, restaurants, banks and insurance offices.

Back on the main trail, you follow the Looking Glass River for a short distance and pass an observation deck and gazebo where you can relax. As the trail continues at the south end of town you pass under the interstate, where the trail turns right and leaves the old railroad bed to become a city trail. The trail continues along separated from the road until you make another right turn and go back under the interstate again. A temporary gap in the trail requires that you follow city sidewalks for about 1 mile with no signage to where the trail picks up behind an elementary school. If you bring a map of the trail, you will be able to find the trail more easily. There are plans to complete this gap.

When you return to the city trail behind the elementary school, it is smooth sailing. Trees lining the trail provide a picturesque tunnel back to the Grand River. Now used exclusively for trail travel, the third steel truss bridge you've crossed transports you across the river. At this point, mile 11, you head back into town within feet of the Grand River and cut through Brush Street and Thompson parks. A fourth steel truss bridge, built at the turn of the century, returns you to the main trail. When you reach the main trail again, turn right (west) and follow the trail back through the tree canopy straight to your starting point.

DIRECTIONS

This trip is a loop. To reach the trailhead, take Exit 77 from Interstate 96. Turn right on Grand River Road and proceed for 1.25 miles to Water Street/Lyons Road. Turn right and follow the road for 1 mile to Portland High School. Turn left into the school driveway and then turn right to stay on the west side of the school. The trail starts on the west side of the school between the football field and tennis courts. Parking is available in the school parking lot. The Bogue Flats Recreation Area has restrooms and parking.

Contact: Portland Parks and Recreation Department
259 Kent Street
Portland, MI 48875
(517) 647-7985
www.portland-michigan.org/parksrec/

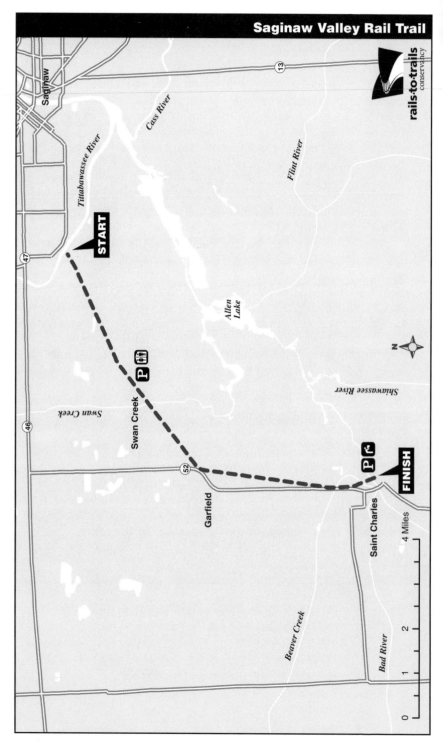

Saginaw Valley Rail Trail

Saginaw Valley Rail Trail

The Saginaw Valley Rail Trail is a perfect summer escape. The foliage-drenched corridor offers respite from the sun. This 9.2-mile trail edges Saginaw's southern boundary before it heads south to St. Charles. Equestrians follow a parallel path that begins at Stroebel Road, where there is plenty of parking and continues all the way to Martin Road at mile 8.1.

From the trailhead, you are in nature's garden. Luscious displays of Queen Anne's lace and wildflowers cluster along the route. Interpretive signs identify many of these species and add a nice touch to your trip. Equally pleasing is the thick carpet of plants flanking much of the trail. The intact canopy of trees makes you feel as if you are in a large forest.

The trail provides views of a mix of agricultural and residential land. About a third of the way through your journey, you will reach a trailhead at the corner of Swan

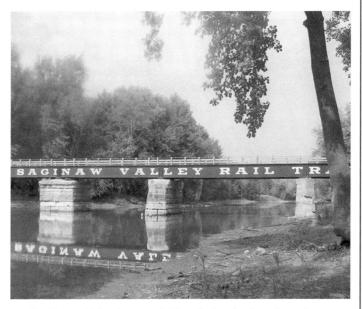

Though the trail bridge above spans Bad River, there's nothing better than a relaxing summer saunter or ride on the Saginaw Valley Rail Trail.

Location
Saginaw County

Endpoints
Saginaw to St. Charles

Mileage
9.2

Roughness Index
1

Surface
Asphalt

Creek Road and Van Wormer Road that has a modern restroom, soda machines, water fountains and parking. Located between Van Wormer and Benkert roads is a fishing platform where you may see anglers hoping to snag a trout, perch or smallmouth bass.

There are three pocket parks, complete with wooden gazebos and benches, along the trail. The first is located between Stroebel Road and River Road, the second between Spencer Road and Lakefield Road and the third between Teft Road and Prior Road. These shelters provide opportunities to relax and further soak in the solace of your leafy green surroundings.

The last half of the trail skirts the Shiawassee River State Game Area. This natural area gives you the chance for some excellent wildlife viewing. You may choose to stop at the viewing platform at Martin Road and take in the scenery. There is a high probability of seeing geese, ducks, swans and white-tailed deer throughout the year.

Lumberjack Park in St. Charles is the end of the line for this straight, wide and smooth trail. The trail ends with a trip across a historical stone railroad trestle bridge and a pretty view of the Bad River.

DIRECTIONS

To start in Saginaw, head south of town on State Highway 46. About 1.25 miles east of State Hwy. 47 turn right onto South Center Road. Go 1.75 miles to Stroebel Road. Turn right and go 1.5 miles to the trailhead and parking lot, which has no facilities.

To start in St. Charles, from the stoplight downtown at Saginaw Street and West Belle Avenue go 1 block west on Saginaw Street to East Water Street. Turn right and proceed 2 blocks to the trailhead and parking on the left.

Contact: Saginaw Valley Rail Trail Friends
Saginaw County Parks and Recreation Commission
111 South Michigan Avenue, LL012
Saginaw, MI 48602
(989) 790-5280
www.saginawcounty.com/parks/page10.html

Traverse Area Recreation Trail

The Traverse Area Recreation Trail (TART) is packed with urban excitement as it winds 11 miles through the infrastructure of Traverse City. The rail-trail cuts a west-to-east path from Carter Road to State Road 22, where it connects with the 15-mile Leelanau Trail (page 157). Twists and turns combined with a mixture of surfaces (wooden boardwalks, asphalt trail and wide concrete sidewalks) could lead to confusion, but red and green TART logo arrows clearly mark the route. Picturesque waterfront views abound as you travel along both the west and east arms of Traverse Bay. You dip down to the water's edge and skirt the swimming beaches and marina on the west side of town and then travel high above the water along 5 Mile Road on the East Grand Traverse Bay side.

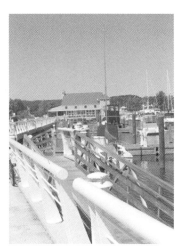

The Traverse Area Recreation Trail makes commuting a breeze with its nearby shops, eateries, marina access, and neighborhood and business center connections.

Starting at Carter Road, a short half-mile trail segment behind restaurants and a major grocery store takes you to the intersection of State Routes 22 and 72. From here you head straight to the waterfront, a 2-mile stretch of trail next to glittering West Grand Traverse Bay with a public marina capped by West End and Clinch beaches on either end. Just past Clinch Park, a bronze sculpture of a parent and child's attempts to ride a bike catches your eye before the trail turns south.

Taking a half-mile jog away from the waterfront, the trail then wends its way through the hustle and bustle of downtown Traverse City, providing easy access to a wide array of shops, boutiques and eateries. An underpass helps you avoid the heavy traffic of State Routes 31

Location
Grand Traverse County

Endpoints
Traverse City to Acme

Mileage
11

Roughness Index
1

Surface
Asphalt and concrete

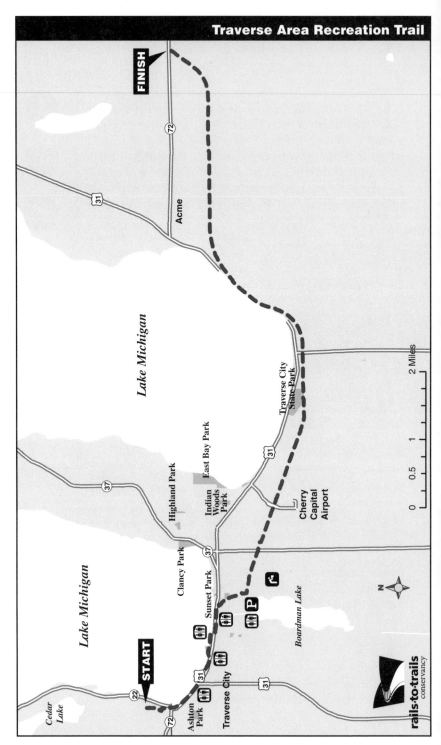

and 72 and eases the transition between the waterfront and downtown.

For the next 6 miles, the trail is a commuter's dream. In fact, statistics show that 17 percent of TART's users report commuting between neighborhoods, restaurants, bike shops, offices, parks, beaches, the marina, the public library and other destinations that are connected along this route.

At mile 3, a restored depot honors the history of railroad days gone by. A bike lane and sidewalks along Woodmere Avenue at this juncture lead you to pretty, paved, 2-mile Boardman Lake Trail along the east side of its namesake, which starts at Hull Park and ends at Medalie Park. If you want to make this connection, travel for a few blocks, pass the library, turn right on Hannah and travel 100 yards to the lake.

Back on TART, the next 4 miles from the depot to Bunker Hill Road is a lightly active rail-with-trail corridor. This is where many of the residential neighborhoods are located. Mile 5 marks the back entrance to Traverse City State Park, where campers enjoy getting out on the trail to access Traverse City's many eateries, miniature golf courses and other tourism attractions located alongside the trail.

Mile 8.5 marks the start of a 2-mile connector on Bunker Hill and Lautner roads until the trail resumes for a final 2-mile stretch from Lautner Road to the end at State Route 72 in Acme. Traffic along Bunker Hill Road is generally light, but use caution as it moves fairly fast. Plans are to connect the last segment of rail-trail between Bunker Hill and Lautner roads in the near future. This last segment crosses wide-open fields to end at State Route 72 in Acme.

DIRECTIONS

To begin in Traverse City, from the south, follow State Route M-31 north to State Route M-37. Turn left onto State Route M-37 and continue 0.5 mile to State Route M-72. Street parking is available along the trail.

To start at Bunker Hill Road in Acme, on the northeast side of Traverse City, follow State Route M-31 west and north through town to Bunker Hill Road. Turn right on Bunker Hill Road and proceed for a quarter mile to the trailhead on your left.

Contact: TART Trails, Inc.
232 East Front Street, Suite 11
Traverse City, MI 49685
(231) 941-4300
www.traversetrails.org

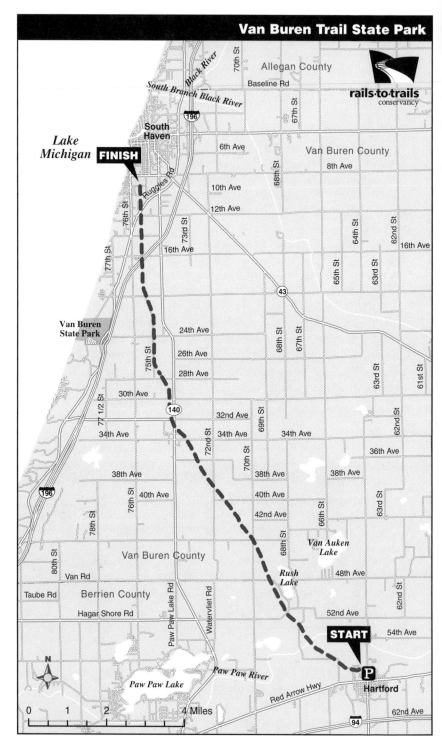

Van Buren Trail State Park

Van Buren Trail State Park

Head for Van Buren Trail State Park and take a walk (or ride) on the wild side. Wildlife abounds on this rural 14 miles between Hartford and South Haven; trail surfaces are plentiful, too. While you might see deer, rabbits, foxes and eagles, this is an undeveloped trail that has rough ballast stones, long sections of sand and grassy two-track. The combined result is a trail suited to hearty mountain bikers, birders and naturalists.

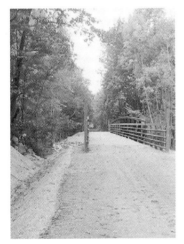

Rough and rural but worth the effort, the Van Buren Trail State Park is best-suited for mountain bikers and hardy trekkers.

Heading north from the grass-covered parking lot in Hartford, which has portable toilets, you glide quietly over a new metal bridge spanning the Paw Paw River. Cruising northwest to South Haven you pass beneath tall pines, maples and various hardwood trees. The scent of pine lingers as you emerge from the woodlands and enter fields of blueberry bushes and vineyards.

At mile 8 the small town of Covert is located one block south of the trail. A convenience store in town has the only refreshments and restroom facilities on this rural trail. You have to navigate a rural State Route M-140 at this point, with no real busy traffic.

The last 8 miles from Covert, the trail passes through woods, open fields and commercial fields of blueberries and grapes. Blueberries grow on treelike bushes and grapes grow on vines tied to fences. This part of Michigan is noted for its wine and fruit. When you arrive at the end of the trail, at Lovejoy Street, next to the water tower in South Haven, there is no parking available.

Location
Van Buren County

Endpoints
Hartford to South Haven

Mileage
14

Roughness Index
3

Surface
Gravel, ballast and dirt

Future plans call for a trailhead here and for a connection to the Kal-Haven Trail (page 147) from this point.

DIRECTIONS

To start in Hartford, from Interstate 94, take the Hartford exit. Head north 2 blocks past the first stoplight. Take a left onto Prospect Street and proceed for 2 blocks. The trailhead has a grass-covered parking lot with portable toilets.

To start in South Haven, take Lagrange Street to Aylworth Avenue (next to South Haven High School, across from McDonald's). Go west on Aylworth Avenue to Kalamazoo Street and then south on Kalamazoo Street to Lovejoy Avenue. The trail is 0.1 mile to the west on Lovejoy Avenue on the south side of the street.

Contact: Van Buren Trail State Park
621 North 10th Street
Plainwell, MI 49080
(269) 685-6851
www.michigandnr.com/parksandtrails

Wadhams to Avoca Trail

The Wadhams to Avoca Trail in southeast Michigan provides a snapshot of scenic rural lands. The trail's name reflects its initial endpoints; it now extends from Avoca 12 miles southeast to the outskirts of Port Huron. This former railroad turned rail-trail is lined with historical mile and half-mile markers that adorn and inform from the sides of the corridor. The trail is a nonmotorized trail open to equestrians.

The rural town of Avoca is a good starting point for those who want to experience the entire route. The trailhead is set among a cluster of businesses, a post office, a restaurant and bar and fire station. It provides trailer parking and hitching posts and restrooms.

The trail is surfaced with limestone fines for the first 1.5 miles to Beard Road. The next 3.5 miles is packed gravel to Cribbons Road. At mile 2 the restored Mill Creek Trestle soars 60 feet through the air and (vertigo

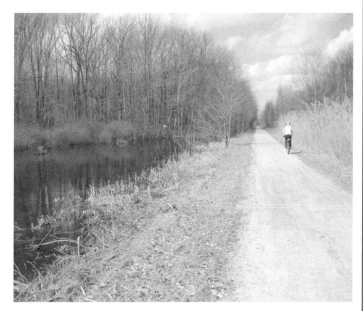

The Wadhams to Avoca Trail, popular with horseback riders, gets high marks for its fall foliage.

Location
St. Clair County

Endpoints
Kimball Township to Emmett Township

Mileage
12

Roughness Index
2

Surface
Asphalt, crushed stone, gravel and ballast

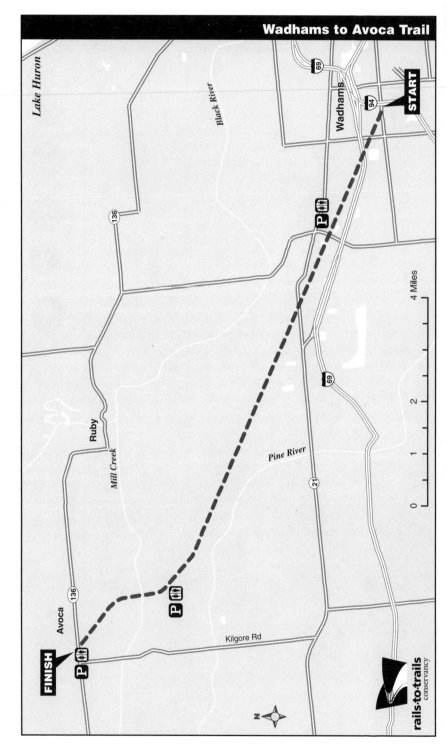

Wadhams to Avoca Trail

Lake Huron

Black River

Wadhams

START

69

94

136

4 Miles

69

Pine River

2

Ruby

1

Mill Creek

21

0

136

Avoca

Kilgore Rd

FINISH

N

rails-to-trails conservancy

sufferers beware) lookout points have been added so that trail users can view the seasons playing out on the waters and woodlands below. As hardwood trees flank much of the trail, autumn is a spectacular time to visit. In addition to the colorful views from the trestle, numerous small ponds and wetlands adjoining the trail mirror the bright colors on the trees. This stretch of trail features a second trailhead at Imlay City Road, which has parking and toilets.

When you reach Cribbons Road, the trail surface is again limestone fines. For the most part the tree-lined trail passes through rural farmland, making for a beautiful walk or ride during any season and a pleasant cross-country ski route. The views change from flat lands to valleys in this area of Michigan.

The last 5 miles, beyond McLain Road, is paved to the Griswold Road, 4 miles from downtown Port Huron. This section of the trail passes through a developing residential area and is used heavily by residents. The last trailhead is at Wadhams Road, where the By-Lo gas station provides additional parking. A fast food restaurant, pharmacy and grocery store are close by.

There are three campgrounds located within 1.5 miles of the trail at various points: one on Imlay City Road (Ruby Campground), another at McLain and Lapeer Road (Fort Trood) and a third (KOA) off of Lapeer Road, between Wadhams and Allen.

DIRECTIONS

The Avoca trailhead is on the south side of State Route M-136 between Kilgore Road and Duce Road. Parking is on the west side of the park.

The Imlay City Road trailhead is at the intersection of Interstate 69 and Wales Center Road. Go north 1 mile to the end of Wales Center Road. Turn right on Kilgore Road. Go 3 miles north and turn right on Imlay City Road. Go east 1.2 miles past Duce Road to the trailhead on the left side.

To reach the Wadhams trailhead, from Interstate 69 take Exit 196 to Wadhams Road and go north a half mile.

Contact: St. Clair County Parks and Recreation
200 Grand River Avenue, Suite 205
Port Huron, MI 48060
(810) 989-6960
www.stclaircounty.org/offices/parks/trails.aspx

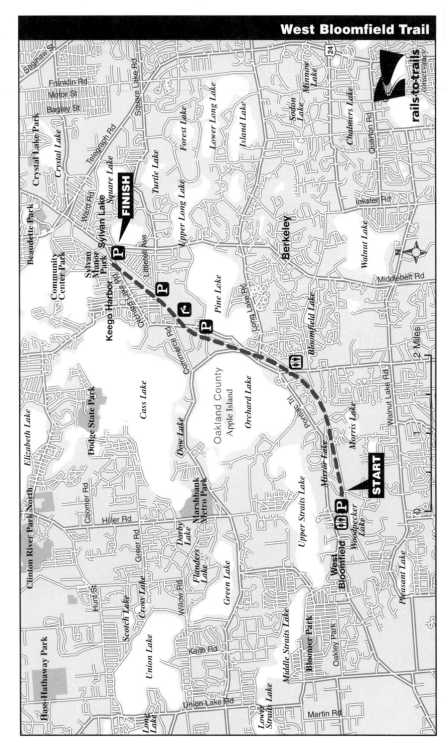

West Bloomfield Trail

Bookended by an established nature preserve and a community park, with plans to connect it to more rail-trail miles, the West Bloomfield Trail measures up to much more than its 4.25-mile length. The southwest trailhead in West Bloomfield Woods Nature Preserve serves up 162 acres with looping hiking trails. The other endpoint may one day connect to the Clinton River Trail and the Paint Creek Trailway (page 169) and the Macomb Orchard Trail (page 163) beyond.

The limestone trail is steeped in nature, aside from some large homes sprinkled around the preserve. Don't be alarmed if what appears to be a lawn ornament suddenly turns and bounds toward the forest—one pass on this trail provides clear sightings of deer, raccoons and rabbits. Turtles, waterfowl and assorted frogs populate the ponds and lakes, and the forests are filled with spruce, hickory, oak and maple trees. Interpretive markers flank the trail, but be sure to pick up a map and brochure at

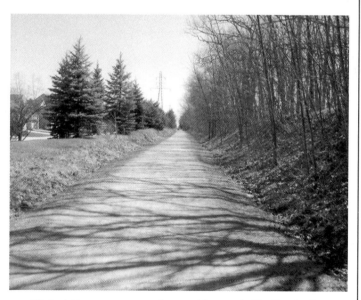

With its start in a nature preserve and its many lake views, the West Bloomfield Trail is as much a nature trail as a rail-trail.

Location
Oakland County

Endpoints
West Bloomfield Woods Nature Preserve to Sylvan Manor Park

Mileage
4.25

Roughness Index
1

Surface
Crushed stone

191

the nature preserve for the real inside scoop on this thriving natural habitat.

Starting from Arrowhead Road in the nature preserve, you can expect to see lots of wildlife such as great blue herons, woodchucks, coyotes and foxes. The trail follows a gentle downhill slope through the communities of West Bloomfield, Orchard Lake, Keego Harbor and Sylvan Lake with many ponds pocketed along the trail. You can expect to see ducks, geese and other waterfowl, as well as turtles parked in a row on logs, soaking up the sun.

Orchard Lake is the first of three large lakes the trail overlooks. At this point the trail follows an old train tunnel under very busy Long Lake Road. Orchard Lake is also home to Apple Island, where Chief Pontiac is thought to have held council with neighboring tribes to plan an attack on Fort Detroit in the mid-18th century. You reach the trail's end at Sylvan Manor Park, the east end trailhead. There are no signs identifying the park from the trail, but an asphalt path with a basketball court signals your arrival in a city park. If you continue from here, you will be following the Clinton River Trail, which connects with Paint Creek Trailway and Macomb Orchard Trail.

DIRECTIONS

To access the Arrowhead Road trailhead in the nature preserve, take State Route M-5 north to where it comes to a T-intersection with Pontiac Trail. Turn right onto Pontiac Trail and travel 3 miles to a right turn on Arrowhead Road. Go 0.5 mile to trailhead parking on the left side.

To access the Sylvan Manor Park, from the intersection of State Route M-24 (Telegraph Road) and Orchard Lake Road, turn west on Orchard Lake Road, go past Middle Belt Road for 2 blocks, turn left on Figa Avenue. Go 1 block, turn right on Woodrow Wilson Road and proceed 4 blocks to Sylvan Manor Park on your right.

Contact: West Bloomfield Parks and Recreation
4640 Walnut Lake Road
West Bloomfield, MI 48323
(248) 451-1900
www.westbloomfieldparks.org

White Pine Trail State Park

The White Pine Trail is Michigan's longest rail-trail, following the former Grand Rapids and Indiana rail bed for 93.5 miles through five counties. This massive trail showcases a variety of landscapes, from swamps to forests to open farmland, plus numerous towns and cities. You will run across existing and in-development trails, too, as this corridor is the backbone of the state rail-trail system.

The trail surface is a mix of ballast and blacktop, so a mountain bike or a hybrid bicycle are best to tackle the distance and terrain. When there are four or more inches of snow on the trail, snowmobiles are allowed from Russell Road (north of downtown Rockford) to the trail's north endpoint in Cadillac.

The southern tip of the White Pine Trail is just north of Grand Rapids in Comstock Park. Heading north from here are 21 miles of paved trail through mostly rural terrain. Several historic railroad trestles along the trail's length have been renovated for stream and river crossings.

Just 8.2 miles from the trail's start, the town of Rockford has a scenic overlook of the Rogue River Dam, with plenty of picnic tables and benches to stop and enjoy the calming sound of the flowing, beautiful water. Heading north from Rockford you pass through small towns such as Cedar Springs, Pierson and Morley.

Big Rapids is located at mile 53.1 and has the distinction of housing the trail's longest bridge. Whites Bridge spans 319 feet over the Muskegon River. Big Rapids is also home to Ferris State University, which boasts an 880-acre campus with state-of-the-art facilities. Just north of Big Rapids is Paris; here the trail runs directly through Paris Park, which features camp-in-cabins, a canoe launch and a fishing concession along the banks of the Muskegon River.

Heading north to Reed City, trail users can catch a view of the Yoplait Yogurt factory. A covered bridge is your ticket over the Hersey River in Reed City. Reed

Location
Kent, Mecosta, Montcalm, Osceola and Wexford counties

Endpoints
Comstock Park to Cadillac

Mileage
93.5

Roughness Index
3

Surface
Asphalt, crushed stone, gravel and ballast

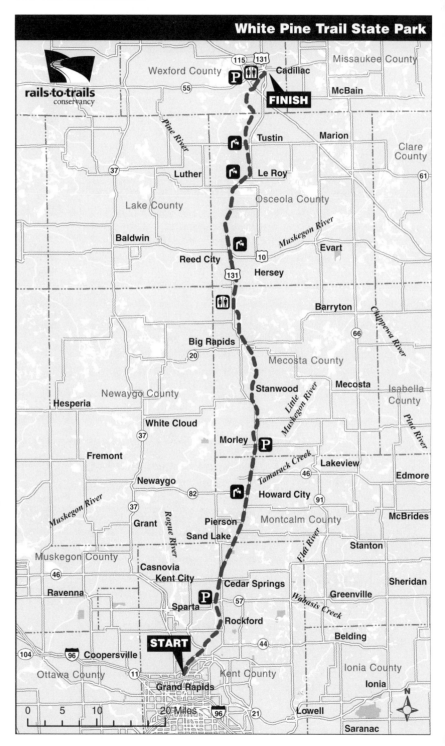

City is also on the east-west route of the 32-mile Pere Marquette Rail-Trail (page 173).

The tiny village of Tustin, at mile 83, has a wonderful railroad museum. Heading north another 11.2 miles takes you to the trail's end in Cadillac but not before circling around Lake Cadillac where you can enjoy swimming beaches and an outdoor amphitheater for concerts.

Only a determined few will ride the White Pine Trail in one fell swoop. A slower approach, using the many campgrounds or bed-and-breakfast inns along the way, allows you to soak up this trail's rural natural beauty and small town charm. Another benefit to taking your time is that it increases your chances of spotting the tiny endangered Karner blue butterfly.

DIRECTIONS

Parking and access to the trail is provided at each community along the trail. Camping is available in Belmont, Cedar Springs, Sand Lake, Morley, Paris, Reed City, Hersey, Evart and Cadillac.

To reach the southern endpoint in Comstock Park, take US Highway 131 north to Post Drive and turn right on Belmont Road. Take Belmont Road to Rogue River Road. The park entrance will be on the left.

To reach the northern endpoint in Cadillac, take US Highway 131 north. Exit onto State Route 115 and go northwest for a half mile. Take North 41 Road 1 mile north to North 44 Road. Go west on North 44 Road approximately a half mile.

To reach the Big Rapids trailhead, take US Highway 131 to Big Rapids, Exit 139. Take State Highway 20 east to Maple Street. Proceed straight for 0.1 mile to the depot staging area and turn south.

To reach the Rogue River Park trailhead in Belmont, take US Highway 131 to Exit 95 (Post Drive). Take Post Drive east to Belmont Road. Take Belmont Road 0.25 mile south to the Rogue River Park entrance and turn left.

Contact: Friends of the White Pine Trail
P.O. Box 159
Belmont, MI 49306
(616) 222-5005
www.whitepinetrail.com

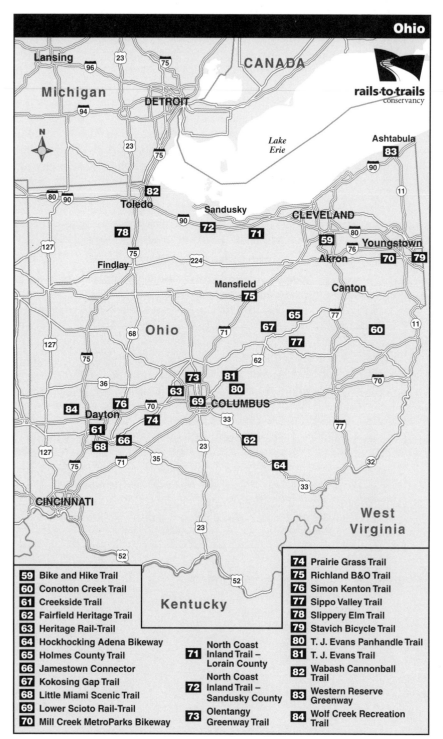

Ohio

rails·to·trails
conservancy

Lansing [96] [23] [75]

CANADA

Michigan

DETROIT

[94]

Lake Erie

Ashtabula [83]

N

[23] [75]

[90] [11]

[80] [90] [82]

Toledo

Sandusky

CLEVELAND

[78] [90] [72] [71]

[59] [80] Youngstown

[127] [75]

Findlay

[224]

Akron [76] [70] [79]

Mansfield [75]

Canton

Ohio

[65] [77]

[60] [11]

[68] [71] [67]

[127] [77]

[75] [62]

[36] [70]

[84] [76] [73] [81]

Dayton [63] [80]

[61] [70] [69] COLUMBUS

[68] [66] [74] [33]

[127] [23] [77]

[75] [71] [35] [62]

CINCINNATI [64]

West Virginia

[23] [33]

[52] [32]

[52] Kentucky

59 Bike and Hike Trail	**74** Prairie Grass Trail
60 Conotton Creek Trail	**75** Richland B&O Trail
61 Creekside Trail	**76** Simon Kenton Trail
62 Fairfield Heritage Trail	**77** Sippo Valley Trail
63 Heritage Rail-Trail	**78** Slippery Elm Trail
64 Hockhocking Adena Bikeway	**79** Stavich Bicycle Trail
65 Holmes County Trail	**80** T. J. Evans Panhandle Trail
66 Jamestown Connector	**81** T. J. Evans Trail
67 Kokosing Gap Trail	**82** Wabash Cannonball Trail
68 Little Miami Scenic Trail	**83** Western Reserve Greenway
69 Lower Scioto Rail-Trail	**84** Wolf Creek Recreation Trail
70 Mill Creek MetroParks Bikeway	
71 North Coast Inland Trail – Lorain County	
72 North Coast Inland Trail – Sandusky County	
73 Olentangy Greenway Trail	

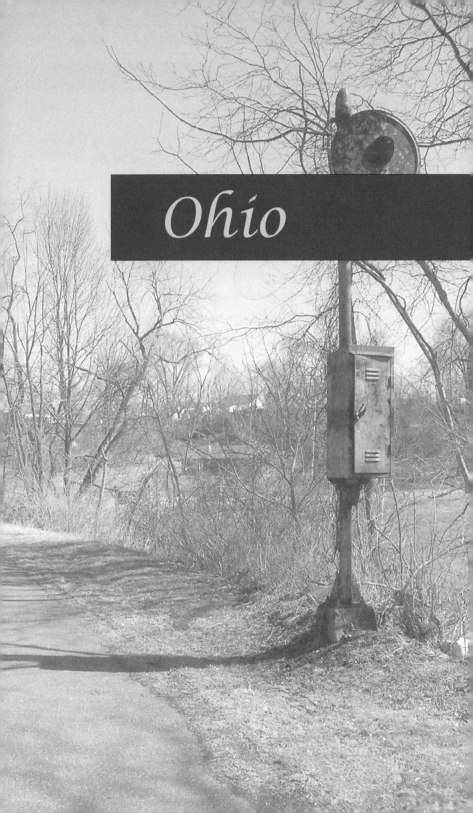

Ohio

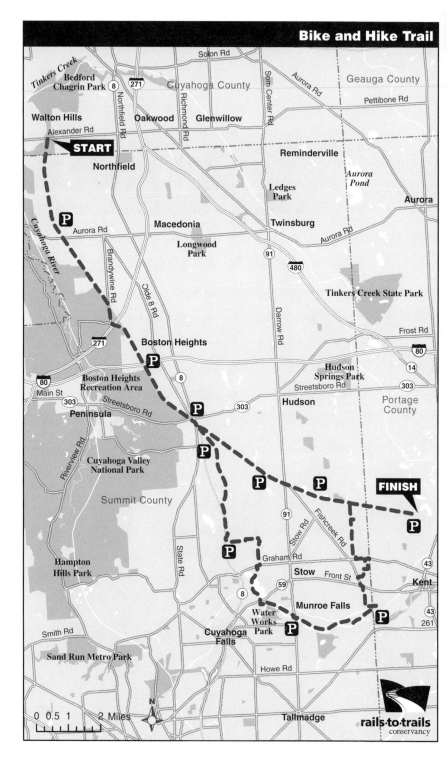

Bike and Hike Trail

The Bike and Hike Trail is a rambling, rolling 33.5-mile rail-trail peppered with bridge crossings and neighborhood road riding in a rural-to-suburban setting. Unlike most flat rail-trails, this route has delightful dips and rises, but small children and level-ground lovers may not enjoy the challenge this trail presents.

This terrific trail offers a ton of green space and fresh air. Playgrounds and restroom facilities are ample too, though you may want to stock up on drinking water and snacks before striking out for the day.

Starting at the northern tip, you experience a beautiful, mostly secluded, multiuse paved trail, much of which borders Cuyahoga Valley National Park. For many miles you are treated to intermittent glimpses of enormous exposed stone ledges. With an early enough start, you might see some deer grazing at the trail's edge. As the trail winds south, it passes through some

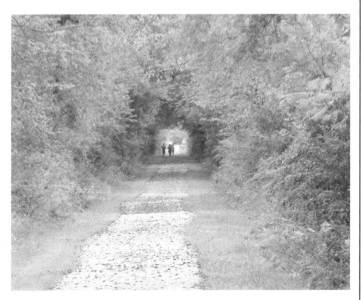

The Bike and Hike Trail is canopied in several places with lush foliage—a real treat in the spring and fall months.

Location
Cuyahoga, Portage and Summit counties

Endpoints
Northfield to Munroe Falls

Mileage
33.5

Roughness Index
1

Surface
Asphalt and crushed stone

beautiful neighborhoods on the way to the more rugged Cuyahoga Valley National Park.

The flatness of the trail falls away as you travel the on-road sections and bikers and inline skaters are treated to a fun descent before the payback of heading uphill. As with all the on-road sections, look for the green trail signs to guide you along the route. An observation deck over on the Cuyahoga River in Munroe Falls is a universally accessed area with lovely scenery and offers fishing in addition to walking, cycling and inline skating.

Once you complete the southern loop you can finish the trail by heading north and back to the trailhead. If you still have energy to burn after the return trip north, complete your day's adventure exploring the Cuyahoga Valley National Park. With miles of hiking trails, breathtaking views and wildlife ranging from bald eagles to coyotes, the national park is the perfect complement to the host of northeast Ohio nature this rail-trail serves up.

DIRECTIONS

To reach the northern trailhead on Aurora Road in Northfield, follow Interstate 271 to State Route 8 and travel north for about three-quarters of a mile. Turn west on Aurora Road and proceed 2 miles to parking on both the left and right sides of the road.

To reach the southern trailhead on North Main Street in Munroe Falls, from Interstate 76 take Exit 27 for State Route 91/Gilchrist Road. Continue north for 0.3 mile to State Route 91 north and turn right. Follow State Route 91 north for 5.3 miles to the parking lot and the trailhead on the right.

In addition to the two endpoints, there are nine other access points, which are listed online at www.summitmetroparks.org/ ParksAndTrails/BikeAndHikeTrail.aspx.

Contact: MetroParks, Serving Summit County
975 Treaty Line Road
Akron, OH 44313
(330) 867-5511
www.summitmetroparks.org

Conotton Creek Trail

The Conotton Creek Trail is 11.4 miles of scenic serenity in northeast Ohio. The trail emanates rustic beauty and its pavement covers a flat, straight route. Several particularly rough spots may bounce you back to consciousness, but the rest of this trail lulls you into a state of relaxation and chases your stress away. If you are searching for rejuvenation, look no further than this trail.

Riding from quaint Bowerston east to Jewett makes your return trip slightly downhill. A multitude of wildlife is found on this trail, as well as animals of a tamer variety; horses and cattle graze on the rolling hills of neighboring farms along the trail's southern edge. East of Bowerston are several ponds that draw beaver, ducks, geese and great blue herons. Lining the sides of the trail between Bowerston and Jewett, more than 40 birdhouses attract tree swallows and bluebirds.

Location
Harrison County

Endpoints
Bowerston to Jewett

Mileage
11.4

Roughness Index
1

Surface
Asphalt

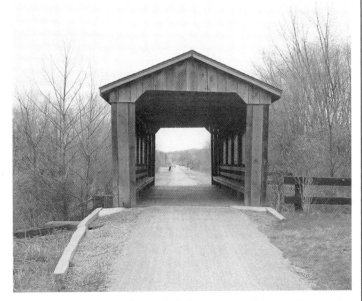

The covered bridge across Conotton Creek—the waterway for which the trail is named—is a popular draw for the pathway.

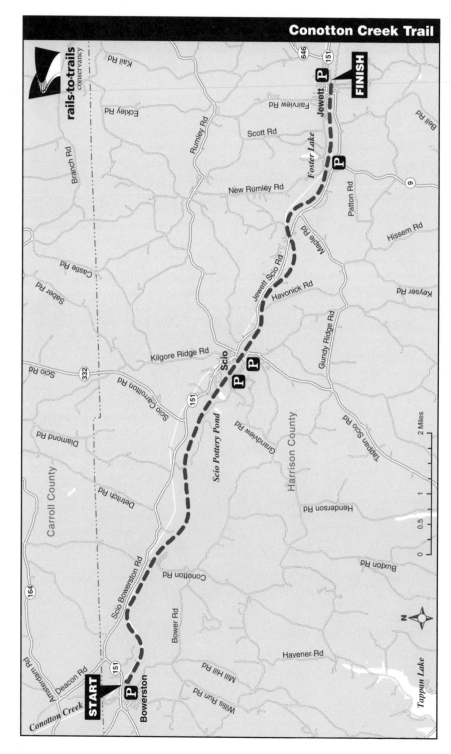

Conotton Creek Trail

The trail's crown jewel is the covered bridge in the town of Scio, the approximate midpoint of the trail. For bridge aficionados this is as good as it gets. This unique covered bridge spans the short section across Conotton Creek, fitting in perfectly in rural Ohio. Pay attention to the fine craftmanship of this structure; it is a true testament to the labor required to span this waterway. The waters below the bridge eventually feed into the Ohio River, as well as into the Mississippi River more than 500 miles away.

The final handful of miles into the town of Jewett is just as calming and refreshing as those from Bowerston to Scio. Jewett, similar to Bowerston is merely a speck on a map but the town was an important cog in the wheel of this region's development. Jewett was not only an important stop on the railroad like the other towns you passed on the trail, but it was also once home to a streetcar manufacturer and an opera house.

DIRECTIONS

To reach the trailhead in Bowerston, from Interstate 77, take the exit for State Route 36. Follow State Route 36 east to State Route 250 east. Take State Route 151 northeast toward Bowerston. Before entering Bowerston, you will see signs directing you to the trailhead on the right side of State Route 151.

To reach the trailhead in Jewett, from Interstate 77, take the exit for State Route 36. Follow State Route 36 east to State Route 250 east. Take State Route 151 into Jewett and to the well-marked trailhead on the east side of town.

Contact: Harrison County Conotton Creek Trail Fund
c/o Crossroads RC&D
277 Canal Avenue, SE, Suite C
New Philadelphia, OH 44663
www.crossroadsrcd.org/hctrail

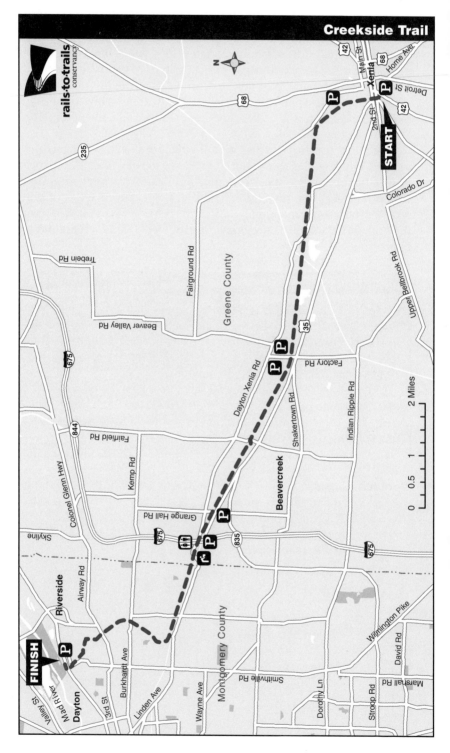

Creekside Trail

Creekside Trail

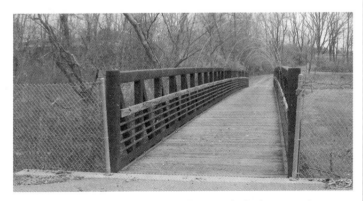

T his 15-mile paved trail cuts a swift route from Xenia to Dayton, passing a variety of sites, including drag racetracks and quiet museums. If you want more trail options, start at the Train Depot in Xenia, where the Little Miami Scenic Trail, the Prairie Grass Trail and the Creekside trails converge. The Creekside Trail used to be called the "H" Connector because of its shape as a link between the Greene County (or Little Miami Trail) and Montgomery County (or Mad River) trails.

To follow the Creekside Trail from Xenia Station, a restored railroad depot, you head north, crossing Cincinnati Avenue, Second Street and Main Street. Main Street is very busy so use caution. If you're interested in a longer trip, you can add a 10-mile side trip to Yellow Springs along the Little Miami Scenic Trail; take Market Street east and follow the signs.

On the Creekside Trail, crossing Market Street makes all the difference. Here you enter a world filled with nature. Shawnee Creek flows along the north side of the trail. At Towler Road you can see the entrance to Sol Arnovitz Park, which offers some parking spaces but no other services. About 1 mile from Xenia Station you reach the James Ranch Spur. This trail heads less than a mile east to the Fairgrounds Recreation Center and Mullins Pool.

Location
Greene and Montgomery counties

Endpoints
Xenia to Dayton

Mileage
15

Roughness Index
1

Surface
Asphalt

Rail-trail and community connections, as well as restored railroad structures, showcase the Creekside Trail's transportation past, present and future.

Before you have traveled 3 miles, be prepared for a shift in your surroundings. The entrance of Kil-Kare Dragway abuts the trail. On race days it is loud and the fragrance of hot rubber fills the air.

Continuing west you reach the William Maxwell Rest Area in Beavercreek Township. Named for the area's first publisher, this park offers a covered picnic table and a nice marble monument to Maxwell.

A bridge over the Little Miami River, about 4 miles from the start, has overlooks at each end that offer beautiful views of the river and its banks in both directions. The Alpha House bed-and-breakfast sits right along the trail in Alpha and is known for its hospitality toward trail users. At mile 6 there is a spur into Beavercreek Community Park, which has restrooms, water and parking facilities. Staying on the trail you find larger Nutter Park, across Factory Road and home to five baseball diamonds, as well as more restroom, water and parking facilities. During games the concessions stands are open and offer trail users an opportunity to stop for refreshments.

At mile 9.5 you reach Fifth Third Gateway Park, which has parking, gardens and other amenities, including restroom facilities. Then the trail crosses Interstate 675 and into Montgomery County via an impressive 465-foot restored railroad overpass.

When you hit a T-junction turn right to continue to the trail's end in Eastwood MetroPark. You cross Burkhardt Road and then busy Airway Road. On your right are the huge, shining silver hangers of the National Museum of the U.S. Air Force. The trail winds down in a serene setting—you would never guess that you are minutes from Wright-Patterson Air Force Base and downtown Dayton.

DIRECTIONS

To reach the Xenia Station trailhead, from US Highway 35, take State Route 380 north for 1.25 miles. Turn left onto South Miami Avenue and look for the restored depot on the right.

To reach the Eastwood Park trailhead in Dayton, from US Highway 35 (between Interstates 675 and 75) follow Wright Brothers Parkway north for 2.8 miles. Turn left onto Springfield Street and look for Eastwood MetroPark on the right.

Contact: Greene County Parks and Recreation
651 Dayton-Xenia Road
Xenia, OH 45385
(937) 562-7440
www.co.greene.oh.us/parks/
multi-use-trails.htm#creekside_trail

Fairfield Heritage Trail

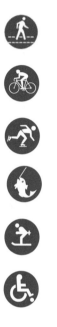

The Fairfield Heritage Trail winds through and connects the community of Lancaster. It links a college, high school, junior high school and elementary school, as well as numerous parks and shopping and dining opportunities along its 5-mile path.

Well-maintained, the asphalt trail begins at the Ohio University–Lancaster campus parking lot and heads south along the edge of campus. A small waterway, Fetters Run, borders the trail to the east. One-third of a mile from the trailhead is the John Bright #2 covered bridge, built in 1881 in nearby Carroll and moved to this site in 1988. Continue on your way to reach John Bright #1, another bridge—this time metal—and historic structure built by the Hocking Metal Bridge Company.

Beyond John Bright #1 you pass Lancaster High School with its many athletic fields and tennis courts, an exercise course and the football stadium, all paralleling Arbor Valley Drive.

After another quarter mile you cross Fetters Run via the donated and painstakingly restored McCleery Covered Bridge and reach Thomas Ewing Junior High School. A well-signed crosswalk guides you across Fair Avenue, where the trail goes through a beautiful grove of trees before coming out in a neighborhood. The route becomes a painted bike lane once you turn south onto Franklin Street. At mile 1.5, cross 6th Avenue and ride through Lanreco Park where the separate paved bike trail begins again.

A quarter mile around the park brings you to a busy crossing of Cherry Street, so use caution at this junction. The trail then passes over Baldwin Run on a bridge, at which point the trail transitions to a sidewalk. Keep an eye out for Goslin Street, which you follow for a short distance until the asphalt trail reappears on the right of the street. A shopping center anchored by a Kroger grocery store dominates the landscape to the left of the trail, which then dips beneath Main Street and continues south to a new bridge crossing of Baldwin Run into Mary Burnham Park, which has baseball fields, a

Location
Fairfield County

Endpoints
Ohio University–
Lancaster campus
to Olivedale Park

Mileage
5

**Roughness
Index**
1

Surface
Asphalt

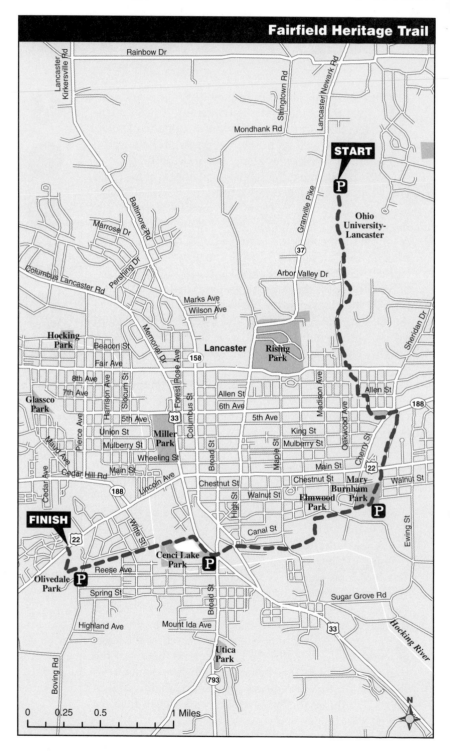

Fairfield Heritage Trail

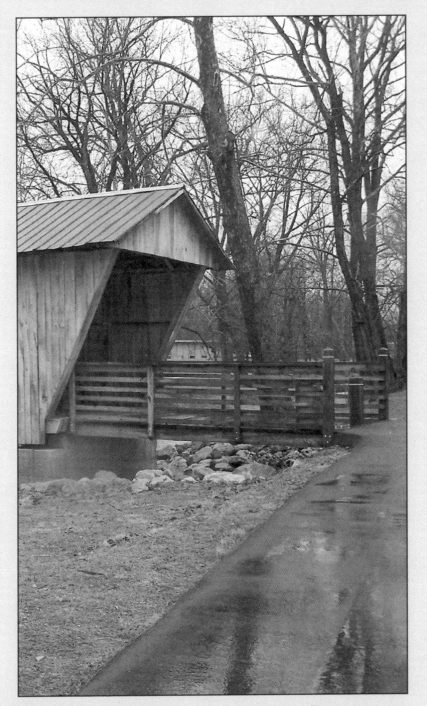

Bridges of both the covered and rail variety put the heritage in the Fairfield Heritage Trail.

basketball court, children's playground equipment, a picnic area and parking for park and trail users.

At mile 2.5 you leave Mary Burnham Park and cross active railroad tracks. For the next quarter mile the trail runs along the same tracks, a nice section of rail-with-trail. The trail then veers off the active corridor and, for the next mile, crosses several streets while hugging the banks of the Hocking River. At mile 3.7 you come to Cenci Park and Cenci Lake where people fish and observe wildlife. There are parking facilities and a half-mile paved loop trail around the lake.

After leaving the park the trail continues for just over another mile past Maher Park, across a well-preserved rail bridge, the Talmadge School and then to Olivedale Park where the trail ends.

DIRECTIONS

To reach the trailhead at Ohio University–Lancaster, from Interstate 270 take US Route 33 south toward Lancaster. After 14.2 miles follow Business Route 33 to Lancaster. Go 7.3 miles and turn left onto Main Street. Take another left after 0.4 mile onto High Street. After 2.1 miles turn right onto College Avenue. The trailhead is on the left at the university campus.

To reach the Olivedale Park trailhead, from Interstate 270 take US Route 33 south toward Lancaster. After 14.2 miles follow Business Route 33 to Lancaster. Go 7.3 miles and turn right onto Lincoln Avenue. After 0.6 mile turn left onto Boving Road. Olivedale Park is a quarter mile down Boving on the right.

Contact: Lancaster Parks and Recreation
1507 East Main Street
Lancaster, Ohio 43130
(740) 687-6651
www.lancaster-oh.com/heritage

Heritage Rail-Trail

More than half of the smooth, flat, 6.1-mile Heritage Rail-Trail has a parallel horse trail. The 4-mile equestrian corridor starts at Hayden Run Road and continues northwest to the Cemetery Pike trailhead.

If you're walking, biking or inline skating, start the trail in downtown Hilliard off Main Street. The trailhead has an abundance of parking, a warm-up area and bike rack; the adjacent Old Hilliard historic district has numerous shops and eateries.

Journeying northwest you immediately come across a lovely fountain and a pond on the south side of the trail. From an observation platform on the banks of the pond you can view Canadian geese. If you prefer art to wildlife, an excellent display of public art includes some very colorful sculptures.

This trail has numerous well-designed connections to soccer fields, tennis courts and the local high school

Location
Franklin and
Madison counties

Endpoints
Hilliard to
Plain City

Mileage
6.1

**Roughness
Index**
1

Surface
Asphalt

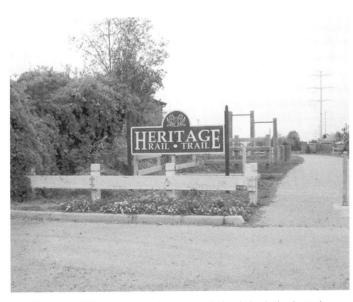

The Heritage Rail-Trail connects local parks, sports fields, a high school and several neighborhoods before meandering toward a finish in the countryside.

211

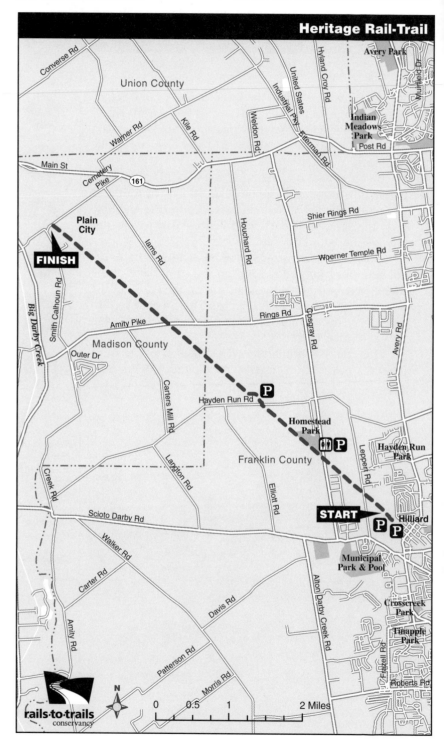

Heritage Rail-Trail

football field. There are also connecting paths to the many housing subdivisions in this rapidly growing part of central Ohio. For example, the Vaniard Trail branches off to the south at Hoffman Farms Drive and connects to a subdivision of homes and Hoffman Farms Elementary School. It ends at Municipal Park and Pool, which has baseball diamonds, soccer fields, a pool and plenty of parking.

The trail links two major parks: Homestead Park in Washington Township and Hayden Run Metro Park. The first, Homestead Park, is approximately 1.3 miles from the start in downtown Hilliard and has a restored Conrail caboose, restrooms, parking, vending machines, public telephones, a 0.75-mile loop trail, playground equipment, an information kiosk, a fishing pond and picnic tables. After Homestead Park the trail continues through the countryside. If you like birding, there are many bluebird boxes along the trail.

Hayden Run Metro Park, on Hayden Run Road, is just 1.1 miles from Homestead Park. The parallel equestrian path begins in this park and the area features a corral and horse trailer parking. The coarse gravel horse trail runs on the east side of the Heritage Trail until Amity Pike, where it switches to the west side. From this point the last 2 miles of tree-lined trail allow glimpses of classic Midwest farmland. The trail ends at Cemetery Pike just over a mile southeast of Plain City. The Heritage Rail-Trail Coalition, in concert with local and state governments, is working to extend the trail into downtown Plain City in the near future.

DIRECTIONS

To reach the trailhead in downtown Hilliard, from Interstate 270 take Cemetery Pike west for 1.5 miles. Turn right onto Norwich Street and after a half mile turn left onto Wayne Street and go another 0.1 mile. Turn right onto Center Street and look for the trailhead on the left.

To reach the trailhead in Plain City from Interstate 270, take US Route 33 west for 2.8 miles and exit onto State Route 161 west toward Plain City. After another 2.8 miles take a left onto Cemetery Pike. The trailhead is on the left.

Contact: Washington Township Parks and Recreation
4675 Cosgray Road
Hilliard, OH 43026
(614) 876-9554
www.heritagerailtrail.org

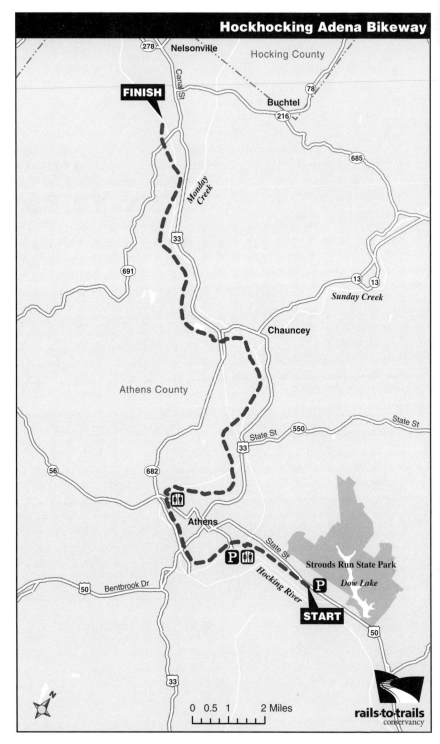

Hockhocking Adena Bikeway

Hockhocking Adena Bikeway

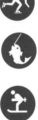

Hockhocking Adena Bikeway traces a beautiful, twisting 16.4-mile course from Athens to Nelsonville along the Hocking River. The rail-trail draws its name from the ancient Adena Indians who lived in this area and called the Hocking, a tributary of the Ohio River, "Hockhocking" or "bottle river" for the tapered bottleneck shape of this river valley in southeast Ohio. The trail is on a canal towpath-turned-railroad corridor that was sufficiently flood damaged in the late 1800s to halt rail service forever. Today the Hockhocking Adena Bikeway is a heavily used rail-trail linking Ohio University with Hocking College and communities in between.

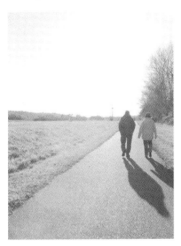

The Hockhocking Adena Bikeway is a popular and collegiate rail-trail, linking two colleges and connecting several communities along its path.

From the southern trailhead on the Ohio University campus in Athens, the trail begins with 1.5 miles of commercial convenience: Many different stores connect to the bikeway, making it a popular venue for college students and shopping. There are three access points to the popular Athens Community Center, which has restrooms, a swimming pool, a volleyball court, tennis courts and a skate park. The trail then connects to the Ohio University bikeway. The path, like the school, borders the Hocking River, part of the reason behind Ohio University's "Harvard on the Hocking" nickname.

Over the next couple miles, the Hockhocking Adena trail crosses a golf course and passes the Athens Public Library, residence dorms, O'Bleness Hospital, a state mental health facility and numerous athletic fields and stadiums. Upon leaving the Ohio University campus,

Location
Athens County

Endpoints
Athens to Nelsonville

Mileage
16.4

Roughness Index
1

Surface
Asphalt

the trail passes a Habitat for Humanity building that provides public restrooms. The trail then crosses to the west bank of the Hocking River and things slow down. In 2.5 miles a short spur trail connects to Eclipse, a former coal-mining town, which has a restaurant that is usually open for dinner. Many of the miner's homes have been renovated and the old company store is still standing.

Back on the rail-trail you wind through rolling Appalachian foothills, the dense woods of Wayne National Forest, wetlands and occasional fields and along the meandering river. In the spring, the wildflowers in the forested areas provide an ever-changing, colorful panorama. Deer are abundant and you may see raccoons amble across your path as well.

Near mile 10 is the Beaumont (also called Salinas) rest area. An early 1900s coal and salt-mining town once stood here; look for the remains of the mines that produced salt and coal. The remaining 6.5 miles is classic Appalachia as you travel along the Hocking River and pass through a portion of the Wayne National Forest. The trailhead on the Hocking College campus in Nelsonville features a spur of the Hocking Valley Scenic Railroad, so you can cap your rail-trail excursion with a ride on the rails. Courtesy of a recently awarded State of Ohio grant, the bikeway will soon continue from Hocking College just over a mile into downtown Nelsonville.

DIRECTIONS

To reach the trailhead on the Ohio University–Athens campus, take the State Street exit east from State Route 33 in Athens. The main trailhead will be on the right in 1.75 miles.

To access the Robbin's Crossing trailhead on the grounds of Hocking College, from State Route 33 just south of Nelsonville turn right on State Route 691. Continue 500 feet to Hocking Parkway, turn right and continue for a half mile. Turn left on Robbin's Crossing to the trailhead.

Contact: Athens County Convention and Visitor Bureau
667 East State Street
Athens, OH 45701
(800) 878-9767
www.seorf.ohiou.edu/~xx088/

Holmes County Trail

If traveling through Ohio's Amish country and sharing space with bicycles, buggies and abundant wildlife sounds like an idyllic day to you, then you will enjoy the nearly 12-mile Holmes County Trail. A good place to start is the trail's southern Hipp Station trailhead in Millersburg, which features the beautifully restored Millersburg train depot. The historic depot, which serves as the trail's headquarters, offers a visitors center with wildlife displays, trail information, restrooms, vending machines, a covered picnic area and a playground.

Millersburg is in the heart of Ohio's Amish country; it is just as common to pass a horse-drawn buggy as it is to pass a cyclist or walker. The trail surface has adjacent paths, one paved and the other of chip-and-seal, which is a bit rougher for bicycles but accommodates horses. Be sure to review the etiquette rules posted at the trailhead so you can share the trail safely with its myriad of users.

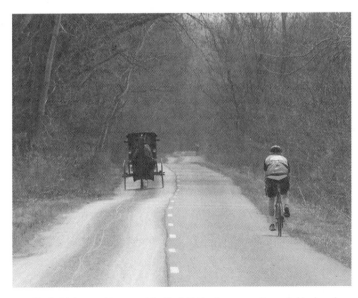

The Amish horse-and-buggy and the "English" bicycling communities amicably share the Holmes County Trail, often cohosting trailside fundraising events and working together to make this a unique and fun rail-trail.

Location
Holmes and
Wayne counties

Endpoints
Millersburg to
Fredericksburg

Mileage
12

**Roughness
Index**
1

Surface
Asphalt

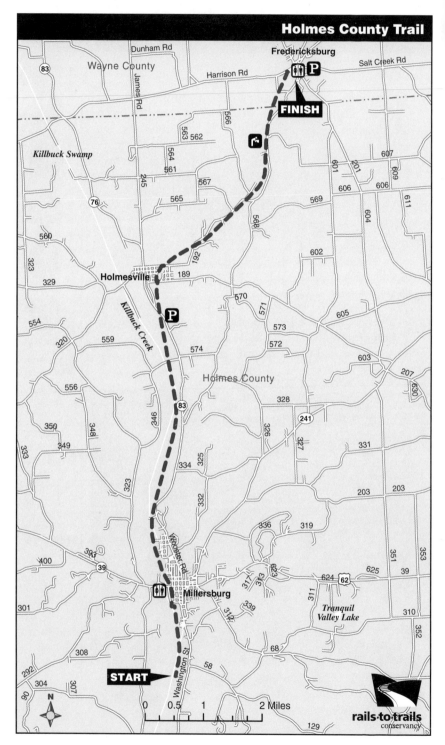

Holmes County Trail

The trail meanders north out of Millersburg at a very easy, even grade. The corridor passes picturesque swamplands for long stretches. Wildlife abounds among the water and trees. You will likely see turtles, snakes and birds, including cardinals, doves and hawks. Given the trail's wet terrain, there are numerous stream crossings, a couple over well-restored railroad bridges.

A well-designed square tunnel takes you underneath County Road 83 at mile 6 just before the small town of Holmesville. When you enter Holmesville, near mile 6.5, you follow quiet community streets for about 1 mile until the rail corridor picks up again. The bypass is very well-marked and the streets are extremely quiet, little used and easy to navigate. Once through Holmesville, the trail continues for another 4 miles along a wonderful mixture of farm fields and tree-lined streams to the Fredericksburg trailhead and the trail's north end.

The Holmes County Trail began its life as a spur of one of Ohio's earliest railroads, the Cleveland and Pittsburgh, and the tracks reached Millersburg in 1854. A catastrophic flood in 1969 washed out sections of railbed and killed 22 passengers and crew members, leading to the line's abandonment. Fortunately, with the conversion of the railway to a rail-trail in 2003–2004 a new generation of users—bicyclists, walkers, inline skaters and horse and buggy riders—can now roll along this picturesque corridor.

DIRECTIONS

To reach the Millersburg trailhead at Hipp Station, begin on State Route 39. Turn on North Grant Street and follow it north for 0.1 mile and then head west on West Clinton Street which dead-ends into Hipp Station Trailhead.

To reach the Fredericksburg trailhead, take State Route 83 to Harrison Road east and go 4 miles. Turn right onto West Water Street; the trailhead is immediately on the right.

Contact: Holmes County Trail
1 Trail Drive, Suite B
Millersburg, OH 44654
(330) 674-0475
www.holmestrail.org

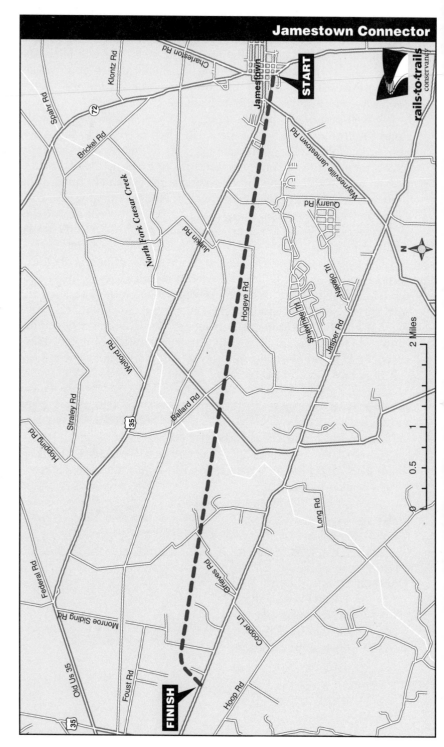

Jamestown Connector

The Jamestown Connector Trail, currently 7.7 miles long, will soon connect all the way to Xenia Station and the network of trails that meet there. Xenia is the hub of Greene Counties trail system where you can head north or south on the Little Miami Scenic Trail (page 227), northwest to Dayton on the Creekside Trail (page 205), or northeast to London on the Prairie Grass Trail (page 247).

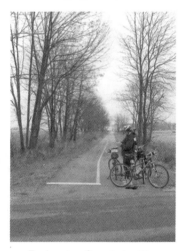

The Jamestown Connector is set to soon be a hub of rail-trail links, living up to its name.

The Jamestown Connector will eventually connect Jamestown to the Washington Court House and the Tri-County Triangle Trail. The trail is relatively new and offers a beautifully maintained asphalt surface suitable for all uses except horses and motorized vehicles.

The trail starts in Jamestown on South Limestone Street where a small parking lot offers a place to leave a car. There are more amenities quickly available along the trail. Just a half mile into the ride a wooden bridge off the right side of the trail leads to Jordan's Supervalu Grocery, which offers beverages, food and restroom facilities. Another trailhead on the left of the trail just 1 mile from the start is at Frank Seaman Park. This park makes for a better starting point than the small parking lot at the beginning of the trail because it offers restrooms and water along with parking facilities. In addition, it has numerous baseball fields, a covered pavilion and picnic area, as well as ample green space to either warm up for your ride or unwind afterward.

Moving west again down the trail brings you to the crosswalk taking you across Quarry Road and officially

Location
Greene County

Endpoints
South Limestone Street to Jasper Road in Jamestown

Mileage
7.7

Roughness Index
1

Surface
Asphalt

221

out of town and into the countryside. The corridor is amazingly well shaded by a thick canopy of deciduous trees. The periodic breaks in the trees over the next 2 miles allow you to get a peek of the vast farm fields that dominate this part of central Ohio. At mile 3.8 the Ballard Road crossing marks the approximate halfway point of the trail.

Just past mile 4 the trail crosses South New Jasper Station Road and less than a half mile past this crossing it comes to the bridge crossing the North Fork of Caesar's Creek. The bridge is a nicely built concrete deck and the view both up and down creek of the meandering waterway and lush vegetation clinging to its banks is well worth a stop.

The remaining 3 miles or so offer a smooth, quick ride through more farm fields and forested canopy. Keep an eye out for South Monroe Siding Road, a half mile from the end of the trail. Just past it on the right is Skydive Greene County, which offers skydiving opportunities; on a nice day it is common to see airplanes taking off and landing. Don't forget to look up as the planes landing will have most likely just had a group of parachutists jump out of them!

The trail ends at Jasper Road, which doesn't have trailhead facilities available. The corridor heading toward Xenia is clearly visible on the other side of the road, promising the much-anticipated link to the Xenia Station Trail hub.

DIRECTIONS

To reach the Jamestown trailhead at South Limestone Street, from US Route 35 take Old US Route 35 east for 1.9 miles. Turn right onto South Limestone Street. After 0.14 miles, look for the small parking lot on the right side of the road that is the trailhead. However, the Frank Seaman Park Trailhead is a better starting point for this trail.

To reach the Jamestown trailhead at Frank Seaman Park, from US Route 35 take Old US Route 35 east for 0.4 mile. Turn right onto Quarry Road; after 0.8 mile turn left onto Cottonville Road. Just 0.2 mile down the road look for Greenview High School on the left. Frank Seaman Park and the trailhead are accessed by going through the high school parking lot and turning right.

Contact: Greene County Parks and Recreation
651 Dayton-Xenia Road
Xenia, OH 43583
(937) 562-7440
www.co.greene.oh.us/parks/multi-use-trails.htm
#jamestown_connector

Kokosing Gap Trail

Part of the 453-mile Ohio to Erie Trail, the 14-mile Kokosing Gap Trail is a straight shot through ravines and farmland and passes a beautifully restored train and a cheerful wood caboose. This outstanding trail connects the towns of Mount Vernon, Gambier, Howard and Danville on a smooth asphalt surface, with park benches about every half mile. The gap between each community is about 4 miles, give or take. Unlike most rail-trails, this one is maintained solely by donations and volunteers.

Starting at the trailhead in Mount Vernon, the first part of the trip takes you along the sunken valley of the Kokosing River. Heading east you pass one of several overlooks of the river and surrounding valley and two old railroad trestles across the river. The bridges have been meticulously restored and are well worth a stop to admire. Shortly after crossing the first bridge you reach the Brown Family Environmental Center at Kenyon College. A visitor center and a butterfly garden beckon you to take a break and come in for a self-guided tour through this wonderful garden area.

Location
Knox County

Endpoints
Mt. Vernon to Danville

Mileage
14

Roughness Index
1

Surface
Asphalt

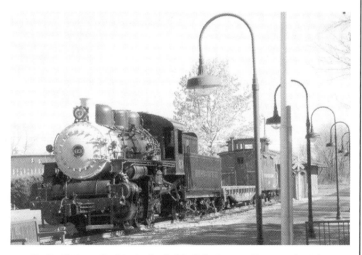

Gambier Station on the Kokosing Gap Trail highlights its past with a restored train locomotive, tender, flat car and caboose.

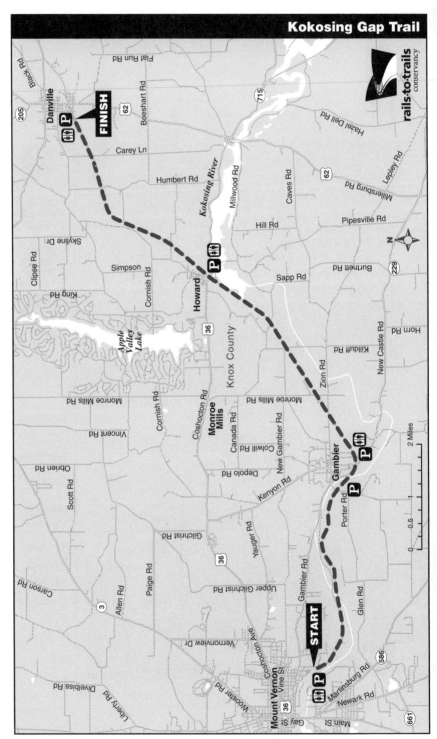

Where the trail intersects busy State Route 229 and enters Gambier, you will want to pay close attention for a safe crossing. The village of Gambier is home to Kenyon College. After passing the campus of this distinguished liberal arts school, you can't miss Gambier Station and its four train cars, a locomotive, tender, flat car and caboose.

The community of Howard, like the rest of the towns along the Kokosing Gap Trail, provides notable diversions. The trailhead has a parking lot, restrooms and a playground donated by the Rotary Club. Just after an arched stone passage under Route 36, an incredible historic barn towers over the trail. Another bridge provides views of a smaller tributary that flows into the Kokosing River, and the trail soon opens up onto farm fields and pastures.

After about a mile more you are back among trees, but you periodically get to peek out of the gaps in the forest to see the farm fields in the distance. There are only four quiet back roads that cause pause in the final 3.5 miles until the trail ends in Danville.

The Kokosing Gap Trail is open 24 hours a day through all seasons. In early morning and twilight hours vintage-looking streetlamps shed light on your journey near the Gambier trailhead. If you visit in fall, be sure to look for the turkey vultures that congregate between Howard and Danville before they head south.

DIRECTIONS

All of the towns along the route provide trailheads with parking and seasonal facilities.

The Mount Vernon trailhead is on Mount Vernon Avenue. From Interstate 71 take State Route 61 north for 1.8 miles. Turn right onto State Route 229, which becomes US Route 35 in Mount Vernon. After about 17 miles turn right onto State Route 13 (South Main Street) and go 0.6 mile and take a left onto Mount Vernon Avenue. The trailhead is on the right side after Cougar Drive just under 1 mile down the road.

To reach the Danville trailhead take US Route 36 to US Route 62 (Millersburg Road) north and go 3.3 miles. Take a left onto West Washington Street, after just over 0.1 mile take a right onto South Richards Street. The trailhead is on the left.

Contact: Kokosing Gap Trail
P.O. Box 129
Gambier, OH 43022
(800) 837-5282
www.kokosinggaptrail.org

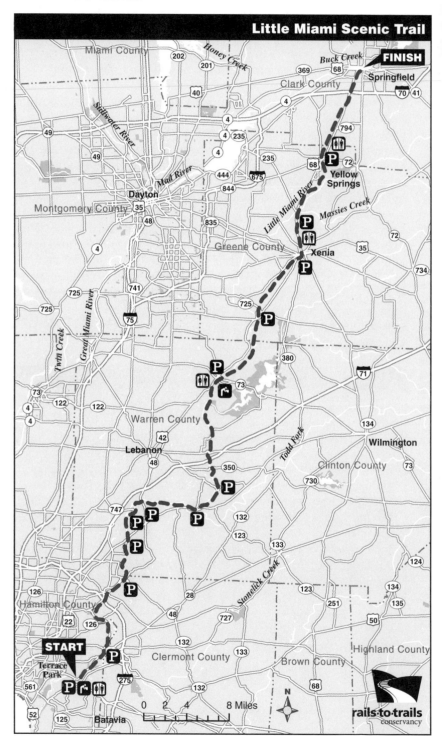

Little Miami Scenic Trail

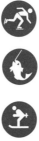

The Little Miami Scenic Trail is a jewel in the crown of Ohio rail-trails. The 72-mile paved path links Terrace Park near Cincinnati to Springfield, a dozen towns and four counties to the north. It passes through quaint small towns, beautiful state parks, picturesque scenery, old and new bridges and natural habitat.

If you are interested in a shorter trip, start at Xenia Station. Trails radiate from Xenia like sunbeams, lending this charming town a reputation as the crossroads of Ohio trails.

Feeling energetic? Take in the Little Miami in one fell swoop, starting and ending at the Avoca Park Trailhead in Terrace Park. This beautiful park has plenty of natural green space to relax in after one of the best rides Ohio has to offer.

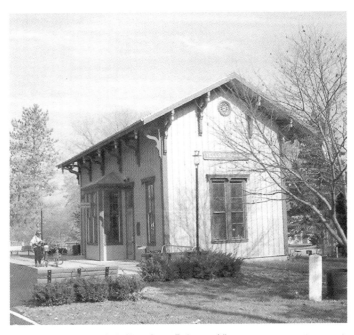

Whether you take the Little Miami Scenic Trail in one fell swoop or space your journey out over a day or so, the trail's historical flair is certain to impress trail users of all ages.

Location
Clark, Clermont, Greene, Hamilton and Warren counties

Endpoints
Terrace Park to Springfield

Mileage
72

Roughness Index
1

Surface
Asphalt and concrete

227

SOUTHERN SECTION

Leaving Terrace Park, a bridge takes you over State Route 50 and you soon come to Milford, until 2005 the trail's southern endpoint. Here and for most of the southern portion, the Little Miami River is your companion. Just north of Milford a lovely 2500-foot-long bridge carries you across the river toward Loveland. "Old Loveland," the quaint older section, is jam-packed with stores, cafes and even a bike shop. The trail is busy here and traffic remains constant all the way past Hamilton Township's Fosters Park, with its parking, restrooms and shady large trees, to the Jeremiah Morrow Bridge. The bridge, named after a former governor, is the highest bridge in Ohio, a twin deck, arch truss bridge, looming 239 feet above the river.

Near the town of Morrow, with its railroad depot and an ancient, but safe, iron trestle, the trail congestion ebbs. There is a lot of ground to cover between Morrow and Xenia, but don't miss Fort Ancient State Memorial, home to a large museum and 3.5 miles of mounds built by the Fort Ancient tribe. Just to the north is Caesar Creek State Park, with more than 70 miles of great hiking and bridle trails as well as canoe rentals.

The town of Corwin at about mile 32 is a pleasant place to stop and recharge. This is the last trailhead before Xenia and Xenia Station, where mileage markers start at 0.

NORTHERN SECTION

Xenia Station to Yellow Springs is an extraordinary 10.25-mile journey. Just 1 mile into the ride, Shawnee Park provides a great fountain, playgrounds, benches and restrooms. There is even a band shell. The trail here begins to see more traffic but remains wide and avoids overcrowding. The Xenia State trailhead is a perfect backdrop for photos to prove the miles you have covered. As you approach Yellow Springs, several 911 call boxes indicate a return to an urban setting. A little farther north a historical marker tells about American abolitionist Moncure Daniel Conway, who briefly spent time in the Cincinnati area. On the left is the Antioch grade school and its impressive contemporary sculpture garden. A little farther along the path is Glen Helen Park and Antioch College.

In downtown Yellow Springs, south of US Route 68, two converted train cabooses function as storefronts; north of the highway Yellow Springs Railroad Station now houses the Chamber of Commerce. The chamber hosts an unusual and fun feature—revolving art exhibits in the public restrooms. Many Little Miami Trail users either turn around or stop here. As it continues north, the trail has multiple road segments and can be confusing.

The final leg of the trail from Yellow Springs Station to Springfield is an approximately 7-mile journey. Start it off with a side trip east on West Jackson Road: The homemade ice cream at Young's Dairy is just 0.8 mile away on Springfield-Xenia Road and is a must for many trail users.

Several street crossings and some road riding are ahead, so take your time and watch for traffic. After you cross Possum Road, the trail curves to the left and turns north next to Springfield-Xenia Road. The road crossing for southbound trail-travelers is unmarked. Bike lanes on the road start just across Leffel Lane, though the official bike lanes start at the Springfield city limit.

After the bike lanes take you right on John Street, cross the street and pick up the rail-trail again. At Johnny Lytle Avenue turn right onto a bike route. Continue traveling east to South Plum Street. At this point go north until you get to Fair Street then turn left. Shortly turn right and go back to the trail. Pass through several underpasses to the corner of Center and Jefferson streets. Here the trail goes north to downtown Springfield's Heritage Center, which houses a library, museum store and the Springfield Arts Society.

The Heritage Center marks the end of the Little Miami Scenic Trail. With all 72 miles under your belt, or even just a sampling, it is plain to see why this trail is traveled by more Ohioans than any other trail in the state.

DIRECTIONS

Avoca Park Trailhead can be accessed by traveling south on State Route 50 toward Terrace Park. On the left side of Route 50 you will see the well-marked entrance.

Xenia Station is located on South Detroit Street (State Route 380) in Xenia, 1 mile south of the US Route 35 and US Route 68 intersection. Take Route 68 south until it becomes State Route 380. Travel 1 mile and look for the caboose on the right. Turn right onto North Miami Avenue at the traffic signal and turn right again into the parking lot.

The Heritage Center Library in Springfield has parking and trail facilities.

Contact: Miami Valley RailTrails
AKA Miami Valley Trails
Miami Valley
Dayton, OH
www.miamivalleytrails.org/miami.htm

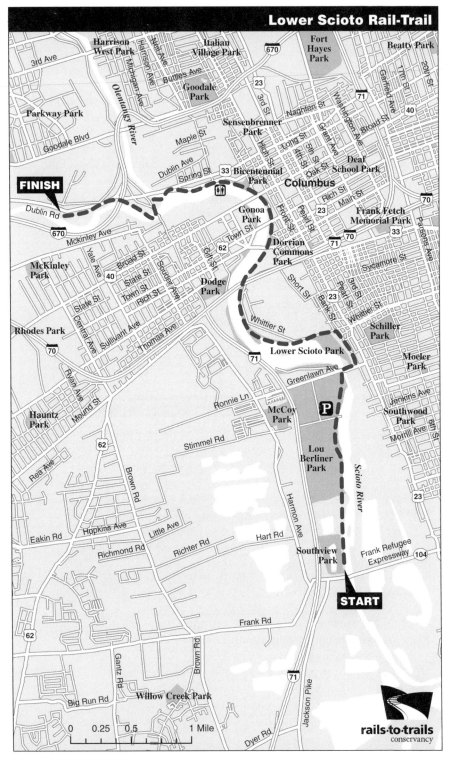

Lower Scioto Rail-Trail

Lower Scioto Rail-Trail

The Lower Scioto Rail-Trail, or Olentangy/Scioto Greenways, is an early urban greenway at its best. The 6.2-mile multiuse trail hugs the banks of the Scioto River as it connects parks, links with other trails and gives fabulous views of downtown Columbus. Portions of the route are considered the state's oldest rail-trail.

The trail starts just north of State Route 104 and follows the west side of the Scioto River. However, the best place to park and access the trail is at Lou Berliner Park, across the river from German Village. The park is a hot spot for team sports, with ball diamonds and athletic fields. From the park you can travel north or south on the rail-trail. If you head south, the trail travels though lush forest all the way to the endpoint near State Route 104.

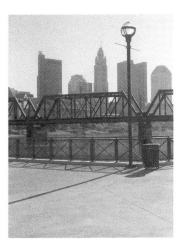

Hugging the Scioto River, the Lower Scioto Rail-Trail is a heavily used corridor for commuters and sightseers alike.

Going north takes you to downtown Columbus. The start of this section is also densely forested, making it easy to forget that you are traveling in a large city.

At Greenlawn Avenue you can ride or walk straight across the street or descend a steep slope below it to get to the other side. Once you get onto Greenlawn Avenue, cross the Scioto River on the Greenlawn Avenue Bridge. The bridge has just been rebuilt with a great bike and pedestrian-friendly path along the edge.

The next 0.3 mile along Front Street alternates between brick and concrete sidewalk. The route here is unmarked. Turn left and head west on Whittier Street to regain the paved rail-trail route. You pass a trailhead at

Location
Franklin County

Endpoints
North of State Route 104 to Confluence Park

Mileage
6.2

Roughness Index
1

Surface
Asphalt

Lower Scioto Park on the left. The trail curves along the river on the Whittier Peninsula, the site for a planned park.

Interstate 70 roars overhead near mile 3, followed by a breathtaking view of the Columbus skyline. First Bicentennial Park and then Battelle Riverfront Park provide vantage points overlooking the river, the urban environment and a replica of Christopher Columbus's sailing vessel the *Santa Maria*.

At North Bank Park, a good stopping point, you can enjoy the million-dollar view of downtown Columbus and the previously mentioned parks that make up its riverfront. Newly constructed restrooms and parking areas are available here, along with an excellent observation deck over the river from which to take in the views.

A short half-mile ride takes you across the river once again and into Confluence Park, on the spot where the Scioto and Olentangy rivers meet. From this park the Scioto River Greenway goes another mile to the northwest, separate from but adjacent to city streets. Confluence Park serves as the northern trailhead, as the endpoint a mile away does not have any public facilities. The park also serves as the southern trailhead for the Olentangy Greenway Trail (page 243), a 13-mile trail to the northern community of Worthington.

DIRECTIONS

Lou Berliner Park is the best southern trail access point. From Interstate 71 take Greenlawn Avenue east for just under a quarter mile. Turn right on Deckenbauch Road. Lou Berliner Park is on the left. Travel east from the parking lot to access the trail.

To reach the Confluence Park trailhead, from Interstate 70, take Route 315 north 1 mile and take the Dublin Road exit. Turn left onto Dublin Road and after just 0.1 mile turn left onto North Souder Road. Take your first left onto Rickenbacker Drive. Confluence Park is at the road's end a quarter mile away.

Contact: Columbus Department of Recreation and Parks
1111 East Broad Street
Columbus, OH 43205
(614) 645-3300
www.centralohiogreenways.com/SciotoTrail.htm
www.centralohiogreenways.com/OlentangyTrail.htm

Mill Creek MetroParks Bikeway

The well-designed Mill Creek MetroParks Bikeway between Canfield Township and Austintown is an 11-mile paved corridor that passes through both suburbs and countryside in northeastern Ohio.

Traveling north from the trail's start at Western Reserve Road, you arrive at MetroParks Farm. This 400-acre working farm sprawls along the western edge of the trail and offers educational programs, tours and agricultural displays. The farm is a popular field trip destination for local schoolchildren. On the opposite side of the trail, the Canfield Fairgrounds holds one of Ohio's largest fairs every year.

About 6 miles into your ride you encounter one of the jewels of this trail: the Kirk Road Trailhead. The well-designed facility provides trailside basics, such as a picnic pavilion and water fountains, as well as an exceptional overall design. This trailhead is not only functional but beautiful as well.

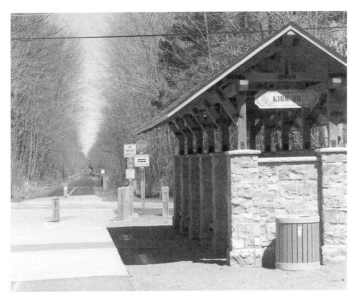

"Functional" and "beautiful" describe how many view the Mill Creek MetroParks Bikeway as it moves smoothly from the suburbs to the countryside.

Location
Mahoning and Trumbull counties

Endpoints
Canfield to Mineral Ridge

Mileage
11

Roughness Index
1

Surface
Asphalt

233

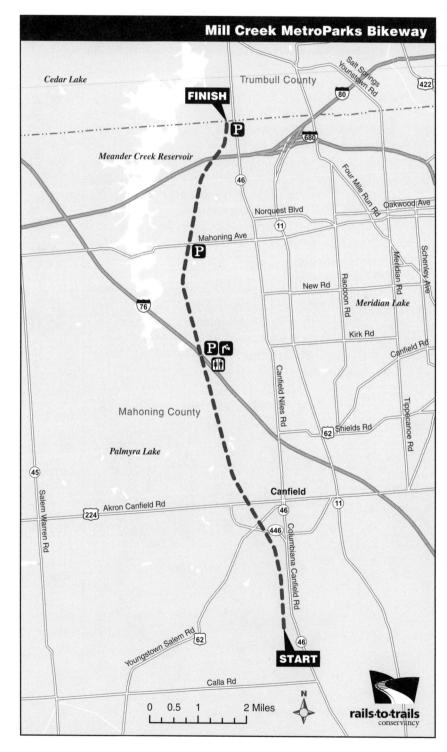

Mill Creek MetroParks Bikeway

Cedar Lake

Trumbull County

Salt Springs Youngstown Rd

422

80

FINISH

P

680

Meander Creek Reservoir

46

Norquest Blvd

Four Mile Run Rd

Oakwood Ave

11

Mahoning Ave

P

New Rd

Raccoon Rd

Meridian Rd

Schenley Ave

Meridian Lake

76

Kirk Rd

P

Canfield Rd

Mahoning County

Canfield Niles Rd

Tippecanoe Rd

Palmyra Lake

62

Shields Rd

45

Canfield

11

Salem Warren Rd

Akron Canfield Rd

224

46

446

Columbiana Canfield Rd

Youngstown Salem Rd

62

46

START

Calla Rd

N

0   0.5   1   2 Miles

rails·to·trails
conservancy

The trail is clean, well maintained and a joy to be on, with a high volume and diversity of users. In the suburban area near Austintown it passes between houses near the trail and takes on a pleasant neighborly feel. At the southern start of the trail near Marquis there are plenty of rural stretches to let you relax and recharge in the natural element.

DIRECTIONS

The trailhead in Canfield Township is at Metroparks Farm. Take US Route 224 to Canfield and turn south on State Route 46. Approximately 1 mile south of 224, the entrance to MetroParks Farm is on the right.

To reach the Kirk Road Trailhead, take Route 224 to Route 46 north. Follow Route 46 to Kirk Road and turn west. The trailhead, with parking for 50 cars, is just over 1 mile on the left.

Contact: Mill Creek MetroParks
7574 Columbiana-Canfield Road
P.O. Box 596
Canfield, OH 44406
(330) 702-3000
www.millcreekmetroparks.com

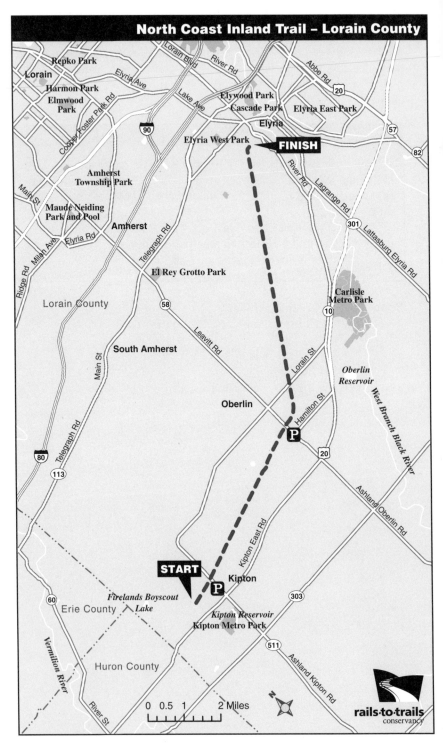

North Coast Inland Trail – Lorain County

Repko Park

Lorain

Harmon Park

Elmwood Park

Lorain Blvd

Elyria Ave

River Rd

Lake Ave

Abbe Rd

20

Elywood Park

Cascade Park

Elyria East Park

Elyria

90

Elyria West Park

57

82

FINISH

Amherst Township Park

Maude Neiding Park and Pool

Amherst

Elyria Rd

Telegraph Rd

River Rd

Lagrange Rd

301

Lattasburg Elyria Rd

El Rey Grotto Park

Ridge Rd

Milan Ave

Lorain County

58

Leavitt Rd

Carlisle Metro Park

10

South Amherst

Main St

Lorain St

Oberlin Reservoir

Oberlin

Hamilton St

West Branch Black River

P

80

Telegraph Rd

20

113

Ashland Oberlin Rd

Kipton East Rd

START

Kipton

P

Firelands Boyscout Lake

60

Erie County

303

Kipton Reservoir
Kipton Metro Park

Huron County

511

Ashland Kipton Rd

Vermilion River

River St

0   0.5   1   2 Miles

N

rails·to·trails
conservancy

North Coast Inland Trail – Lorain County

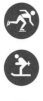

The Kipton to Elyria rail-trail is a 13-mile paved path and part of the 65-mile North Coast Inland Trail. The corridor is classic rail-trail: flat and straight. Heading northeast from Kipton's downtown community park and restored depot, you travel only 50 feet before encountering a plaque commemorating the Great Kipton Train Wreck. This was the scene of an 1891 train collision in which eight people died. The wreck was blamed on the station engineer's watch, which was slow by four minutes and caused him to delay moving one of the trains to a separate track. Railroad officials hired prominent Cleveland jeweler Webb Ball to investigate railroad timekeeping and institute precision performance and inspection standards. Locals credit Ball's capable work with the origin of the much-used idiom "on the ball."

Heading toward Oberlin you pass rural homes and take in sweeping views of a community golf course.

Location
Lorain County

Endpoints
Kipton to Elyria

Mileage
13.1

Roughness Index
1

Surface
Asphalt

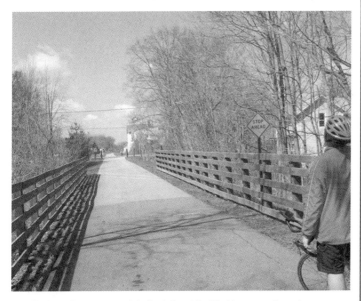

The Lorain County section of the North Coast Inland Trail has a storied past that you can read about on interpretive trailside signs along the way.

Before entering Oberlin the trail turns off the rail corridor and onto country roads for less than 1 mile. The on-road bike lanes are well defined, traffic is light and the route is easy to negotiate. The rail line picks up again in the beautiful small college town of Oberlin. The trail travels through the town's central park, with water fountains and a playground and passes Oberlin's restored historic train depot.

Leaving Oberlin, the vista becomes rolling farmland with herds of cattle and roaming horses. You also pass rural homesteads and are welcomed by the baying of kenneled hounds. Bird life along the trail is impressive. You may see cardinals, turkey vultures, bluebirds, warblers, vireos and other varieties common to northern Ohio.

The trail ends in Elyria when it hits Industrial Parkway. Plans are afoot to extend this trail in both directions to form the 65-mile North Coast Inland Trail between Elyria and Toledo.

DIRECTIONS

The Kipton trailhead is easy to reach from US Route 20 by taking State Route 511 north for just over a half mile to downtown Kipton. Park on the left in Kipton Community Park on Rosa Street.

To reach the Oberlin trailhead from Route 20, follow State Route 58 north to downtown Oberlin. There is a parking lot on the left at the Oberlin Depot. Kipton and Oberlin are the preferred access points for this trail.

Contact: Loraine County MetroParks
12882 Diagonal Road
LaGrange, OH 44050
(800) 526-7275
www.loraincountymetroparks.com/ncit.htm

North Coast Inland Trail – Sandusky County

The 8.5 miles from Fremont to Clyde on this paved section of the developing 65-mile North Coast Inland Trail serves up a slice of corporate America—Whirlpool and Heinz have factories here—with a heaping side of down-home Ohio countryside. The corridor is open all year, with cross-country skiing a popular winter activity.

Much of the corridor is a rail-with-trail, with an active rail line paralleling your path. Begin in Fremont just over 0.5 mile north of the Rutherford B. Hayes Presidential Center and Library. A visit to the Center and Library and then a trail ride would make a perfect Saturday. A beautiful bicycle and pedestrian bridge carries you to the east bank of the Sandusky River. In the early spring when walleye run the river, you will see eager fishermen in the waters below. If the town of Fremont triggers memories of hot dogs and French fries, blame it on the familiar fragrance wafting on the breeze from the Heinz Ketchup factory.

Location
Sandusky County

Endpoints
Fremont to Clyde

Mileage
8.5

Roughness Index
1

Surface
Asphalt

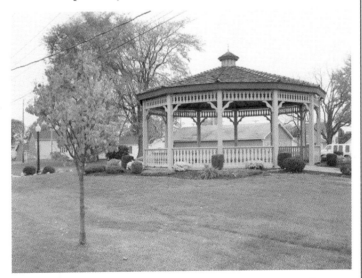

The Sandusky County section of the North Coast Inland Trail mingles corporate America and Ohioan countryside in pleasing harmony—local factory workers often use the trail for lunchtime workouts and commuting.

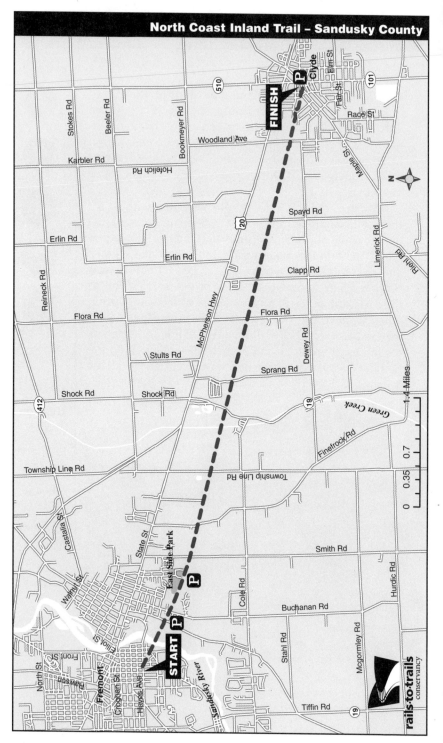

North Coast Inland Trail – Sandusky County

Just 1.5 miles into the trip you reach the picnic shelters, ball fields and playground in Biggs-Kettner Memorial Park. The park is the main access point for the trail and the site of the Fremont Community Recreation Complex. Refill water bottles or take a shade break beneath the many mature trees. If you are starting here, you have the option of heading west to the Sandusky River bridge and the presidential library, or turning east toward Clyde. Heading directly east from Fremont, you can look forward to 6.5 miles of rail-with-trail that is flat, paved and sprinkled with rural farms. Wildlife and natural wildflowers are abundant along the trail and you may see many birds, squirrels, rabbits and even an occasional deer.

Arriving in Clyde you are greeted by the world's largest Whirlpool washing machine factory on the left side of the trail. Nearby bicycle parking areas are used by Whirlpool employees who commute to work via the rail-trail. The remaining mile of the trail winds through neighborhoods and ends in a quaint park near the historic downtown. There are a few restaurants available if you want an out-and-back trip with a lunch stop in the middle.

DIRECTIONS

The only official trail access in Fremont is at the Fremont Community Recreation Complex at 600 St. Joseph Street. It can be accessed from State Route 20 by turning south on St. Joseph Street and continuing about 0.75 mile until it ends at the park and recreation center. Trail access and parking are in the southeast corner of the park's parking lot.

To reach the trail endpoint in Clyde take State Route 20 to Vine Street. Take Vine 0.5 mile south until it crosses the trail just after Eaton Road. Parking is available in multiple areas.

Contact: Sandusky County Park District
1970 Countryside Place
Fremont, OH 43420
(888) 200-5577
www.scpd-parks.org/index.htm

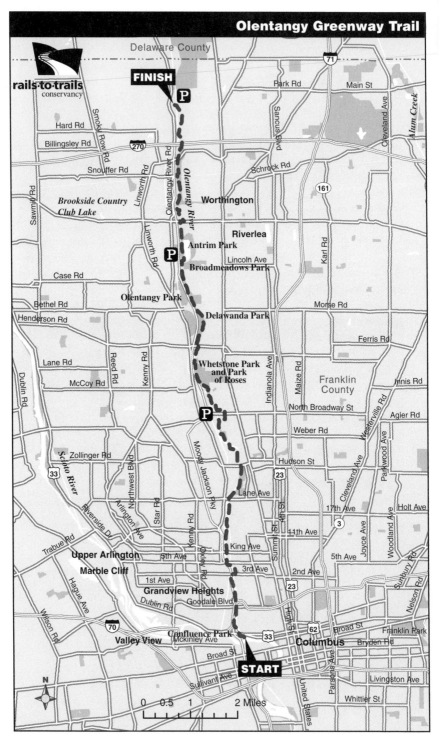

Olentangy Greenway Trail

The Olentangy Greenway Trail (a.k.a. Olentangy River Greenway) picks up near the north end of the Lower Scioto Rail-Trail (page 231) and heads 13 miles north through several parks and Ohio State University. Portions of the trail are rough going, but for the most part it is serene and scenic.

From Confluence Park, head north and use the crosswalk at Dublin Road. Once across the road, the trail travels north on the west side of the Olentangy River. At some points the trail is very close to the river and flood warnings are posted. After passing under several freeways the trail becomes quieter as you meander along the bank of the river with some light tree cover and the sound of the water drowning out some of the city sounds.

At Third Street a bridge takes you to the east side of the Olentangy River, and at Fifth Avenue you must choose between a lower trail along the riverbank or an

Location
Franklin County

Endpoints
Downtown
Columbus to
Worthington

Mileage
13

**Roughness
Index**
1

Surface
Asphalt and
concrete

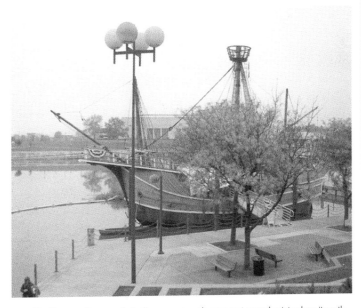

The Olentangy Greenway Trail offers easy riverside access at several points along its path.

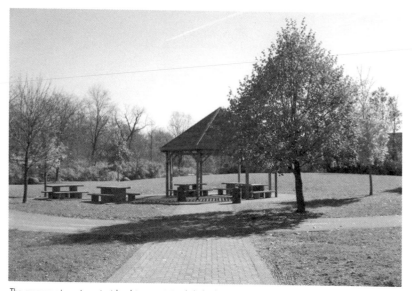

The greenway is an important local transportation link, hooking into the campus of Ohio State University and the city and outskirts of Columbus.

upper trail with access to Fifth Avenue and part of the Ohio State University campus. Between Fifth and King avenues there is an overlook with a large concrete deck jutting over the river's edge that allows a good look at the lowhead dam spanning the river there.

The campus area of the trail—roughly 1 mile—is in transition and a university bikeway plan has been recently released and can be accessed on the Ohio State University website. Bicyclists are cautioned to dismount and walk through the rough sections, or, at the very least, slow their speed considerably. The rough ride is due to deteriorating asphalt, which poses a real hazard to riders. A local landmark arises on the right side of the trail in this section. Ohio Stadium, or the Horseshoe, as locals call it, is the home of the Ohio State Buckeyes football team.

The trail then passes under the new Lane Avenue Bridge, a striking structure, with an amazing cable-stayed design. The anchorages for the bridge cables are 47 tons each, making them the largest pieces of steel ever galvanized. Unmarked neighborhood trails feed into the bikeway periodically. Near mile 4 the university's wetland research area flanks the west side of the route. Feel free to take a self-guided tour of the native plants and wetland habitat.

A short stretch takes you on a well-marked route over city streets in Clintonville before you travel though Whetstone Park and the Park of Roses. Whetstone Park offers playgrounds, picnic pavilions, baseball fields, basketball courts and 136 acres of facilities and nature areas. The 11-acre Park of Roses is a park within a park, with more than 11,000 rose bushes. After these parks you return to the river's west edge via a challenging, narrow sidewalk lane along the bridge at Henderson Road.

You soon arrive at Antrim Lake and Antrim Park. There is an excellent overlook on the lake and a 1.2-mile loop trail around the lake that is popular with trail users as well as park visitors. A short trail connection takes you under the highway west to Antrim Park.

A short time later you cross back to the east side of the river at State Route 161 in Worthington over a highway bridge that has a bike pedestrian lane on the south side. From this point it is another 3 miles to the end of the trail, with half of that distance coming between the Route 161 bridge and Interstate 270. The scenery in this stretch is very relaxing as you wind your way upriver amongst beautiful hardwoods, with a periodic neighborhood park opening up to the east.

The imposing elevated lanes of Interstate 270 mark the final crossing of the river over a nicely constructed trail bridge. After crossing underneath the interstate, it is a short, 1-mile ride through a small section of forest and then on a narrow strip of land between the river and some of Worthington's new development. A small circle of green grass with a nice gazebo greets you at the endpoint in Worthington.

DIRECTIONS

To reach the southern trailhead at Confluence Park, take Interstate 70 to Route 315, turn north 1 mile and take the Dublin Road Exit. Turn left onto Dublin Road, after 0.1 of a mile turn left onto North Souder Road. Take the first left onto Rickenbacker Drive. Confluence Park is at the end of this road a quarter mile away.

. To reach the northern trailhead in Worthington Hills Park, take Interstate 270 to State Route 315 north. Look for Worthington Hills Park on the right.

Contact: Columbus Recreation and Parks Department
200 West Greenlawn
Columbus, OH 43223
(614) 645-3300
www.centralohiogreenways.com/SciotoTrail.htm
www.centralohiogreenways.com/OlentangyTrail.htm

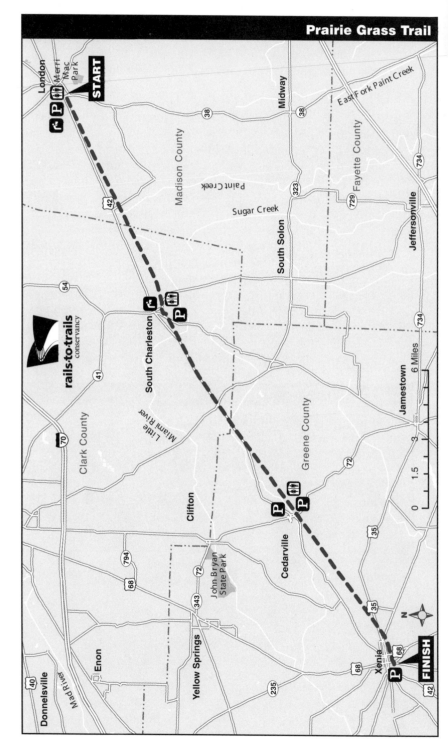

Prairie Grass Trail

Prairie Grass Trail

This beautifully maintained asphalt rail-trail stretches 29 miles from London to Xenia, generally following US Route 42. The northern trailhead is located in London, behind the senior citizen's center and has a picnic pavilion and public restroom. The first mile west of London has several benches and another small picnic pavilion for trail users.

The trail takes a rural flavor immediately upon leaving London. The corridor has been planted with natural prairie grasses, surrounded by flat, open farmland. In keeping with the prairie grass landscape, there are few trees, which makes it important to keep your water bottles full.

After 10.4 miles you reach the small town of South Charleston. As it passes through town the trail diverts onto sidewalks for a half mile. The South Charleston trailhead is highlighted by the wonderfully restored historic train depot; it also offers picnic tables, water and restrooms. The community park surrounding the trailhead is also home to a red and a blue caboose that are being restored for public enjoyment.

The almost 10 miles between South Charleston and Cedarville are dominated by huge fields of corn and soybeans as far as the eye can see. There is virtually no tree cover, so you should protect yourself against wind and sun. The trail travels close to US Route 42 for much of the way and also shares the corridor with power lines owned by Dayton Power and Light (which allowed an easement on the corridor that made the trail possible). About 7 miles after leaving South Charleston you cross the county line from Clark into Greene County.

In Cedarville, the trail travels beside Massie Park, with parking, playground equipment, water and restrooms available. The Hearthstone Inn directly beside the trail on Main Street is accommodating to weary trail travelers, as is Main Street Station just across the street from the inn, which offers food and other refreshments.

The trail runs another 9 miles from Cedarville to the endpoint in Xenia. As you head out of town you pass

Location
Clark and Greene counties

Endpoints
London to Xenia

Mileage
29

Roughness Index
1

Surface
Asphalt

a good-sized lake off to the right that is separated from the trail by a high chain-link fence. Just before the crossing at Murdock Road 1.7 miles out of Cedarville, there are a couple of benches and a nice overlook. This is a great rest stop, offering views of a small creek and the farms that surround the corridor. Keep an eye out as well for the monarch butterflies that are prevalent in the area. At about the halfway mark the trail becomes shaded by trees growing up to the edges of the route, a welcome respite from the summer sun. There is a busy crossing of Business Route 35 coming into the town of Xenia. Note that the bridge just across Jasper Road is made of fiber-reinforced composite materials, the first of its kind in Ohio. The final mile or so has many road crossings; follow the well-placed signs.

The trail's endpoint is at Xenia Station, a wonderfully restored train depot. The station is also the hub of Greene County's extensive trail system. From here you can head east to Dayton on the Creekside Trail (page 205), south to Cincinnati or north to Springfield on the Little Miami Scenic Trail (page 227).

The Prairie Grass Trail is an important piece of the Ohio-to-Erie Trail, the extensive cross-state, 453-mile trail that is more than halfway built.

DIRECTIONS

The trailhead in London is behind a senior center that allows overflow parking in their lot. If you plan to park here overnight you must inform either the London City Police at (740) 852-1414 or the Madison County Sheriff at (740) 852-1212 of your plans and give them your license plate number. Take Interstate 70 to Urbana-London Road south. Turn right onto West High Street, then turn left onto Midway Road. The trailhead is on the right.

The Cedarville trailhead can be accessed from US Route 42. As you enter Cedarville go straight across Route 72. Take a right onto East Street and look for Massie Park and the trailhead on the left.

Contact: National Trail Parks and Recreation District
1301 Mitchell Boulevard
Springfield, OH 45503
(937) 328-7275
www.ntprd.org/trails.htm#Grass

Richland B&O Trail

Carving a semicircular route from Butler to Mansfield, the Richland B&O Trail zigzags across the same several roads and weaves in and out of rural landscapes as it moves northwest from Butler. With an aggressive maintenance program in the past few years, the 18.4 miles of asphalt trail are in excellent condition.

From Hitchman Park in Butler, commemorative benches depict the history of the Baltimore and Ohio Railway that operated on the route. Your first of several crossings of State Route 97 is just 1.5 miles into the trip.

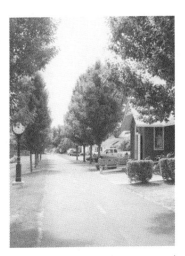

The Richland B&O Trail features a restored railroad depot built in 1906.

Continuing on, cross Elm Street and leave the town of Butler. After traveling through a wooded area you cross the clear fork of the Mohican River via a bridge offering beautiful views of the river valley. On the far side of the slow-moving river, the trail takes you into quiet, rural fields. At the next crossing over Route 97 trail users have a stop sign and motorists have a warning sign, though it is slightly unorthodox: BIKE ROUTE.

Crossing the river again on a unique curved-deck iron trestle bridge brings you into Bellville, about 5 miles from the start. Just over the bridge, the Bellville Trailhead is located in a restored railroad depot built in 1906. The depot offers restrooms, parking and some wonderful historic information. Several more road crossings are ahead, as is a view south toward downtown Bellville, with its classic small-town main street shopping district. After crossing Route 97 again, the trail crosses Alexander Road. If you need a refreshment stop, there are a plethora of restaurants; just take a right at this crossroads. Going straight, take the

Location
Richland County

Endpoints
Butler to Mansfield

Mileage
18.4

Roughness Index
1

Surface
Asphalt

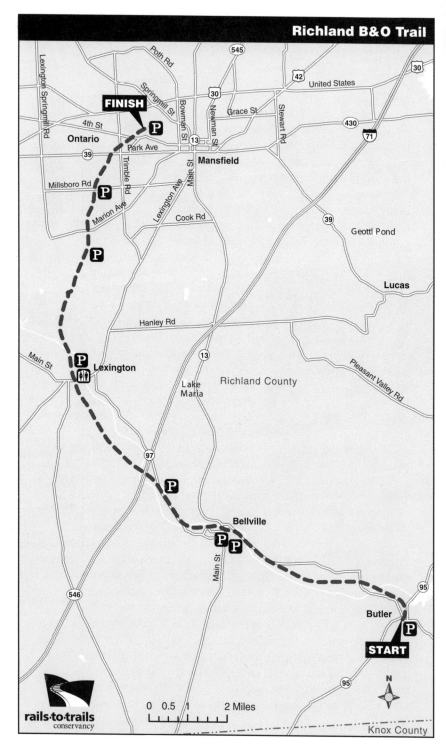

Richland B&O Trail

trail and sail below Interstate 71. The following 2-plus miles are very serene, with only one rural road crossing and a few farm fields breaking up the pleasant forested environment.

Coming out of the forest, the trail parallels South Mill Street for about a mile and passes a water treatment plant just before arriving in Lexington. The Lexington Senior Center Depot on the left side of the trail offers a restroom break and water fill-up that is your last opportunity for nearly 7 miles. Soon the trail becomes a forested area again and passes a small lake, though some road crossings will keep you on your toes. Deer Park, at mile 15, has basic trailhead amenities, and shortly after the park you reach Home Road Marsh. The marsh is home to an abundance of bird species, from swallows to hawks, as well as an assortment of other animals, including turtles, snakes, deer and raccoons. There are benches where you can sit and observe all that the marsh has to offer.

A trailhead at Millsboro Road with parking and emergency call phones welcomes you to Mansfield. Crossing Millsboro Road you enter a wooded area with a creek flowing at your left. The trail dips under Park Avenue West. You can access the trail here but the approaches are very steep. Another underpass carries you under West 4th Street.

The northern end of this trail is lovely. North Lake Park, with a shallow pond, attracts geese and even a few anglers trying for the fish that are stocked in the pond. (To fish here you need an Ohio fishing license.) With clean new restroom facilities, a year-round heated pavilion, playground equipment, tennis courts, the lake and bird life, this park is a wonderful endpoint.

DIRECTIONS

The trailhead in Butler is in Hitchman Park. From Interstate 71 take State Route 97 east toward Bellville. After about 8 miles Route 97 becomes Main Street in Butler. Cross Elm Street and look for Hitchman Park, just south of the BP gas station, on the right.

The Mansfield trailhead, in North Lake Park, is accessible by taking I-71 to State Route 13 for 5 miles to downtown Mansfield. Turn left on West 4th Street, go 1.2 miles, then turn right onto Parkway Drive. You will be forced onto a one-way to the right on Hope Road. North Lake Park is to the right around this loop.

Contact: Mansfield & Richland County Convention
& Visitors' Bureau
124 North Main Street
Mansfield, OH 44902
(800) 642-8282
www.mansfieldtourism.com

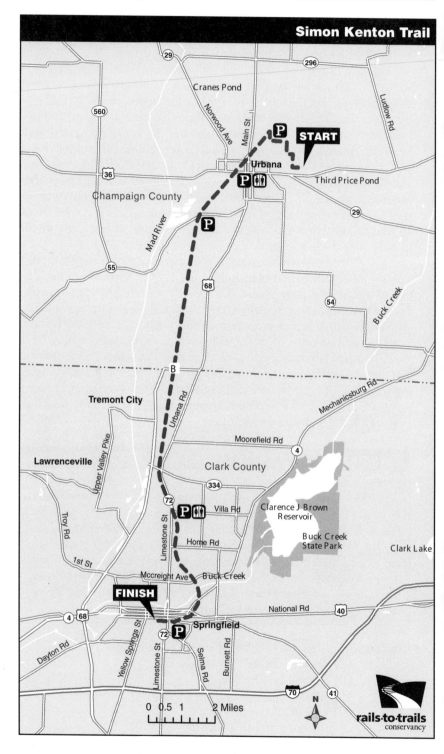

Simon Kenton Trail

The Simon Kenton Trail is a tribute to the hardworking volunteer group that built and maintains the 16.6-mile corridor. The rail-trail is well designed, has extensions and improvements in the offing and has excellent signs throughout the trip connecting Urbana to Springfield.

Beginning at the Urbana YMCA, head into town, intersecting a short bike route to Melvin Miller Park. This southbound stretch offers an excellent strip of rail-with-trail, where freight trains mainly hauling grain travel next to the path before you enter Urbana proper. While the trail passes through many of Urbana's industrial tracts, downtown is just a couple of blocks to the east.

Heading out of the more populated part of Urbana, cross busy Miami Street. Trail signs are just a half mile ahead. At the intersection of Edgewood Avenue and State Route 55, there is a trailhead with benches, a bike rack and parking lot. South of here the trail is nicely shaded and a short trip west on Woodburn Road will take you to Cedar Bog Nature Preserve. The preserve has an ADA-accessible boardwalk that allows visitors to walk through the unique environment without harming it. The preserve is home to hundreds of plant and animal

Location
Champaign and Clark counties

Endpoints
Urbana to Springfield

Mileage
16.6

Roughness Index
1

Surface
Asphalt

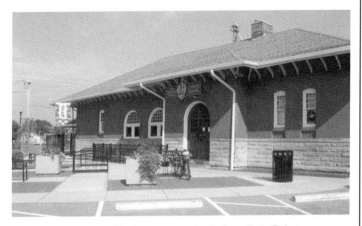

Volunteer dedication and local appreciation makes the Simon Kenton Trail a true community asset.

species, including more than 50 that are rare or endangered. Cedar Run, a small tributary of the Mad River, from which the bog takes its name, is one of the few Ohio streams that has a native population of brook trout.

Cross County Line Road and enter Clark County. At Tremont City Road, pass the Clark State Community College Truck Driver Training Institute. After crossing the railroad tracks and several creeks you reach a connecting trail to the west that accesses the Eagle City soccer fields a half mile away. Just south of the soccer field connection is a new, 1,000-foot trail connection to the sparkling new SplashZone water park.

Though the trail crosses several more busy roads, including State Route 72, there are still pleasant views, especially of some of the beautiful old homes as you begin to get closer to downtown Springfield. After you cross Buck Creek on a trestle bridge, you'll reach a connecting trail that heads to Buck Creek State Park almost 4 miles to the east.

Across Warder Street you begin to travel with another rail-with-trail. This continues for three-quarters of a mile past East Main Street and to Linden Avenue where the trail turns into bike lanes on both sides of East Washington Street. The rail-trail picks back up after crossing East Limestone Street. At this point you have entered the Clark State Community College campus. Cross Fountain Avenue and you have reached the endpoint at South Center Street by the Heritage Center and Clark County Library.

DIRECTIONS

To reach the Urbana Trailhead at the YMCA, take US Route 68 to US Route 36 east (Scioto Street) for 1.5 miles. Turn left onto Commercial Drive and look for the YMCA in front of you.

The Springfield trailhead is at the intersection of South Center Street and West Washington Street. From Interstate 70 take State Route 72 north for 1.7 miles. Bear left onto South Limestone Street. After a little more than a tenth of a mile take a left onto West Pleasant Street for another quarter mile. Turn right onto South Center and look for the trail on the far side of the intersection with West Washington.

Contact: Simon Kenton Pathfinders
P.O. Box 91
Urbana, OH 43078
(937) 484-3335
www.simonkentonpathfinders.org

Sippo Valley Trail

The Sippo Valley Trail is a nearly 10-mile trail with flat, gentle grades from Dalton to Massillon. It takes its name from Sippo Creek, which cascades along the side of the trail for nearly its entire length. There are numerous small bridge crossings, as well as 12 road crossings. All road crossings are well marked for both trail and road traffic and are easily navigated.

The rail-trail begins in Dalton at Village Green Park, where open green space (bordered by ball fields and a playground) and trail amenities are plentiful. After leaving the trailhead you traverse fields, forests and streams. Trail mileage markers, with the zero point originating in the eastern terminus at Massillon, are provided every half mile.

The scenery is a beautiful mix of rolling farmland, forests and small-town homes, starting with a close-up ride along the creek banks.

Location
Stark and Wayne counties

Endpoints
Dalton to Massillon

Mileage
9.6

Roughness Index
2

Surface
Asphalt and crushed stone

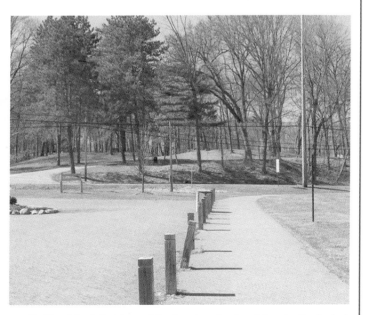

The Sippo Valley Trail retains a parklike atmosphere along its path through rolling farmland and woodlands and along the banks of Sippo Creek.

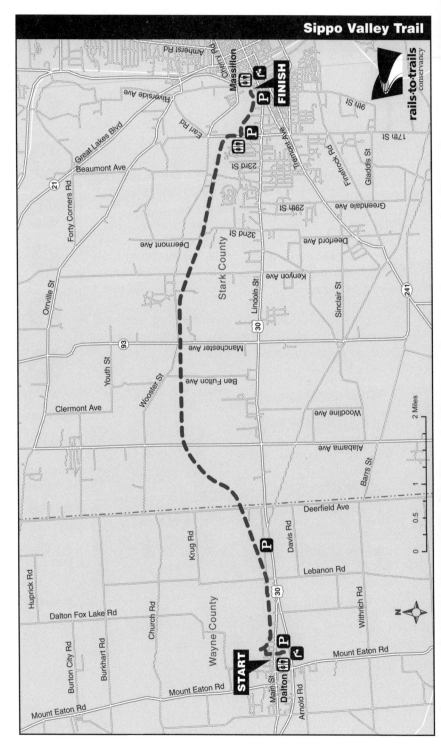

After the first road crossing leaving Dalton, the view opens onto the farm fields that dot the horizon.

At mile 2.75 on the Wayne-Stark County line, you begin a 3-mile section of crushed stone surface that makes up the trail's midsection. The stone portion of the trail is in great condition and in dry weather is easily passable. In wet conditions the stone surface gets slick and may be difficult for road bikers and wheelchair users. Pockets of forest create pleasant shade along the trail corridor. The rural feel of the trail begins to change around mile 9 as you enter Massillon. The crossing at 17th Street brings you to a very steep descent on the east side of the road along the trail. The hill takes you down to Oak Ledges Park and its beautiful setting next to Sippo Creek. Two bridge crossings take you over the creek and once you leave the park a short 0.75-mile stretch remains on the trail.

Arriving at trail's end in Massillon, the Sippo Valley Trail intersects with the 70-plus mile Ohio-Erie Canal Towpath on 6th Avenue. If time permits, venture onto the towpath for a scenic side trip. The formal trailhead is just 450 feet back the way you came on the south side of Bottoms Park.

DIRECTIONS

The Dalton trailhead can be reached by taking US Route 30 to State Route 94 north for a quarter mile. Turn left onto Main Street after just 0.2 mile, turn right onto Freet Street. Freet dead-ends at Village Green Park.

To reach the trailhead in Massillon take US 30 to State Route 21 (Great Lakes Boulevard) north for 2.6 miles. Take a left onto Lincoln Way NW/Route 172 after 0.2 mile, take a right and head north on 6th Street NW for one block. Take the first left and head west on Water Avenue NW, which dead-ends at Bottoms Park.

Contact: Stark County Parks Department
5300 Tyner Street NW
Canton, OH 44708
(330) 477-3552
www.starkparks.com

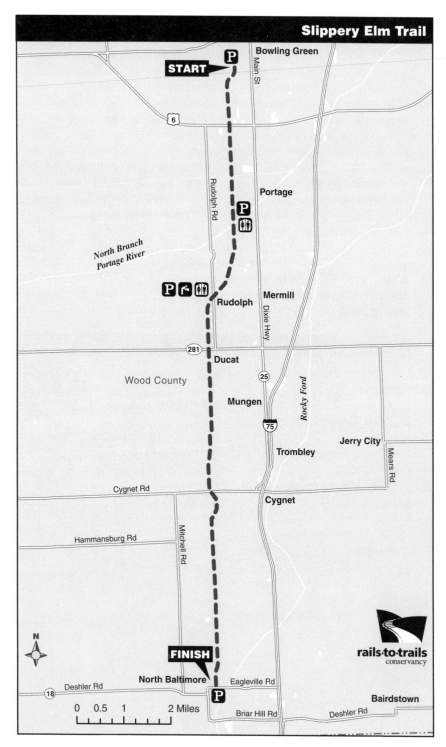

Slippery Elm Trail

Bowling Green

START

Main St

6

Rudolph Rd

Portage

North Branch
Portage River

Rudolph

Mermill

Dixie Hwy

281

Ducat

Wood County

25

Rocky Ford

Mungen

75

Jerry City

Trombley

Mears Rd

Cygnet Rd

Cygnet

Hammansburg Rd

Mitchell Rd

N

FINISH

North Baltimore

Eagleville Rd

18   Deshler Rd

Bairdstown

0   0.5   1   2 Miles

Briar Hill Rd   Deshler Rd

rails·to·trails
conservancy

Slippery Elm Trail

T he mileage slips by on the Slippery Elm rail-trail as you take in the flat, fast and scenic northwest Ohio countryside. The 13-mile paved path runs south from Bowling Green through the small town of Rudolph and finishes in North Baltimore. Its half-marathon length is ideal for runners in training and the smooth surface is a joy for cyclists and inline skaters. Between Rudolph and the southern endpoint, expansive agricultural landscapes offer the quiet charm visitors have come to expect from this area of the country.

Start at the Sand Ridge Road Trailhead in Bowling Green and head south. After mile 1 the trail ducks under US Route 6. As you emerge on the other side the urban surroundings melt away and the countryside takes over.

With a keen eye and light foot (or wheels), you may catch sight of red-tailed hawks, white-tailed deer, red squirrels or the many birds found here. Be sure to take

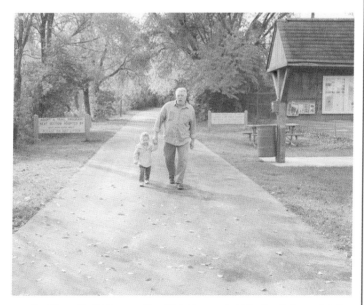

The Slippery Elm Trail is a smooth and fast ride or run for high-octane trail users, but also makes a cheerful place for a family stroll.

Location
Wood County

Endpoints
Bowling Green to
North Baltimore

Mileage
13

**Roughness
Index**
1

Surface
Asphalt

note of the unique terrain. As far as the eye can see the land here—as in much of northern Ohio—is as flat as a pancake, thanks to the glaciers that moved south through Ohio, leveling everything in their path. This area used to be the Great Black Swamp, but by the mid-1800s the swamp was drained, leaving the rich, fertile farmland that now yields corn, soybeans and livestock.

As you pass through the small village of Rudolph you encounter arguably one of the best signs you will ever see on a rail-trail: WELCOME TO RUDOLPH, THE DEEREST LITTLE VILLAGE IN WOOD COUNTY. There is a trailhead and restrooms in the village. After Rudolph you are about halfway along the trail. The southern half is extremely rural and quiet, with serene country vistas all the way to North Baltimore. At the endpoint there is a very nice playground and small park, a nice place for a picnic. Here, if you like, you can turn around and head back to Bowling Green.

If you do return to Bowling Green, be sure to take the time to explore this small college town. Bowling Green State University has more than 21,000 students and is among Ohio's top universities. Bowling Green itself is brimming with great little restaurants and cafes and the shops in town make for fun exploring.

DIRECTIONS

The Bowling Green trailhead is accessed by taking Interstate 75 to the Bowling Green Route 64/Wooster Street exit. Head west on Wooster for 1.75 miles and turn south on South Main Street. Continue on South Main for just over 0.75 mile to Sand Ridge Road and head west 0.5 mile. Trail access is from the Montessori school on the left.

To reach the southern trailhead in North Baltimore, take I-75 to the North Baltimore Street/State Route 18 exit west. Follow Route 18 just over 1 mile to South Main Street and turn north for 0.75 mile. Turn onto East Broadway Street and the parking lot will be on the left after 0.25 mile. This trailhead has parking and restroom facilities, as well as a playground.

Contact: Wood County Park District
18729 Mercer Road
Bowling Green, OH 43402
(419) 353-1897
www.woodcountyparkdistrict.org/SET_files/set.htm

Stavich Bicycle Trail

T he Stavich Bicycle Trail is not your ordinary bike ride. The 10-mile paved trail parallels a very active rail line; expect to see at least one train on your adventure. There is no fence separating the trail and rail line, but there is enough space to eliminate safety concerns.

The trail is built on an old trolley track. Trolleys tolerated steeper and more uneven slopes than traditional rail lines. What that means for you is a mostly level trail with several short steep hills. Just remember: What goes up must also come down.

The quiet, rolling trail starts on a nice downhill from the town of Struthers and runs through some small agricultural communities. At mile 1, you pass the local high school and stadium in the town of Lowellville, where a small stretch of the trail travels on a side street. This street is little used and offers access to a trailside restaurant.

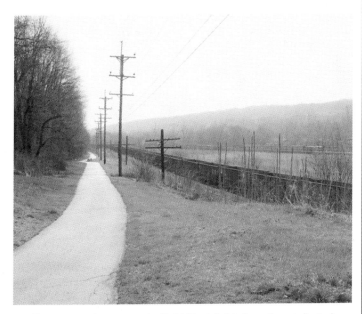

Train-spotting enthusiasts enjoy the Stavich Bicycle Trail, built on a former trolley track and parallel to an active rail line.

Location
Mahoning County

Endpoints
Struthers, OH, to New Castle, PA

Mileage
10

Roughness Index
2

Surface
Asphalt

261

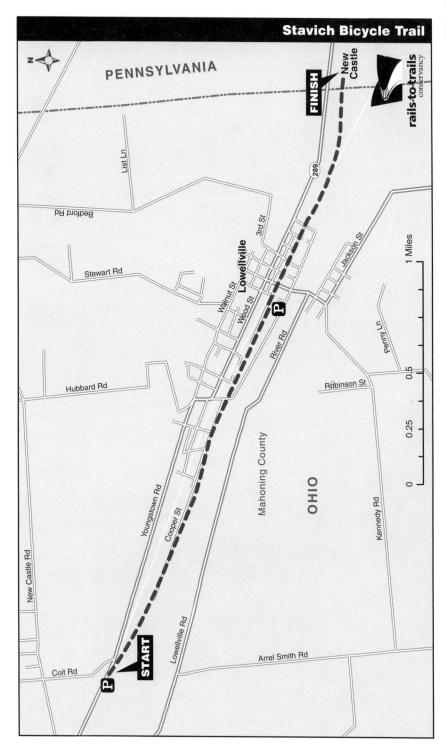

After Lowellville the trail starts to climb again. From the top of the hill you have beautiful unobstructed views of some of the best scenery in eastern Ohio and western Pennsylvania. You can catch your breath while taking in rolling hills, a lazy meandering river and an abundance of trees (fall colors can be spectacular). A nice downhill coast brings you near to the trail's end just south of New Castle. After one more slight uphill punctuated by a pleasant overlook with a picnic table and some benches, the trail comes to a close at the trailhead along Covert Road.

The trail in general could use some maintenance, as there are some bumpy portions and a few areas that take you close to the edge of steep drop-offs. But if you are up for a little adventure, or even just a leisurely bike ride or a bird-watching walk, the Stavich Bicycle Trail fits the bill.

DIRECTIONS

To reach the Struthers trailhead take State Route 224 to Poland, Ohio. Turn onto State Route 616 north and follow it across the Mahoning River. After just over 3 miles and immediately after the bridge, turn right onto Broad Street. A large sign marks the trailhead, which is on the right in about 1 mile.

To reach the trail outside of New Castle, take State Route 422 west to State Route 224 west. At 0.9 mile beyond the intersection of Routes 422 and 224, turn left onto Covert Road. Follow Covert Road south for 1.3 miles. The trailhead is along the road, on the right side.

Contact: Falcon Foundry
6th and Water Streets
P.O. Box 301
Lowellville, OH 44436
(216) 536-6221
www.theneonweb.com/trails/stavich.html

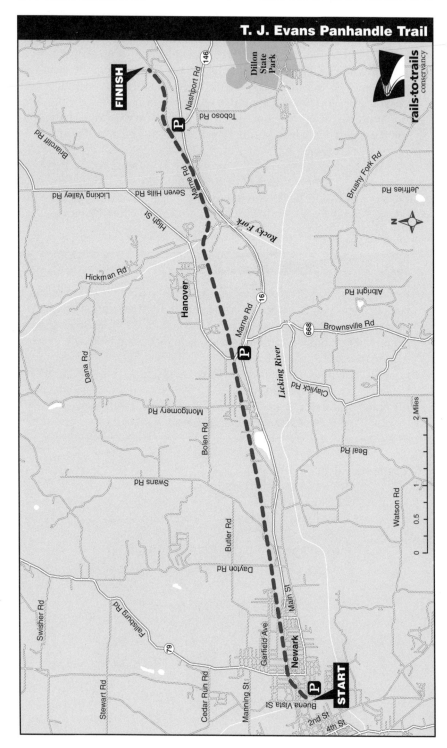

T. J. Evans Panhandle Trail

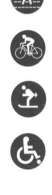

Beginning just east of downtown Newark, the T. J. Evans Panhandle Trail runs parallel to active tracks of the Ohio Central Railroad, making this trail a nice example of rail-with-trail. Built and funded by the Thomas J. Evans Foundation, the trail is primarily used as a recreational corridor by the families living along the trail. The first miles of this nearly 10-mile trail are tucked behind neighborhoods and businesses and run along State Route 16 and the rail line, illustrating how much urban activity and transportation can fit along a single corridor.

Looking south around mile 3.5, you can't miss the home office of The Longaberger Company, maker of handcrafted baskets. This seven-story office building is a replica of the company's Medium Market Basket. Longaberger employees designed the picnic-basket exterior and interior, managed the entire project and constructed

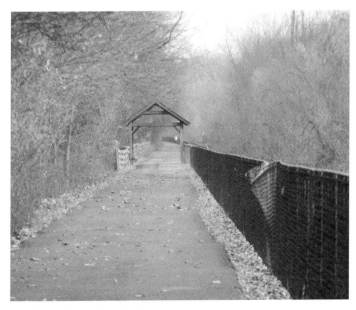

The T. J. Evans Panhandle Trail is a true backyard park, drawing many of its users from trailside residences.

Location
Licking County

Endpoints
East Newark to Licking/Muskingum County Line

Mileage
9.9

Roughness Index
1

Surface
Asphalt

more than 50 percent of the building. The interior has cherry woodwork harvested from Longaberger Golf Club property and milled, sawed and shaped by Longaberger employees.

For the next handful of miles the trail winds through the rural landscape of eastern Licking County. Here in Amish County, horse and buggy caution signs are as prevalent as cornfields. You sail past grazing cows and hear frogs croaking in marshy areas along the trail. Summer days find turtles sunning on logs and creek banks. American sycamores, slippery elms and bittersweet grow in the surrounding woods, and white-tailed deer visit isolated ponds along the route. The best time to visit this trail is early October, when the leaves are bright and the air is crisp.

The last 2 miles of the trail mark the southern border of the Longaberger Golf Club property. The course is one of most coveted in the state, with 12-month-long waiting lists.

DIRECTIONS

To reach the trail's west end in Newark, take State Route 16 east to the Buena Vista exit in downtown Newark and go south 500 feet. Turn left onto Main Street for 300 feet, then left onto North Morris Street. After crossing the railroad tracks veer right and turn left into the parking lot.

To reach the eastern endpoint in Hanover, take State Route 16 east to the Nashport Road/State Route 146 exit and go north. Turn right onto State Route 585/Marne Road NE. Take Marne about 1 mile to Felumlee Road and turn left. Go across the railroad tracks; the end of the trail will be on your left.

Contact: Licking Park District
4309 Lancaster Road, SE
P.O. Box 590
Granville, OH 43023
(740) 587-2535
www.lickingparkdistrict.com

T. J. Evans Trail

The T. J. Evans Trail is a very popular route, drawing locals and visitors, as well as through-travelers on the Ohio to Erie Trail that counts this rail-trail among its 200-plus miles from the Ohio River to Lake Erie.

The southern trailhead at Cherry Valley Road in Newark has a kiosk with a pay phone, drinking fountain and user guidelines. Just after you leave you pass a connecting trail to new ranch-style condominiums. This is the first of several residential developments that tie in to the trail. After passing a second parking lot, you come to a connecting trail going east. Although unsigned, it takes you a couple miles to the Ohio State University– Newark campus and to the Newark YMCA.

Rapids in Raccoon Creek keep the pace on the trail's east side as you trek through a beautiful shaded ravine area. A bridge across the creek has a marker discussing the trail's rail history. After passing under State Route 16 cow-filled fields extend from both sides of the trail.

Location
Licking County

Endpoints
West Newark to Johnstown

Mileage
14.2

Roughness Index
1

Surface
Asphalt

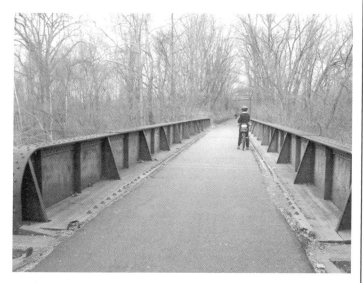

A popular rail-trail with locals and visitors alike, the T. J. Evans Trail connects rural scenery with local colleges and charming towns.

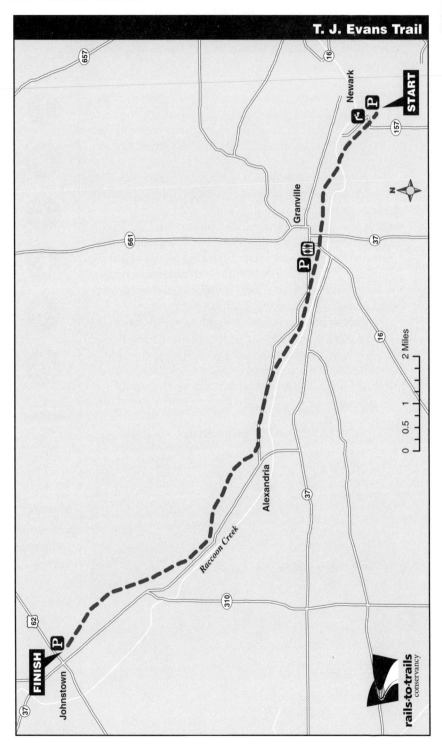

T. J. Evans Trail

At about 4 miles you come to Granville. There is a sign directing you off the trail to downtown Granville for shops, dining and overnight options. A short climb brings you to the quaint and amazingly beautiful downtown, where you can find many restaurants, as well as Denison University (a noted liberal arts school that counts Hollywood's Jennifer Garner as a graduate).

Continuing along the trail, a pedestrian crossing guides you over State Route 37 at the former Granville Railroad Station, which now houses a realtor's office. If you're looking for a break, stop at Wildwood Park near mile 3.5, with open fields and an incredible, wooden castle-shaped play area. Continuing north, you shortly arrive at the ruins of Clemons Railroad Station. There are several bridges spanning small creeks between here and Alexandria, about 2 miles northwest.

When you cross Raccoon Valley Road you are in the village of Alexandria. A marker at the trailhead describes the founding of Alexandria. The remaining 6.3 miles of trail to Johnstown pass alternately though woods, ravines and farm fields. The setting is remote and relaxing, but many rural road crossings require caution.

Just before Johnstown you pass another housing subdivision with connectors to the trail and a new subdivision being built on the other side of the trail. Then the Jersey Street trailhead signals the trail's end. The beautiful T. J. Evans rail-trail only gets better on the return trip, as a slight grade gives you a downhill advantage.

DIRECTIONS

To start the trail in Newark, take Interstate 70 to State Route 79 and travel north for 6 miles. Turn left onto Irving Wick Drive, go west for 2 miles, then turn right onto Thornwood Drive southeast. Thornwood becomes Reddington Road after about 1.4 miles. Turn right onto Cherry Valley Road and look for the trailhead on the right.

To reach the Jersey Street trailhead in Johnstown from I-270 on the northeast side of Columbus, take State Route 161 east for 6 miles to US Route 62 (Johnstown-Utica Road) then turn left and head north for almost 8 miles. Turn right onto State Route 37 for 0.3 mile and take a left onto Jersey Street. Jersey Street dead-ends in the trailhead parking lot after 0.25 mile.

Contact: Licking Park District
4309 Lancaster Road, SE
P.O. Box 590
Granville, OH 43023
(740) 587-2535
www.lickingparkdistrict.com

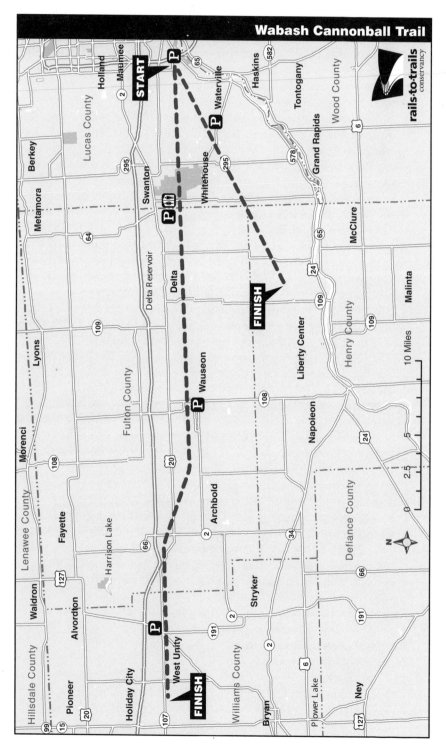

Wabash Cannonball Trail

Wabash Cannonball Trail

The Wabash Cannonball Trail in northwest Ohio is actually two trails in one: The North Fork runs east-west for 46 miles and the South Fork makes up the balance of this 63-mile trail. The trails converge in the eastern city of Maumee, then jackknife away on their separate routes.

Both trails begin at Jerome Road within sight of Fallen Timbers Shopping Center. Don't be confused by the sign labeled WABASH CANNONBALL TRAIL NORTH FORK; just a quarter mile west the South Fork breaks off to the left while the North Fork continues straight. By following the bicycle and pedestrian bridge over State Route 24, you can visit the Fallen Timbers State Memorial (recognizing the 1794 battle that helped open the Northwest Territory) and Side Cut Metropark, an offshoot of the Miami and Erie Canal.

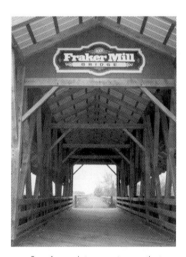

One of several river crossings on the two-trails-in-one Wabash Cannonball Trail.

The first 9.5 miles of the North Fork are nicely paved. This section travels through Oak Openings Metropark. Several bridges cross small creeks, marshy wetlands and deeper ravines before the pavement ends and the smooth paved trail gives way to crushed stone, grass and dirt for the remainder of its length, with the exception of 2 paved miles in the town of Wauseon. Before you reach Wauseon, though, the trail is closed at County Road 11. For most users this is the unofficial end of the trail. To navigate around this closure, turn north on County Road 11 for 0.2 mile and west on County Road F for 2 miles before turning south on County Road 13 for another 0.2 mile. The trail appears again on the

Location
Fulton, Henry, Lucas and Williams counties

Endpoints
Maumee to Montpelier (North Fork) and Liberty Center (South Fork)

Mileage
63

Roughness Index
2

Surface
Asphalt, crushed stone and cinder

271

right. Back on the trail you come to the town of Wauseon. Rotary Park on the right-hand side of the trail offers parking, restrooms and plenty of shade. West from here, some sections of the trail are open and many are closed. The trail group opens more miles each year, so check back often.

The South Fork is a beautiful trail about 17.5 miles long through western Lucas County. The first 10.5 miles are paved and a fun, flat and fast ride. The final 7 miles are similar to the unpaved section on the north fork. The crushed-stone section is best suited to walkers, equestrians, hybrid and fat-tired bikers. In the village of Whitehouse a park on the left of the trail has a large playground and baseball diamonds. This park is only 6 miles from the start of the trail and makes a perfect turnaround.

DIRECTIONS

The main trailhead is at Jerome Road in Maumee. From Interstate 475 on Toledo's west side, take the Route 24 exit and head east 0.75 mile to Monclova Road. Turn left on Monclova for 1.3 miles, then turn left on Jerome Road. The trailhead and parking are on the right.

To reach the North Fork's Wauseon Trailhead, take US Route 20A toward Wauseon to Route 108/West Linfoot Street south for 1 mile. Turn right and head west on County Highway F and then turn left to go south on Krieger Street. Rotary Park and the trailhead are on the left.

The North Fork's West Unity Trailhead is accessible by taking Route 20A to West Unity and turning left to go south on Main Street. The trailhead is in the park on the left.

The best trailhead for the South Fork is in Whitehouse. Take State Route 64 into the town of Whitehouse, to the park adjacent to the trail on Saint Louis Avenue where there is a parking lot.

Contact: Northwestern Ohio Rails-to-Trails Association, Inc.
P.O. Box 234
Delta, OH 43515
(800) 951-4788
http://home.tbbs.net/~norta/index.htm

Western Reserve Greenway

The Western Reserve Greenway is a 43-mile, mostly rural rail-trail that cuts a north-south course from Ashtabula to Warren, Ohio. The greenway's start is only a few miles from Lake Erie, and a planned extension will bring it right to the shoreline. For now you can start at Herzog Rotary Park, where signs detail the importance of northeast Ohio in the Underground Railroad.

Heading south, you cross the historic King Bridge, a steel railroad trestle built in 1897 that now spans Clay Street. Ahead is Austinburg, with a trailhead and plenty of options for refreshments and nourishment. South of town you reenter the trail's rural surroundings and

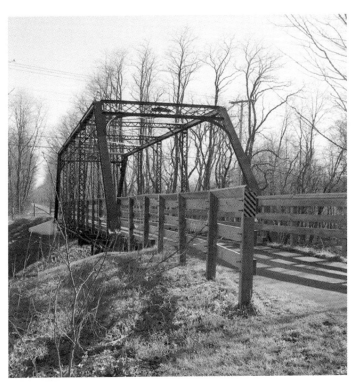

Get your fill of restored railroad bridges on the Western Reserve Greenway.

Location
Ashtabula and Trumbull counties

Endpoints
Ashtabula to Warren

Mileage
43

Roughness Index
3

Surface
Asphalt and ballast

273

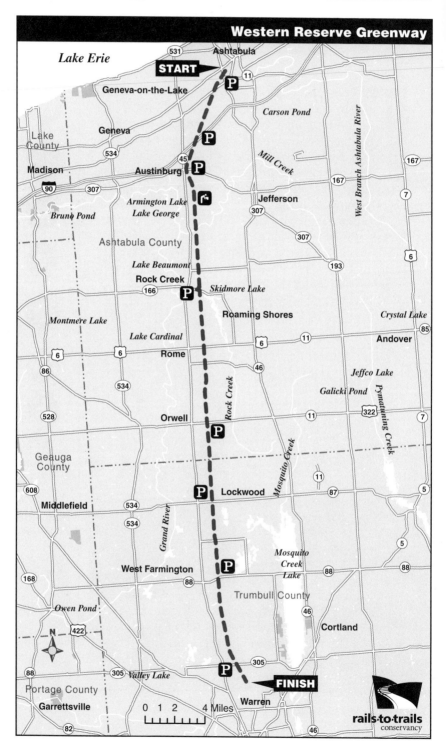

Western Reserve Greenway

Lake Erie

531 Ashtabula

START

P 11

Geneva-on-the-Lake

Carson Pond

Geneva

Lake County

534

P

Madison

90 307

Austinburg 45

P

Armington Lake
Lake George

Bruno Pond

Jefferson

307

Mill Creek

167

167

7

West Branch Ashtabula River

Ashtabula County

307

307

6

193

Lake Beaumont

Rock Creek

166

P *Skidmore Lake*

Roaming Shores

Crystal Lake

Montmere Lake

Lake Cardinal

6

11

Andover

85

6

6

Rome

46

Jeffco Lake

86

534

Galicki Pond

Pymatuning Creek

528

Orwell

P

11

322

7

Rock Creek

Geauga County

Mosquito Creek

11

608

P **Lockwood**

87

5

Middlefield

534

534

Grand River

Mosquito Creek Lake

168

West Farmington

88

P

88

88

Owen Pond

422

Mosquito Creek

46

Cortland

88

305 *Valley Lake*

P

305

FINISH

Portage County

Garrettsville

0 1 2 4 Miles

Warren

82

46

rails·to·trails
conservancy

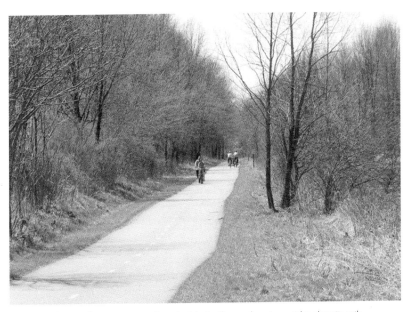

The Western Reserve Greenway is a mostly rural rail-trail with several must-see sights along its path.

enjoy the company of deer, beavers and a multitude of birds, including wild turkeys and waterfowl.

In the small town of Rock Creek you are directed off the trail for approximately 1 mile of road riding. Back on the greenway's rail corridor, the Rock Creek Trestle spans the river. The bridge features bump-outs that give a bird's-eye view of the river and scenery below. In about 1 mile you leave the smooth asphalt behind and spend the next 6 miles bouncing over an as-yet unpaved section. This is great mountain biking territory, but not suitable for road bikes.

When the pavement picks up again, you sail beneath sheltering trees and past the tiny village of Orwell, with a trailhead located below a water tower. In North Bloomfield at about mile 30, the Mosquito Lake wetlands area has a must-see observation deck. Take a break and marvel at the breadth of wildlife, particularly birdlife, found here. Red-tailed hawks, marsh and sparrow hawks and bald eagles have been spotted here. The Stone Arch Bridge in Trumbull County is a true highlight of the Western Reserve Trail. To further explore this superb tribute to time and engineering, hit the road on the north side of the bridge for 0.25 mile and take in the magnificent side view of the bridge. Back on the trail you will come to the Sunside Trailhead at State Route 305. The rail-trail continues a short distance beyond here to Champion Street in Warren, but the best access is from this trailhead.

DIRECTIONS

To start at Herzog Rotary Park trailhead, located on the west side of Woodman Avenue in Ashtabula Township, take State Route 20 to Woodman Avenue and turn south for 0.75 mile. The trailhead will be on the right-hand side.

The trailhead in Austinburg can be reached from Interstate 90 by taking Exit 223 for State Route 45 south. In approximately 1 mile, turn left and head east on State Route 307 for about 1,000 feet. The trailhead is on the left at the edge of town.

To reach the Sunside Trailhead in Warren from State Route 45 in Warren, travel north to State Route 305. Turn right and head east on 305, then look for the trailhead on your left.

Contact: Ashtabula County MetroParks
25 West Jefferson Street
Jefferson, OH 44047
(440) 576-0717
www.ashtabulacountymetroparks.org/trail.htm

Wolf Creek Recreation Trail

The Wolf Creek Recreation Trail in suburban Dayton is a well-maintained asphalt trail stretching 13 miles from Trotwood in Montgomery County to Verona in Preble County. Reflecting the nature of the densely settled areas, there are many street crossings. However, the trail redeems itself, passing through spacious expanses of cornfields and pasture.

The Trotwood Depot, with historical exhibits, an information kiosk and restored railroad cabooses, is a good place to kick off your adventure. There is a bus stop in front of this old railroad station, a convenience for bike and bus commuters. Traveling northwest from the depot you cross Broadway, then Main Street, reaching the trail—and several more road crossings—after a short stretch of sidewalk. Houses and apartments backing up to the trail soon give way to cornfields. At Snyder Road you will see an entrance to Sycamore State Park.

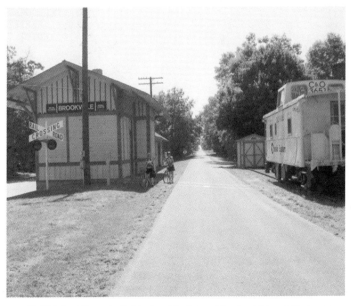

The Wolf Creek Recreation Trail begins at the Trotwood Depot and links neighborhoods to expanses of pastures and farmland.

Location
Montgomery and Preble counties

Endpoints
Trotwood to Verona

Mileage
13

Roughness Index
1

Surface
Asphalt

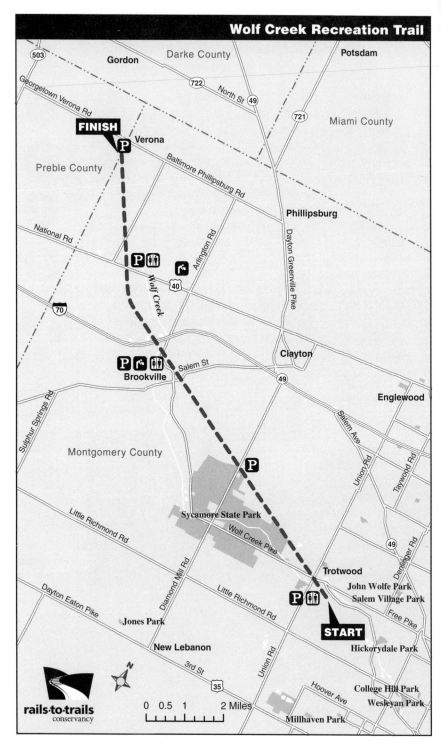

Wolf Creek Recreation Trail

The park has miles of hiking and bridle trails under canopies of giant sycamore trees.

A strip of wildflowers decorates the trail just before the Air Hill Rest Area. You can nestle your bike into the racks here and settle yourself into a bench to rest up for two tricky road crossings ahead. At Shiloh Springs Road and Diamond Mills Road, sight lines are tight and there are no crosswalks. Traffic is minimal here, but be cautious nonetheless.

Busy Westbrook Road signals your arrival in Brookville, a sleepy town of 5200. You pass a skateboard park and Brookville Station. A real gem in Brookville is Golden Gate Park, with picnic shelters and a kids park that resembles a scaled-down castle and even hosts the local theatre productions.

An underpass at Interstate 70 returns you to farmland for the trail's remaining 5 miles. Shortly after Dull Woods you reach a trailhead at US Route 40. The busy crossing is unmarked for motorists so take care.

Wengerlawn Rest Area is also known as "Pete's Station," in honor of trail builder Peter Smith. The trail comes to an end after Sweet Potato Ridge Road and the Preble County line in Verona. Aside from parking, there are no facilities, but you can imagine someday continuing the final 20 miles west to Indiana along the same old railroad corridor that serves up the Wolf Creek Recreation Trail.

DIRECTIONS

The Trotwood Depot Trailhead is located at the intersection of Wolf Creek Pike (Main Street) and Broadway. From Interstate 70 take State Route 49 south for 5.3 miles. Turn right onto East Main Street toward Trotwood and look for the depot after 1.75 miles.

To reach the Verona Trailhead from I-70, follow Route 49 north for 1.8 miles to Wengerlawn Road. Turn left onto Wengerlawn and look for the trailhead just past Number 9 Road after 4.5 miles.

Contact: Five Rivers MetroParks Administrative Offices
1375 East Siebenthaler Avenue
Dayton, OH 45414
(937) 275-7275
www.metroparks.org

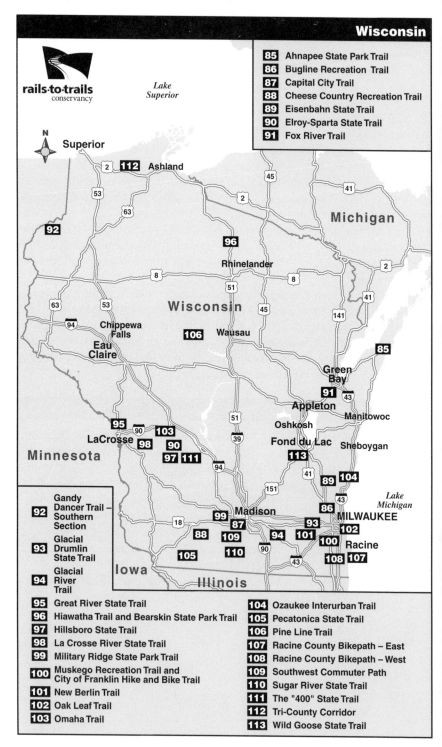

Wisconsin

85	Ahnapee State Park Trail
86	Bugline Recreation Trail
87	Capital City Trail
88	Cheese Country Recreation Trail
89	Eisenbahn State Trail
90	Elroy-Sparta State Trail
91	Fox River Trail

Lake
Superior

N

Superior

112 Ashland

Michigan

Rhinelander

Wisconsin

Wausau

106

Chippewa
Falls

Eau
Claire

Green
Bay

91

Appleton

Manitowoc

Oshkosh

95

LaCrosse

103

98

90

97 **111**

Fond du Lac

Sheboygan

113

Minnesota

89 **104**

Lake
Michigan

92	Gandy Dancer Trail – Southern Section
93	Glacial Drumlin State Trail
94	Glacial River Trail

Madison

99

87

86

MILWAUKEE

93

102

88

109

94

101

100

Racine

105

110

108 **107**

Iowa

Illinois

95	Great River State Trail
96	Hiawatha Trail and Bearskin State Park Trail
97	Hillsboro State Trail
98	La Crosse River State Trail
99	Military Ridge State Park Trail
100	Muskego Recreation Trail and City of Franklin Hike and Bike Trail
101	New Berlin Trail
102	Oak Leaf Trail
103	Omaha Trail

104	Ozaukee Interurban Trail
105	Pecatonica State Trail
106	Pine Line Trail
107	Racine County Bikepath – East
108	Racine County Bikepath – West
109	Southwest Commuter Path
110	Sugar River State Trail
111	The "400" State Trail
112	Tri-County Corridor
113	Wild Goose State Trail

rails·to·trails
conservancy

Wisconsin

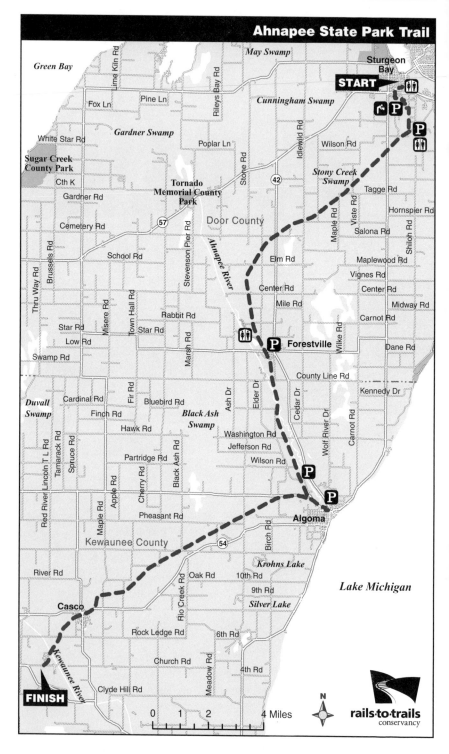

Ahnapee State Park Trail

Ahnapee State Park Trail

Take a trip on the Ahnapee State Trail for an excursion through farmland, forest and, for about 5 miles, along the Ahnapee River as it flows to Lake Michigan. The 27.7-mile trail runs from Sturgeon Bay in the north to 2 miles beyond Casco Junction in the south, with a short, 0.75-mile spur at mile 16 that heads east to Algoma. Summer months see hikers, bikers, horseback riders and horse-drawn carts and wagons, so expect a crowded ride in parts. When the snow flies cross-country skiers and snowmobilers zip along the line.

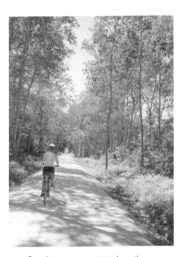

Bicyclists can expect to share the Ahnapee State Park Trail with a variety of users, including those in horse-drawn carriages.

The Ahnapee State Trail follows the corridor of the Ahnapee and Western Railroad, which served as an industrial link between Door, Brown and Kewaunee counties. The steam- and diesel-powered locomotives hauled dairy goods, cherry crops and lumber until the early 1970s.

Begin the Ahnapee State Trail just south of Sturgeon Bay where white-barked birch trees, colorful lilies and daisies line your way to the small community of Forestville. At mile 10, a pleasant lake formed by the Forestville Dam gleams in the sunlight, surrounded by cattails, phlox and high grasses. The trail runs through Forestville Dam Park, which offers restrooms, picnic tables and an opportunity to watch kayakers and fishermen enjoy the lake. The section of trail in Forestville is steeped in history. Here, in 1871, the Great Peshtigo Fire ravaged the area. Though overshadowed by the Great Chicago Fire, which occurred at the same time, historians cite the Great Peshtigo blaze as the largest and most

Location
Door and Kewaunee counties

Endpoints
Casco Junction to Sturgeon Bay

Mileage
27.7

Roughness Index
2

Surface
Asphalt and crushed stone

devastating in American history. More than 1000 people perished and 1.25 million acres were destroyed.

The Ahnapee River, teeming with perch and bass, is your companion for the next 5 miles. A bridge at mile 12.5 affords a wonderful view of the river's twisting course toward Lake Michigan.

Soon after the river the trail meets a crossroads. Turn east and in less than a mile you arrive in the picturesque lakeshore community of Algoma (an Indian name meaning "park of the flowers"). Historic warehouses along the trail mark this quaint town's woodworking past. The Ahnapee State Trail is not clearly defined here, but you can follow it by looking for trail-sized stop signs and telltale railroad tracks still embedded in intersecting streets.

Heading west at the crossroads will take you to Casco Junction through a landscape dominated by red board-and-batten barns, dairy farms and wheat fields. Reaching the very small town of Casco Junction, the trail parallels old manufacturing buildings. The trail ends at County Road A.

DIRECTIONS

To reach the Sturgeon Bay endpoint from Green Bay, take Hwy. 42/57 north to Sturgeon Bay. Shortly before entering the city limits take a right on South Neenah Avenue. Follow this road for less than a mile and make a left at the sign for the Ahnapee State Trail to the parking lot and restroom.

If you choose to start at the midpoint in Algoma, from Green Bay take State Route 54/57 North. After approximately 7 miles, follow State Route 54 east (right exit) where it breaks from State Route 57. Upon reaching Algoma (about 23.5 miles) merge left onto Lake Street and staying right go six blocks to Navarino Street and turn left. Go three blocks to reach the trailhead and parking on the right (between 4th and 5th streets). There is a short on-road route to reach the trail, which is shown on a big map in the parking lot.

There is no parking at the Casco Junction endpoint. To reach it from Casco, take State Route 54 west. Turn left on Hawthorne Road. Turn left onto County Road A. The trailhead is on the left, denoted by a sign.

Contact: Friends of the Ahnapee
E4280 County Road F
Kewaunee, WI 54216
(920) 487-3822
www.ahnapeetrail.org

Bugline Recreation Trail

Broad blue skies strung with white cloud wisps; gem-green fields harboring cattails and butterflies; canopied glens giving way to cavernous quarries. It's all part of the ride on the 12-mile Bugline Recreation Trail in and around Menomonee Falls, Wisconsin, just 20 miles northwest of Milwaukee.

Begin at the Menomonee Falls Post Office adjacent to the trailhead, where you will find an 8-foot-wide surface of compacted crushed Lannon stone—a limestone mined from nearby quarries.

Tall trees envelop the first mile of the trail before it enters a tranquil residential area. Residents in one-story ramblers have fashioned makeshift trail-access points all along the Bugline, and you'll be sharing the trail with local walkers, hikers, bikers and runners who flock to this recreation corridor.

Out of the neighborhood after mile 2, the trail dips back into a forest of forked barr oak and linden trees. Dappled light laces the mostly straight, white path until a clearing opens up to an active limestone quarry. The sheer, white sides of the excavation site dwarf enormous

Location
Waukesha County

Endpoints
Menomonee Falls
to Merton

Mileage
12

Roughness Index
1

Surface
Crushed stone
and dirt

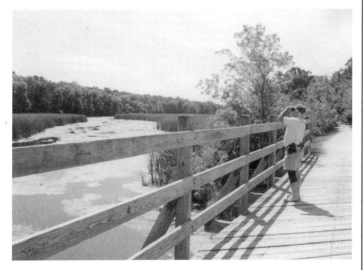

Birding is a popular activity on the Bugline Recreation Trail, particularly near Mill Pond.

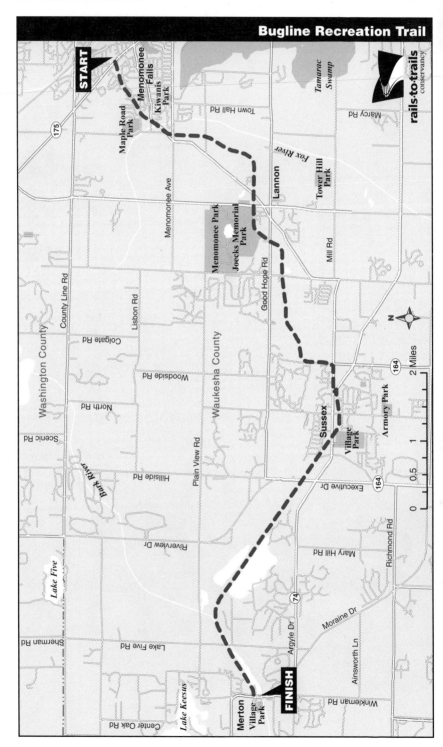

Bugline Recreation Trail

construction vehicles. About 1.5 miles past the quarry is a short rail-trail spur leading to Menomonee Park, site of the stone quarrying that was this area's significant industry from 1880 to 1900. Today, remnants from that time remain in Menomonee Park, including an old stone crusher and a public swimming beach at the now-flooded quarry.

Signs and crosswalks mark the several points where the trail crosses moderately busy roads, though it pays to be alert as some of the crossings are at odd angles to the road. In suburban Sussex, at the trail's halfway point, the Bugline makes a short jaunt south along Route 164. Follow Silver Spring Drive west toward Sussex Village Park, a green swath of sports fields and resting places.

Near mile 8, the vista widens into peaceful farmland and small prairies of Joe-Pye weed, sunflowers and swamp thistle. Red barns and silver silos dot the landscape. When a light breeze gathers over the fields, it carries the quintessential country scents of wildflowers and farm animals.

An industrial rail line, still in use, runs adjacent to the trail through several miles of prairie and farmland. Keep a lookout for gopher holes at the edge of the trail—they can make for a suddenly bumpy ride. At mile 11, prairie gives way to wetlands. The trail skirts the edge of Mill Pond and rounds out its route on Main Street in Merton. In addition to Lannon stone architecture, Merton offers up another Wisconsin specialty—frozen custard. Grab a creamy cone before turning back on the Bugline to enjoy the slightly downhill return journey.

DIRECTIONS

The trail begins at Appleton Avenue in Menomonee Falls and ends at Main Street in the village of Merton. Access Appleton Avenue from State Road 74 and park at Menomonee Falls Post Office.

Access the Merton trailhead from State Road 74, to West Highway VV, which turns into Main Street in Merton. You'll find the trailhead on your right off of Main Street.

Contact: Waukesha County Department of Parks and Land Use
Park System Division
1320 Pewaukee Road, Room 230
Waukesha, WI 53188
(262) 548-7801
www.waukeshacounty.gov/page.aspx?
SetupMetaId=10888&id=10924

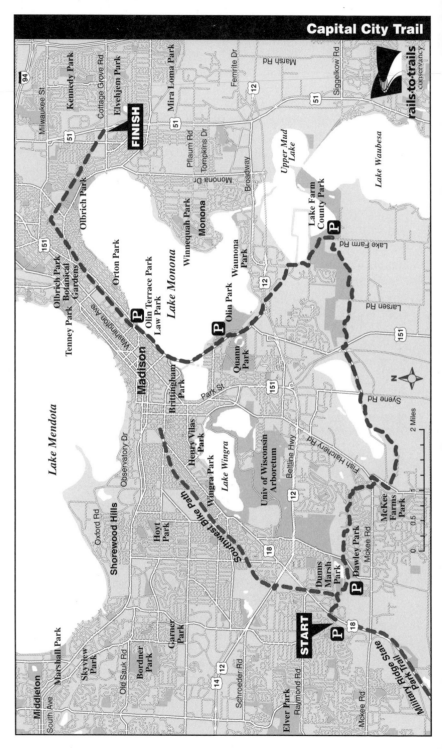

Capital City Trail

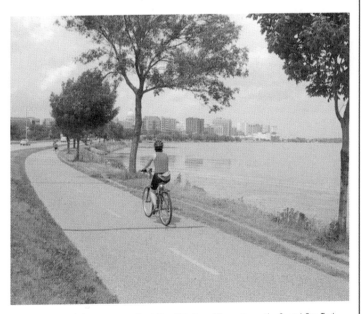

I f you want to get to know Madison, Wisconsin, ride this trail! The trail-progressive metropolis recently renamed the Nine Springs E-Way, the John Noland, Isthmus and the East Side bike paths the "Capital City Trail." The newly anointed, 17-mile trail meanders around and through the heart of Madison, giving you a keen understanding of the natural and urban beauty of this city.

Beginning from the southwest, the first 5 miles are lush with a heavy tree canopy lined with raspberry bushes. This opens up into marshland filled with echinacea flowers and the bright flashes of red-winged blackbirds. At Fish Hatcher Road, the trail disappears for 0.2 mile. (To find it again, turn left at Fish Hatcher Road, right on Glacial Valley and veer to the right.) At 8.5 miles the trail passes through the Capital Springs Centennial State Recreation Area, with the Monona Conservancy Wetlands, a fish hatchery and a wildlife observation area.

Enjoy a crash-free course on the sights of Madison, Wisconsin, on the Capital City Trail.

Location
Dane County

Endpoints
Madison to
Fitchburg

Mileage
17

**Roughness
Index**
1

Surface
Asphalt

The terrain is rolling golden hills dotted with trees and picnic benches with scenic valley views.

After 12 miles of pastoral views you reach Olin Park, with breathtaking views of downtown Madison. Here you have a choice: Follow the signs for Wingra Creek Trail to the arboretum, Henry Vilas Zoo and beaches at Vilas Park, or continue north on the Capital City Trail and veer into the heart of Madison over a bridge affording exceptional views of the capitol and along Lake Monona. Turning off the trail away from the lake onto city streets takes you into the historic center of Madison. Along the lake you pass Monona Terrace, the Frank Lloyd Wright-designed convention center, which is open for tours and noted for its exceptional lake views.

Continuing on the trail you skip back and forth over a street traveling through historical Madison neighborhoods including Schenk-Atwood at mile 16, where the trail is flanked by community garden plots, bungalow-style homes and shops where you can pick up a bite to eat or a cup of joe. The northern mile of the trail takes you along Olbrich Botanical Gardens, with 16 acres of plants and paths, a tropical paradise in the conservatory and a Thai pavilion that is easily recognizable from the trail.

The trail ends at mile 17, but you can keep on exploring. At the southwest end you can connect via a short on-road segment with the 40-mile Military Ridge State Trail (page 327). Eventually the northeast end of the Capital City Trail will link with the 52-mile Glacial Drumlin State Trail (page 307).

The Wisconsin Department of Natural Resources requires a trail pass for this trail (visit the WDNR website for information) but Dane County provides free passes for frequent commuters.

DIRECTIONS

To reach the Capital Springs Centennial State Recreation Area trailhead from Interstate 90, take the West Beltline (US Highway 12/18) to the South Towne Drive Exit (Exit 264) and go south. Continue for almost 1 mile and then turn left on Moorland Road, which turns into Lake Farm Road. Look for trailhead parking on your right. The trail is generally accessible from downtown Madison.

Contact: Madison Area Transportation Planning Board
121 South Pinckney Street, Suite 400
Madison, WI 53703
(608) 266-4336
www.madisonareampo.org

Cheese Country Recreation Trail

If you're looking for an invigorating motorized trail experience, the Cheese Country Trail (a.k.a. the Tri-County Trail) will not disappoint. The 47-mile trail meanders through the heart of southwest Wisconsin's Driftless Area, a massive tract of land noted for the rolling hills and rocky outcroppings left untouched by glaciers. The Cheese Country Trail traverses Iowa, Green and Lafayette counties, intersects with the Pecatonica State Trail (page 347) near Calamine and crosses a total of 57 small bridges and overpasses, including the 440-foot bridge at Brownstown as it winds from Monroe to Mineral Point.

This is primarily used as an ATV and snowmobile trail, though bicyclists, horseback riders and cross-country skiers share the corridor. The surface in many areas is quite rough; if you plan to bike, opt for the sturdy tires of your mountain bike. You should also be prepared to share the trail with loud and heavy ATV traffic.

Monroe, the Cheese Country Trail's southern end is—quite fittingly—known as the "Swiss Cheese

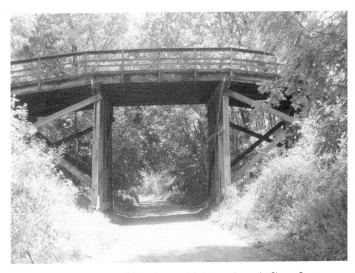

Year-round motorized use (ATVs and snowmobiles) is popular on the Cheese County Recreation Trail, so fatter tires are recommended for bicyclists.

Location
Green, Iowa and Lafayette counties

Endpoints
Monroe to Mineral Point

Mileage
47

Roughness Index
3

Surface
Crushed stone

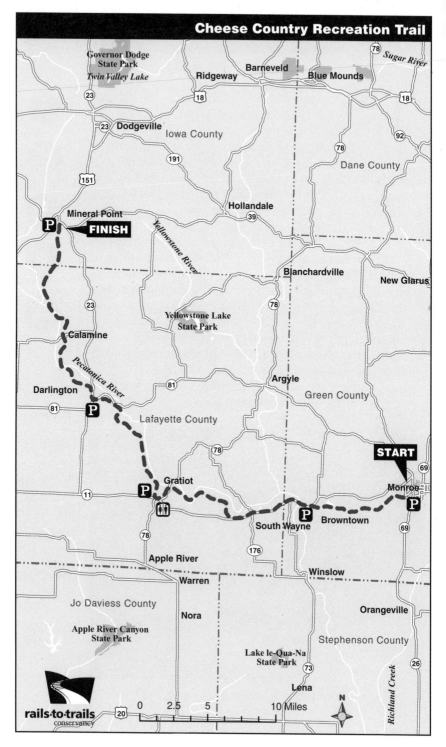

Cheese Country Recreation Trail

Governor Dodge State Park
Twin Valley Lake
Ridgeway
Barneveld
Blue Mounds
78 Sugar River
23
18
18
Dodgeville
23
Iowa County
92
191
78
Dane County
151
Hollandale
Mineral Point
P
FINISH
39
Yellowstone River
Blanchardville
New Glarus
23
Yellowstone Lake State Park
78
Calamine
Pecatonica River
Darlington
81
Argyle
Green County
P
Lafayette County
81
78
START
69
Monroe
11
Gratiot
P
P
South Wayne
Browntown
P
69
78
176
Apple River
Winslow
Warren
Jo Daviess County
Nora
Orangeville
Apple River Canyon State Park
Stephenson County
26
Lake Ie-Qua-Na State Park
73
Richland Creek
rails·to·trails
conservancy
0   2.5   5   10 Miles
20
Lena
N

Capital" of the United States. The trailhead, with parking, is just 6 miles from the Illinois border. Heading northwest from Monroe, you follow Highway 11 through Brownstown and South Wayne. After passing through Brownstown, the trail crosses a 440-foot bridge spanning the Pecatonica River. Here the trail runs through wooded areas and marshes, all the while hugging the scenic farmland of the local dairy farms. If you want to take a break, Gratiot, at mile 20, is a good bet. Restaurants and shops are found here, as well as ATV rentals in case you want to start your motorized adventure.

From Gratiot the trail continues northwest along stretches of farmland and wooded ridges for about 11 miles to Darlington, right off Highway 81. Refreshments, supplies and ATV rentals are plentiful in this community.

Another 5 miles on the trail brings you to Calamine. As you approach Calamine you run into the Pecatonica rail-trail, which runs west for 10 miles to Belmont. Finally, from Calamine the Cheese Country Trail heads north for an additional 10 miles until it ends in the lovely town of Mineral Point at the old Railroad Depot Museum. Mineral Point is among Wisconsin's oldest communities and this historic mining village is today rich with artists' studios and galleries. Many of the old homes in Mineral Point have been restored and some of them have been made into restaurants and bed-and-breakfast inns that will allow you to stay awhile.

A state trail pass is required for bicyclists, horseback riders and cross-country skiers 16 years and older and registration is necessary for ATVs. Visit the Wisconsin Department of Natural Resources website for more information.

DIRECTIONS

The Monroe endpoint is accessible from Highway 11/81 by taking Hwy. 69 south. Turn right at the third stop on 21st Street. It's about a half mile to the parking lot on 4th Avenue west.

To reach the Mineral Point endpoint from Highway 151, take Exit 40, then turn left on Commerce Street. Turn left again on Old Darlington Road to the parking spaces available 200 feet at the bottom of the hill and to the left of the Mineral Point Railroad Depot Museum.

Contact: Tri County ATV Club
201 South Chestnut
Mineral Point, WI 53565
(608) 574-2911
www.tricountytrails.com

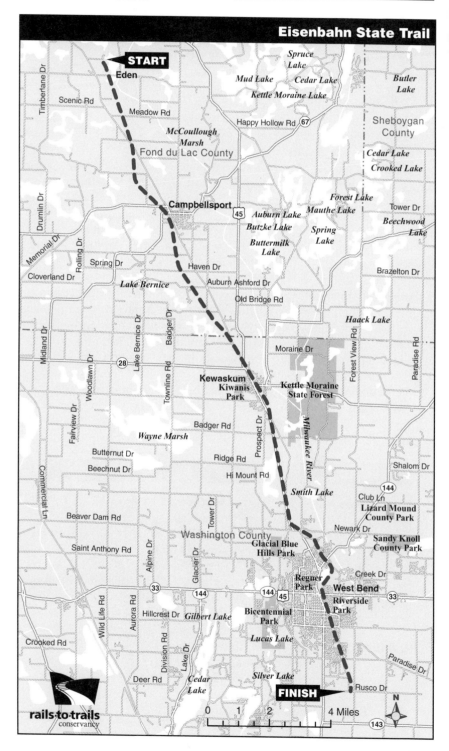

Eisenbahn State Trail

START
Eden

Spruce Lake
Mud Lake
Cedar Lake
Kettle Moraine Lake
Butler Lake

Timberlane Dr
Scenic Rd
Meadow Rd

Happy Hollow Rd 67

Sheboygan County

McCoullough Marsh
Fond du Lac County

Cedar Lake
Crooked Lake

Campbellsport 45

Auburn Lake
Butzke Lake
Buttermilk Lake

Forest Lake
Mauthe Lake
Spring Lake

Tower Dr
Beechwood Lake

Drumlin Dr
Rolling Dr
Memorial Dr
Spring Dr
Cloverland Dr
Lake Bernice

Haven Dr
Auburn Ashford Dr
Old Bridge Rd

Brazelton Dr

Haack Lake

Midland Dr
Woodlawn Dr
Lake Bernice Dr
Badger Dr
Townline Rd

28

Moraine Dr

Forest View Rd
Paradise Rd

Kewaskum
Kiwanis Park

Kettle Moraine State Forest

Fairview Dr

Badger Rd
Wayne Marsh

Prospect Dr
Milwaukee River

Butternut Dr
Beechnut Dr

Ridge Rd
Hi Mount Rd

Shalom Dr

Commercial Ln

Smith Lake

Club Ln
144

Beaver Dam Rd
Tower Dr

Lizard Mound County Park
Newark Dr

Washington County

Saint Anthony Rd
Alpine Dr
Glacier Dr

Glacial Blue Hills Park

Sandy Knoll County Park

Creek Dr

33
144
144
45

Regner Park

West Bend
Riverside Park

33

Wild Life Rd
Aurora Rd
Hillcrest Dr
Gilbert Lake
Lake Dr
Division Rd

Bicentennial Park

Lucas Lake

Crooked Rd

Deer Rd
Cedar Lake

Silver Lake

FINISH

Rusco Dr

Paradise Dr

rails·to·trails
conservancy

0   1   2   4 Miles

N

143

Eisenbahn State Trail

The Eisenbahn State Trail (a.k.a. the Eden to West Bend Trail) occupies a former Chicago and North Western Railroad corridor that was originally called the "Air Line" because of its direct-route passenger service between Chicago and Green Bay. The trail name pays tribute to this region's heritage: *Eisenbahn* is German for "iron road."

The northern section of the trail was recently opened. It starts just south of Eden in Fond du Lac County and runs for 10 miles to the Washington County line, passing through the community of Campbellsport. This section of the trail is remote and surrounded by beautiful farmland. It is a peaceful, flat ride and the corridor is slightly elevated from the surrounding landscape for nice views. There are plans to extend this section 1.5 miles north to Eden, which would dramatically improve the accessibility of this trail.

The southern section in Washington County begins at the county line and runs 12.4 miles to Rusco Drive in West Bend. This section is considerably less rustic,

Location
Fond du Lac and Washington counties

Endpoints
West Bend to Eden

Mileage
22.5

Roughness Index
1

Surface
Crushed stone

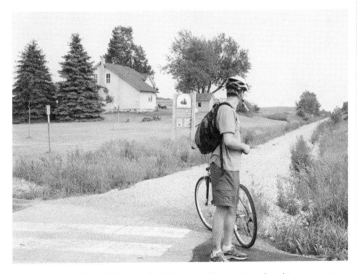

The Eisenbahn State Trail is one of multiple personalities: rustic and rural in some spots, suburban and industrial in others, and enjoyed by all types of trail users.

passing through the village of Kewaskum and then running right along US Route 45 for 4.5 miles.

Approaching the city of West Bend, the trail veers southwest through some green countryside before passing a short stretch of industrial and residential development. The first major intersection is at Barton Avenue, marking the entry to downtown. In the city, the trail intersects with several major roads and all crossings are well marked. At the 7.5-mile point of this southern section, you'll enjoy some nice views as the trail runs along the Milwaukee River. Here the trail passes the LacLawrann Conservancy to the east. The conservancy, a 136-acre nature preserve at 300 Schmidt Road, is worth a visit. At the southern end of West Bend after crossing Decorah Road, Ziegler Park is off a path to the right,with picnic tables, restrooms and drinking fountains available. The trail again becomes rural in its last mile from Paradise Road to Rusco Drive.

Expect to share the trail with bicyclists, hikers, dog walkers (leashes required) and other nonmotorized uses in summer. The 6-mile section of trail north of Lighthouse Lane to the Fond du Lac County line is open only to snowmobiles during winter; cross-country skiing, snowshoeing and hiking are allowed in the 5-mile stretch of trail south of Lighthouse Lane.

DIRECTIONS

To reach the northern trailhead, take County Road V south from Eden for 1.5 miles. Turn left on Tracks Road (note that the street sign is very difficult to read; it is the first left turn coming south from Eden that isn't private property). The road dead-ends at the trailhead.

To reach the southern endpoint, take US Route 45 south to West Bend. Take Exit 7 on US Route 33/144 and follow Route 33 east to County Road G. Take County Road G south for 2 miles, through one traffic circle, then turn left on Rusco Drive. The trail starts on the right at the unused railroad tracks.

There is no public parking at the north and south trailheads, but multiple access points where the road crosses the trail may provide on-street parking.

Contact: Washington County Golf & Parks Division
432 East Washington Street
West Bend, WI 53095
(262) 335-4400
www.co.washington.wi.us/departments.
iml?mdl=departments.mdl&ID=PAR

Elroy-Sparta State Trail

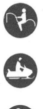

The history of the Elroy-Sparta rail-trail is almost as fun as the ride. In its prime this section of Chicago and North Western Railroad supplied markets in Chicago and Madison with goods from Minnesota, northern Iowa and the Dakotas. Countless numbers of cattle traveled this track from the heartland to the Chicago stockyards. Six passenger trains and 40 to 50 freight trains once passed daily through the corridor's three historical tunnels and over its 34 bridges that today are used by more than 60,000 cyclists each year.

The 32-mile trail celebrated its 40th anniversary in 2007, and towns along the Elroy-Sparta proudly lay claim to the rail-trail as the oldest in the state. It is an easy ride between the quiet country towns of Elroy and Sparta. Here and in the towns between them—Norwalk, Wilton and Kendall—there are rest areas, restrooms, drinking water, camping areas and snack concessions. The trail's hard-packed crushed limestone base is comfortable for

Location
Juneau and
Monroe counties

Endpoints
Sparta to Elroy

Mileage
32

Roughness Index
1

Surface
Crushed stone

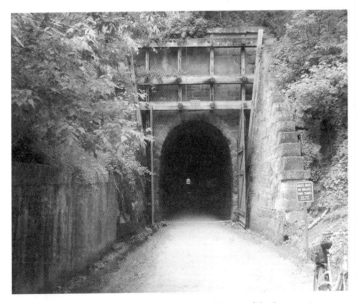

Bring your flashlights and your courage as you head into any of the three massive, carved rock tunnels on the renowned Elroy-Sparta State Trail.

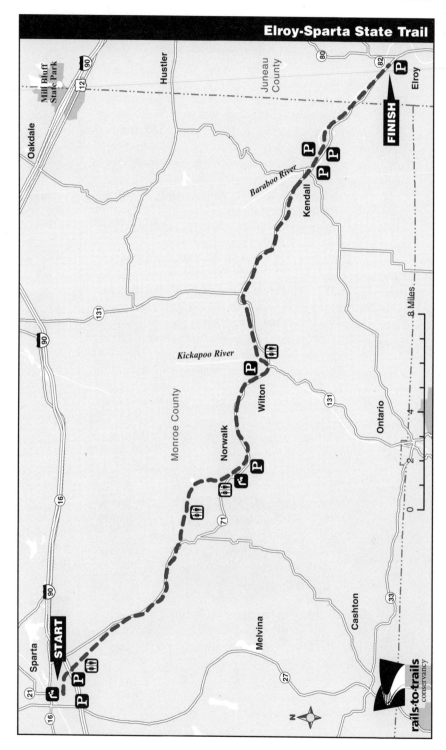

Elroy-Sparta State Trail

walking and running and suitable for most bicycle tires. Both end-points offer more riding: Pick up the 21-mile La Crosse River Trail (page 325) in Sparta, or the "400" State Trail (page 365) and Omaha Trail (page 341) in Elroy. These trails can all be pieced into 100 miles of rail-trail adventure from the mighty Mississippi into the heart of beautiful cheese country.

Heading east from Sparta you come to the longest and most dramatic of the trail's three tunnels. The tunnels are fascinating, at times seeming more like caves. Water drips down the walls and pools at your feet. The temperature in the tunnels is a cool 50 to 60 degrees, regardless of the outside temperature.

Tunnel No. 3 is located 9 miles from Sparta. It is 3,810 feet long—more than 10 football fields—and completely dark. Without proper lights and a fearless companion, this tunnel is impassable. From either direction there are seasonal kiosks where you can purchase flashlights. Tunnel No. 3 cost more than a million dollars to build and was a three-year engineering feat, opening in 1873. The tunnel was dug by hand through solid rock. A shaft was dug from the top of the hill into the center of the tunnel, allowing workers to dig from the center out, as well as from both ends. It is just over 3 miles from Tunnel No. 3 to Norwalk.

The highlight of the 5 miles between Norwalk and Wilton is Tunnel No. 2. Like the others, Tunnel No. 2 has gigantic 20-foot-tall wooden doors at its entrances. These doors were opened and shut between traveling trains in the winter, to prevent snow from accumulating inside the tunnels. They are still used for this purpose when snowmobiles use the trail in the winter. When entering the tunnels look for the small doorway-sized indentations in the walls near the doors. This is where the tunnel watchmen were stationed, opening and closing these massive doors up to 50 times each day.

From Wilton, Tunnel No. 1 is 5.5 miles along the trail. At 1694 feet (the exact same length as Tunnel No. 2), it runs a similar straight-arrow path through the rock, with the pin-prick of light visible at the other end. That tunneling effect is mirrored by the trees along the trail as well, as it continues 3.3 miles to Kendall, home to the trail's headquarters at the restored Kendall Depot. From here, it's another 6 miles to the trail's conclusion in Elroy.

All along the trail, the scenery is sweetly rolling hills, farmland, crops and pastures. And despite the trail's popularity, you will undoubtedly see more cows than people on your journey, which may be exactly the kind of Wisconsin getaway you're seeking.

DIRECTIONS

The five major towns of this trail—Elroy, Sparta, Norwalk, Wilton and Kendall—each have parking, restrooms, food and water. For a straight ride and trail information, head to the endpoints of Elroy or Sparta. Wheelchairs can access the trail easily from all towns and parking lots.

In Elroy the trailhead is located between Main Street and Railroad Street. To get to Elroy from Interstate 90 east, take State Hwy. 80, Exit 61 toward New Lisbon. Stay on Hwy. 80 for 12 miles, until it intersects Hwy. 82 in Elroy. Once in Elroy there are signs to the trail. (From I-90 west, take State Hwy. 82, Exit 69 toward Mauston. Stay on Hwy. 82 until it joins Hwy. 80 in Elroy.)

To reach Sparta take I-90 to Exit 25 and head north on Blackriver Street. Take a right onto West Wisconsin Street, in downtown Sparta, then a right onto South Water Street. The trail depot and parking are on the corner of Milwaukee Street and South Water Street.

Contact: Elroy-Sparta State Trail Headquarters
P.O. Box 297
Kendall, WI 54638
(608) 463-7109
www.elroy-sparta-trail.com

Fox River Trail

The Fox River looms large in the life and landscape of Green Bay, Wisconsin. Along its east side the Riverwalk follows the contours of the downtown shoreline like two friends on an evening stroll. Then, just south of the Mason Street Bridge, it merges seamlessly into the 25-mile Fox River State Recreational Trail. Historically this has been a well-traveled route: first by Native Americans, then French explorers and traders and later the Milwaukee and Northern Railway.

For the initial 5 miles the wide and forceful river flows beside the trail. You might notice some industry and maybe a large ship unloading on the far side. In this urban segment the trail is just out the back door of riverfront homes, restaurants and even a bike shop. About a half mile from the start is the Hazelwood Historic House Museum and the Brown County Historical Society. Take some time to enjoy this mighty river—there are benches, an overlook and a dock to choose from. The weekend

Location
Brown County

Endpoints
Green Bay to Greenleaf

Mileage
25

Roughness Index
1

Surface
Asphalt and crushed stone

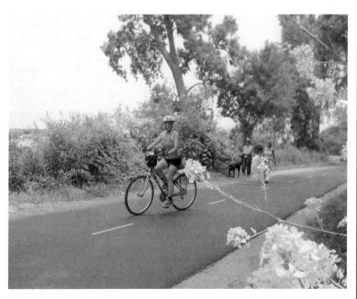

The Fox River Trail is no stranger to travelers—the pathway has been used by Native Americans, early French explorers and the Milwaukee and Northern Railway.

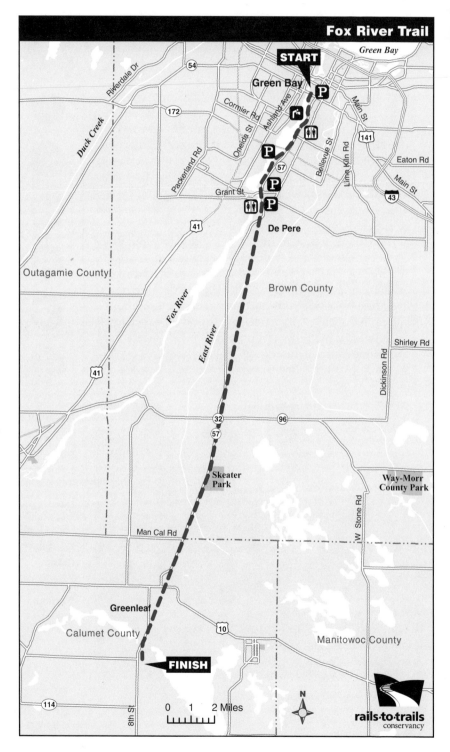

Fox River Trail

trail traffic is a lively blend of ages and transportation modes. If you are looking for more of a workout, hit the fitness challenge course in the Allouez section at 1.25 miles. Also here is St. Francis Park, where a charming gazebo, river views and picnic tables invite you to take a break.

In the town of De Pere, at 4.2 miles, the trail passes a popular fishing spot at Voyager Park before it bends away from the river. By Rockland Road (about 6.5 miles), the number of people diminishes, the surface changes from asphalt to crushed stone and the route remains rural. It passes through several small communities before reaching Greenleaf, where the southern tailhead is located. The trail continues about 6 more miles to Ott Road. The trail's popularity has led to additional paving and there are plans to extend the trail 2 miles south to Hilbert in Calumet County. Equestrians use accompanying bridle paths from Heritage Road in De Pere south to the trail's end.

A Wisconsin State Trail Pass is required for trail users (except walkers) over 16 and passes are available at self-registration stations and other locations along the trail.

DIRECTIONS

From Milwaukee, take Interstate 43 north to Green Bay (about 120 miles). Take Exit 180 and right after that take the WI-172 W ramp. Go for 3.7 miles and take the exit for County Road X. Turn right onto WI-57 N (Riverside Dr). Go 2.3 miles and turn left onto Cass Street. Turn right onto South Adams Street. The Fox River Trail begins at the junction of Porlier Street and South Adams Street in Green Bay. Parking is available on South Adams Street and on weekends in the lot under the Mason Street Bridge.

To reach the southern trailhead in Greenleaf, take Route 32/57 south from Green Bay to Route 96 or Day Street, turn left and go one block to Follett Street. Turn left and go one more block. The trailhead is on the right.

Trail access and parking are also available at the Fox Point Boat Launch facility, Voyager Park, Bomier Boat Launch and the corner of Klaus and Follett Streets in Greenleaf.

Contact: Brown County Park Department
305 East Walnut Street
Green Bay, WI 54301
(920) 448-4466
www.foxrivertrail.com

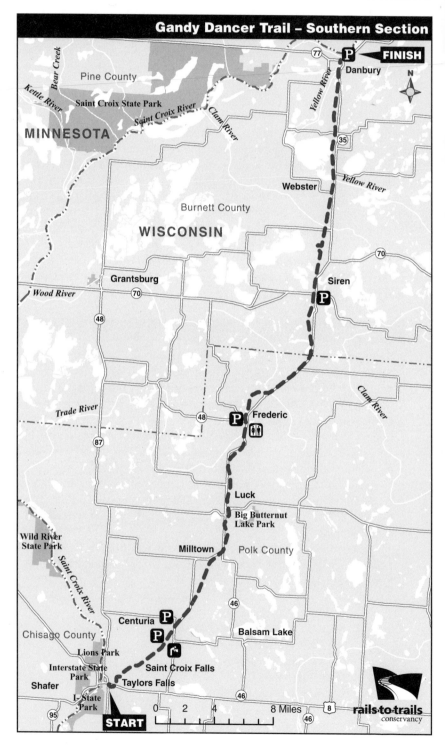

Gandy Dancer Trail – Southern Section

Gandy Dancer Trail – Southern Section

The 98-mile Gandy Dancer Trail runs along the old Minneapolis, St. Paul and Sault Ste. Marie railroad corridor from St. Croix Falls north to Superior. The Gandy Dancer Trail can be separated into two sections: The 51-mile northern section (between Superior and Danbury) is primarily a snowmobile/ATV trail, while the 47-mile southern section (between St. Croix Falls and Danbury) offers trail users a more traditional and leisurely rail-trail experience. This trail review covers the southern section of the Gandy Dancer Trail, with a well-maintained, crushed limestone surface and scenic views of northwestern Wisconsin.

The name "Gandy Dancer" is derived from the trail's historic use as a railroad corridor. In the 1880s, work crews building and maintaining the corridor used tools manufactured by the Chicago-based Gandy Tool

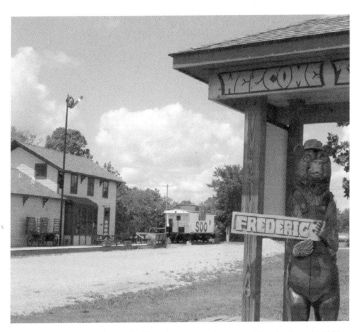

When on the Gandy Dancer Trail's southern section, be sure to take advantage of trailside treats and other amenities offered in the towns along the way.

Location
Burnett and Polk counties

Endpoints
St. Croix Falls to Danbury

Mileage
47

Roughness Index
2

Surface
Crushed stone

Company and could often be found working in unison to a vocal and mechanical beat, much like a well-rehearsed dance.

Beginning in St. Croix Falls, the Gandy Dancer Trail travels north for a total of 47 miles through the communities of Centuria, Milltown, Luck, Frederic, Lewis, Siren, Webster and Danbury. Before heading off down the trail, consider a side trip to Interstate State Park (just down the road from the Polk County Information Center), where you can marvel at the beauty of the St. Croix River and the unique glacial heritage of the area. Once on the trail, be sure to take advantage of the many sights and amenities in each of the friendly towns along the way. For railroad buffs, the restored railroad depot and area museum in Frederic are a must-see. Also, don't miss the fabulous food and genuine staff found at Cafe Wren just off the trail in Luck.

DIRECTIONS

From the intersection of US Route 8 and WI 35 near St. Croix Falls, go south a quarter mile to the Polk County Information Center. Parking is available.

A Wisconsin State Trail Pass is required of all bicyclists 16 years of age or older riding the trail between St. Croix Falls and Danbury. Trail passes are available at the Polk County Information Center and from business vendors in communities along the trail. Fees are $4 for a daily pass and $15 for an annual pass.

Contact: Polk County Visitors Center
Highway 35
St. Croix Falls, WI 54024
(800) 222-7655
www.polkcountytourism.com/gandydancer.html

Glacial Drumlin State Trail

It is common on a rail-trail to be reminded of railroading history; it is quite another experience to be taken back thousands of years and witness the effects of ancient ice flows on the landscape. This is the case with the nearly 52-mile Glacial Drumlin State Trail, particularly at its western end. As gigantic sheets of ice bore down on this area, they created wetlands, ponds and rivers and hundreds of low, cigar-shaped hills called drumlins. This landscape was a challenge for the railroad builders, since bridges had to be built over the extensive wetlands, but many of the wood pilings sank in the deep muck and created often dangerous passage for trains.

These wood-planked bridges now provide great viewpoints for the wetlands, where a host of wildlife thrives. You may spot large sandhill cranes, an ancient

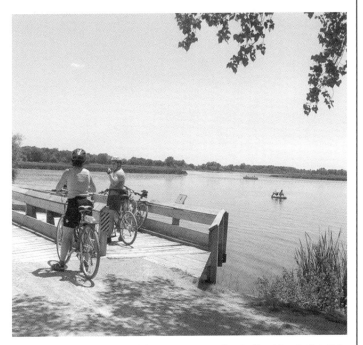

Broad wetlands are a feature of the entire region as well as the Glacial Drumlin State Trail itself.

Location
Dane, Jefferson and Waukesha counties

Endpoints
Cottage Grove to Waukesha

Mileage
51.6

Roughness Index
1

Surface
Asphalt and crushed stone

307

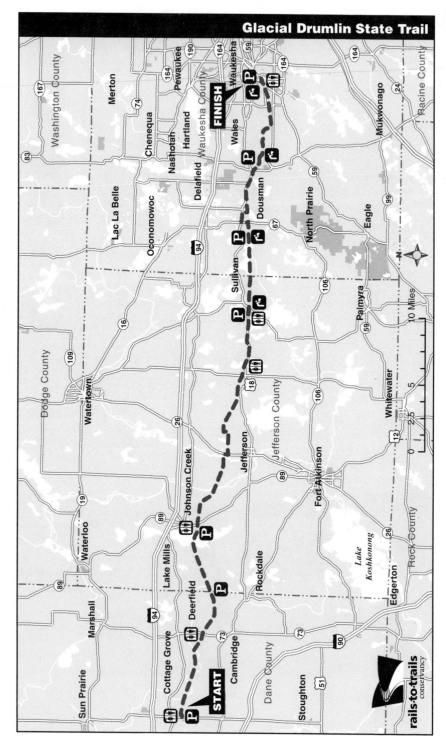

Glacial Drumlin State Trail

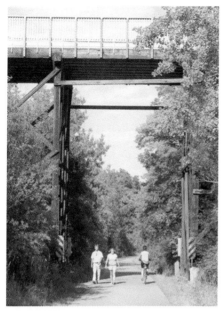

The scale of the former rail corridor is nicely illustrated along the Glacial Drumlin State Trail.

species with bright red adorning the tops of their heads, or hear spring peepers and chorus frogs announcing their presence.

From Cottage Grove, the openness of the early miles (be prepared for headwinds) alternates with wooded sections as the trail travels east through mostly serene countryside. This is periodically broken up by towns and villages along the former rail line, with varying amenities if you are willing to go explore. Passing Deerfield and London, you reach Rock Lake, at nearly 15 miles. You sail over a quarter-mile-long bridge that separates upper and lower Rock Lake. The beautiful view of the two lakes begs to be savored, which you can easily do by pulling off onto fishing and picnicking platforms away from the main trail traffic.

In the 5-mile stretch between Lake Mills and Jefferson the trail tunnels under thick tree canopy in the summer and crosses Crawfish River and Rock River (a fishing haven for locals). In Jefferson, at about 22 miles, signs guide you through an easy 1.5-mile on-road section before reconnecting with the trail. As you journey through the small towns and communities of Helenville, Sullivan, Dousman and Wales (you can almost hear the conductor listing them), you'll find restaurants and grocery stores close to the trail for a meal or provisions. Before reaching Sullivan the trail parallels US Highway 18 for a couple miles, then a stream and wetland populated with yellow finches and purple thistles. Here, outside of Dousman, the crushed stone surface ends and the final 13 miles to Waukesha are smooth pavement. Near the trail's end in the Fox River Sanctuary, you are reminded of the journey's past: There beside the new bridge across the Fox River lies the framework of the venerable iron railroad trestle.

Trail passes, required for ages 16 and up, can be purchased at self-registration stations on the trail or at select parks and private businesses.

DIRECTIONS

The trail has multiple trailheads, with parking, over its nearly 52 miles.

The western trailhead, in Cottage Grove, can be reached from Madison by taking US 90 south to Route 147 (Stoughton/Cottage Grove/ County N). Turn left in 4.5 miles onto County North Drive. The trailhead is on the right in the center of town.

The Jefferson trailhead is closest to the trail's midpoint. Follow US Highway 18 east to Jefferson. In town, Highway 18 becomes West Racine Street and after several blocks crosses the Rock River. Turn left on Route 26 (the first street just after the bridge), heading north. Go a couple of miles to West Junction Road and turn right. The trailhead is just past the intersection on the left. This is the location of the one on-road section of the Glacial Drumlin Trail, but signs guide you to the trail.

The eastern trailhead is in the Fox River Sanctuary in Waukesha. From Interstate 94, take Highway 164 (North Street) for 3.1 miles to St. Paul Avenue. Turn right on St. Paul and go to Prairie Avenue (0.2 mile). Turn left on Prairie Avenue and, in 0.4 mile, turn right on College Avenue. Look for the Fox River Sanctuary parking lot and the trailhead.

Contact: Glacial Drumlin Trail – West
1213 South Main Street
Lake Mills, WI 53551
(920) 648-8774

Glacial Drumlin Trail – East
W329 N846, County Highway C
Delafield, WI 53018
(262) 646-3025

www.glacialdrumlin.com

Glacial River Trail

The Hoard Historical Museum is a good place to kick off a visit to Fort Atkinson. The museum is named after the Hoard family behind the nationally distributed dairy farm magazine *Hoard's Dairyman*. Exhibits of tools, textiles and Native American artifacts will get you up to speed on the area's early fort history, European settlers and American Indian culture.

Then hop on the Glacial River Trail and see the sights. The 6.5-mile rail-trail begins in downtown Fort Atkinson. Travel south a couple of blocks to the beautiful metal archway announcing the trail. A bridge crossing the Rock River brings you to the River Walk, which is off the trail and under the bridge and offers quaint shops and restaurants. The trail shoots through the city, crossing busy Janesville Avenue. A low stone wall next to the path marks the Glacial River Rotary Depot, which offers a water fountain and covered picnic area. The paved

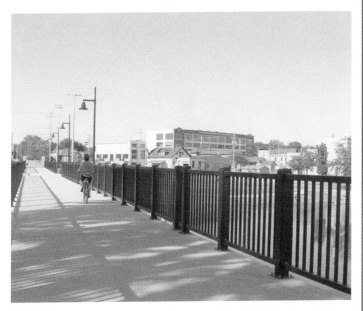

For those seeking a quick urban-to-rural escape, the Glacial River Trail packs in sights on its 6.5-mile path.

Location
Jefferson County

Endpoints
Fort Atkinson to
Jefferson County/
Rock County Line

Mileage
6.5

Roughness Index
1

Surface
Asphalt and
crushed stone

311

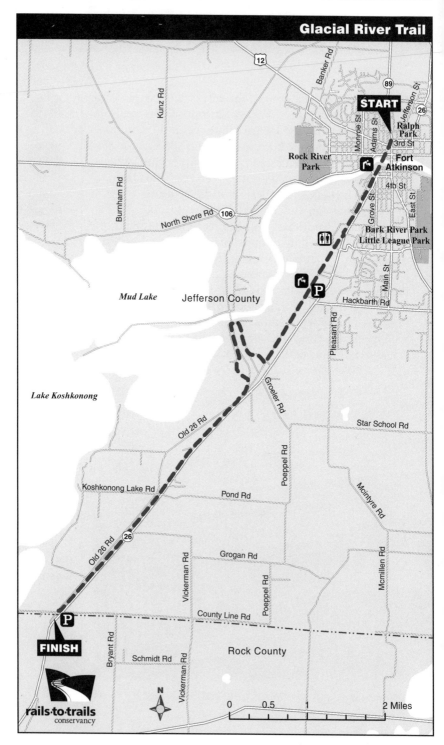

trail continues through the Fort Atkinson business district and then, at mile 2, enters quiet woodlands, where the surface changes to crushed stone.

At the intersection with lightly traveled Groeler Road, the path detours from the old rail corridor for about 1.5 miles. Turn right on Groeler Road to head northwest to a long, nearly 1-mile downhill slope that brings you to a T-intersection with an unmarked town road. Follow the town road under the Highway 26 bridge along the Rock River. Immediately after passing under the highway bridge, turn left onto Schwemmer Lane. Follow this quiet, dead-end town road south for about a half mile. The trail has left the railroad grade at this point. It rolls gently downhill between farm fields before joining an un-named town road for another short on-road section. As the route connects with Old 26 Road, the railroad grade trail picks up again. Take a worthwhile side trip by turning right on Old 26 Road and following it southwest for 1 mile. Here you will find Indian Mounds Park, a collection of 11 Indian mounds and an old Indian trail. The mounds, large earthworks with religious or ceremonial origins, can be seen from the trail. Look closely to see the turtle and bird shapes identified by experts. The mounds are thought to have survived about 1,500 years.

Back on the trail you travel through patches of woods and open areas, with Highway 26 nearby. The trail ends at the Jefferson County and Rock County line.

DIRECTIONS

To reach the Fort Atkinson trailhead from the north, follow State Route 26 south until it turns into North High Street in Fort Atkinson. Turn left on North 4th Street and continue until Main Street. Street parking is available.

To reach the southern trailhead, take Route 26 north, turn left on East County Line Road to a small parking area.

Contact: Jefferson County Parks Department
320 South Main Street
Courthouse Room 204
Jefferson, WI 53549
(920) 674-7260
www.travelwisconsin.com/item_detail/
Glacial_River_Bike_Trail.aspx

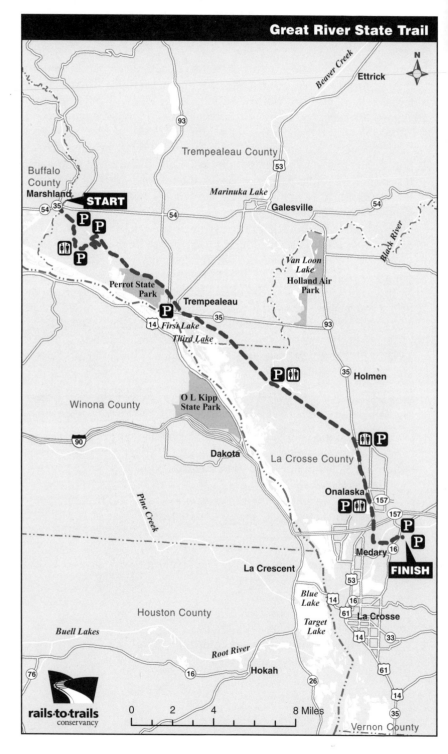

Great River State Trail

The Great River State Trail follows the shores of the majestic Mississippi River in western Wisconsin. The trail meanders through 24.4 miles of river marsh, thick hardwood forests and quiet farmland. It is a wonderful nature escape and a reflection of easy Midwestern life along the river and its many tributaries early in its long journey to the Gulf of Mexico.

Starting from the northern trailhead in Marshland, the limestone surfaced trail points you southeast along the river and immediately enters the Trempealeau National Wildlife Refuge. This is the first of three wildlife refuges on the route. The region is on the Mississippi flyway, so if you time your visit right, you'll be in the company of a vast assortment of waterfowl, wading birds and migratory songbirds. Pay attention to the signs for the Great River State Trail, because the refuge provides a number of offshoot trails.

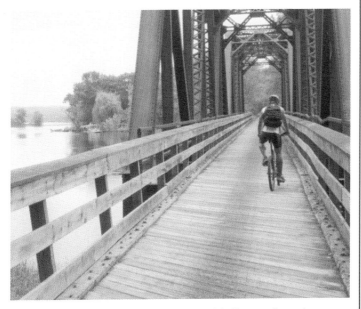

The Great River State Trail aptly follows the course of the Mississippi River and crosses several tributaries along the way.

Location
Buffalo, La Crosse and Trempealeau counties

Endpoints
Marshland to Medary

Mileage
24

Roughness Index
1

Surface
Crushed stone

As you exit the national refuge, you briefly pass through Perrot State Park, a wildlife area with hiking, skiing and boating trails. The small town of Trempealeau at mile 9.3, with its several cafes and parks, provides a nice break point. The trail travels through peaceful wooded areas that provide shade on a warm summer day, then leads you over a series of bridges that spans several small tributaries within the Upper Mississippi River Fish and Wildlife Refuge. There are wonderful wildlife viewing opportunities here and a dizzying array of small streams that all flow into the Mississippi just a few hundred yards off the trail.

Next up, at mile 14.5, is Lytles Landing. This park area provides parking and trail access, as well as a rusting steel train trestle over the Black River. Continuing south the trail cuts through miles of small neighborhoods and pockets of wooded areas. Spring and summer there is a beautiful selection of wildflowers nodding in the breezes along the trail.

Onalaska, at mile 22.5, is about 5 miles north of the industrial city of La Crosse and situated on a ridge overlooking the Mississippi and Black rivers. A bit of on-road travel in this bustling community requires attention. Follow trail signs for about three-quarters of a mile to the center of town, where restaurants, bike shops and resting spots will suit your fancy. To reach the trail's end at the very small town of Medary, you must carefully cross busy Route 35. If you plan to end your trip here, pay close attention: A seamless transition to the delightful La Crosse River State Trail (page 325) could take you all the way to Sparta!

DIRECTIONS

To reach the Marshland trailhead from Interstate 90, take the WI 35 exit (3B) and head north all the way to Marshland. Take a left on the unpaved Marshland Access Road immediately east of the railroad track crossing and the WI 35/County Highway P junction at Marshland.

To reach the Medary trailhead from I-90, take the WI 157 Exit 4, travel south for less than 1 mile and take a right on State Route 16. Take a left onto County Highway B, and you will see parking for the trailhead approximately 0.5 mile down the road on the left.

Contact: Great River State Trail
W26247 Sullivan Road
P.O. Box 407
Trempealeau, WI 54661
(608) 534-6409

Hiawatha Trail and Bearskin State Park Trail

Shimmering lakes and Wisconsin's beautiful North Woods wilderness await you on the Bearskin State Park Trail and Hiawatha Trail. The two trails are currently separated by a 5.5-mile gap, but taken together or alone they provide a splendid journey along an old Milwaukee Road rail corridor that hauled white pine to the Midwest and later carried a passenger train named the *Hiawatha*.

The trails traverse an area that has one of the densest concentrations of lakes in the world. Converted railroad trestles help you glide across long spans of lilypad-covered lakes. On the Bearskin trail, eight of 13 trestles cross the trail's namesake, Bearskin Creek, and act as lookout landings for bald eagles, loons and other wildlife. Watch for snapping turtles basking in the sun.

Bearskin State Park Trail starts in Minocqua, where a long boardwalk across shimmering Lake Minocqua is the beginning of an 18.3-mile venture south where you

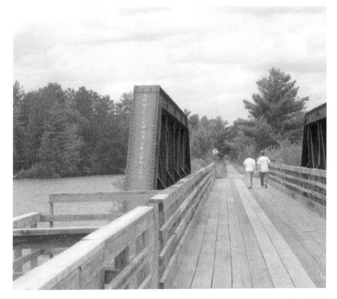

Part of the multistate Milwaukee Road corridor, the Hiawatha Trail and Bearskin State Park Trail features 13 railroad trestles.

Location
Lincoln and Oneida counties

Endpoints
Minocqua to Tomahawk

Mileage
32.8

Roughness Index
2

Surface
Crushed stone

Hiawatha Trail and Bearskin State Park Trail

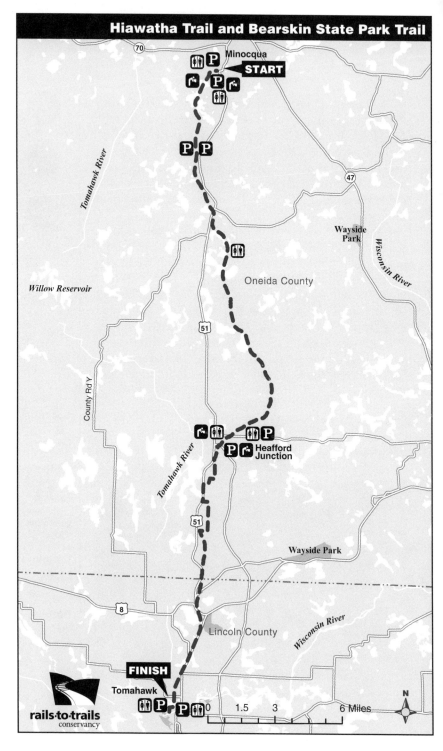

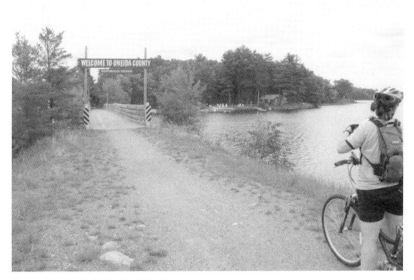

The lake-dotted trail links Oneida and Lincoln counties.

encounter a beautiful, remote wilderness—plus a few picnic tables and portable restrooms at various trailheads.

Several interpretive signs and old railroad structures provide a glimpse into the rich history of this railroad corridor. A century-old railroad line shed approximately 9.5 miles from Minocqua attests to the rustic living conditions of some railroad workers, and historic photographs illustrate the challenging nature of railroad labor. During the warmer months hikers and bikers hit these trails and take in the astounding lake vistas. Snowmobiles are permitted in the winter months and many connecting trails provide endless hours of exploration.

The 9-mile Hiawatha Trail hooks up with the Bearskin via a 5.5-mile on-road connection for a 32-mile one-way journey. Traveling north from Tomahawk on the Hiawatha Trail you are surrounded by glistening lakes and travel over expansive trestle bridges.

The Hiawatha Trail peters out after 9 miles. There are no clear signs indicating you have hit the end of the line, so be on the lookout for bike route signs where the trail intersects with Lake Nokomis Road. At this juncture, follow the on-road bike route and snowmobile signs east and then north along quiet neighborhood streets and the busier County Road L. Passing under a Highway 51 overpass signals that you will soon arrive at the trailhead for the Bearskin Trail on County Road K.

The allure of these north woods trails lies in their isolated, scenic charm. If you want to explore both trails, plan accordingly; besides one remote restroom facility on the Bearskin, there are no other amenities or easy access to food and water.

Parking and restroom facilities are located at each trailhead at Sara Lake Park in Tomahawk and the trailhead in Minocqua. You won't have problems finding a motel or a good meal in the tourist towns of Minocqua and Tomahawk. After a day on the trails, treat yourself to a cold glass of homemade root beer at the local brewery in Minocqua and watch the sun set across the lake.

DIRECTIONS

To access the Hiawatha Trail from US Hwy. 51, take Exit 229 for State Route 86 west/CR-D toward Tomahawk. Route 86 becomes East Somo Avenue. After passing through town, continue on Somo Avenue until you reach Sara Lake Park, which will be on your left after crossing the intersection of North Railway Street and West Somo Avenue. Continue to veer right after passing the park facilities to reach the large parking lot. The Hiawatha Trail will be on your left.

For the Bearskin trail, there are two trailheads. For the southern terminus, take US Hwy. 51 south from Minocqua to County Road K and turn left. The trailhead will be on the left, approximately 0.75 mile from the turn. The northern terminus is in the town of Minocqua. From the south, take US Hwy. 51 north. Before entering the downtown area, turn left onto Park Avenue, continuing until the road veers right, then becomes Front Street. The trailhead parking lot is located off of Front Street behind the Post Office.

Contact: Wisconsin Department of Natural Resources
518 West Somo Avenue
Tomahawk, WI 54487
(715) 453-1263
http://dnr.wi.gov/org/land/parks/specific/bearskin/
index.html

Hillsboro State Trail

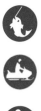

The 4.3-mile Hillsboro State Trail makes you feel instantly at home. Easy and flat, a short excursion on this trail takes you from Hillsboro to Union Center on a smooth gravel surface. But this trail is more of a draw for what it connects you to than for the trip itself.

In Union Center you can hook up with the "400" State Trail (page 363), which connects to the Elroy-Sparta(page 297) and Omaha rail-trails (page 341) to the north. Access this longer trail system for amenities such as campsites, trail information kiosks, picnic rest areas and restroom facilities.

In Hillsboro you have your pick of activities. Outdoor types will find hiking opportunities in Wildcat Mountain State Park, canoeing on the Kickapoo River, bird-watching at the Wildcat Mountain State Park Wildlife Reserve or trout fishing at Hillsboro Lake. Shoppers will enjoy the farmer's market (May to October), with

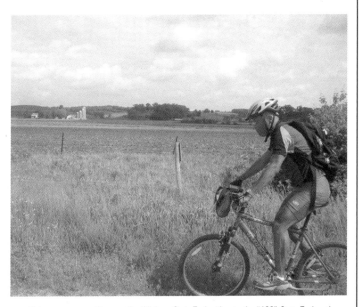

Make some connections on the Hillsboro State Trail, either to the "400" State Trail or the food and festivities of the local Czech and Amish communities.

Location
Juneau and
Vernon counties

Endpoints
Hillsboro to
Union Center

Mileage
4.3

Roughness Index
1

Surface
Crushed stone

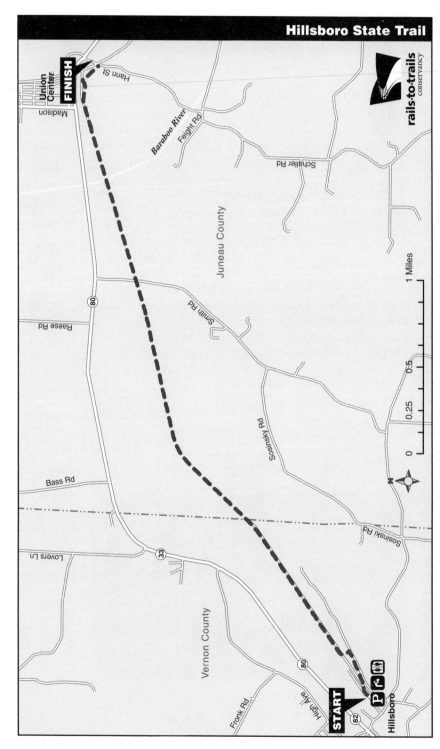

local produce and Amish baked goods brought to market by buggies from the surrounding Amish community. History buffs will want to stop by the Field-Veteran's Memorial Park to pay tribute to local veterans. And architecture enthusiasts can explore one of the largest concentrations of round barns in the United States. Many were built and designed by Alga Shivers, an African-American settler and son of a slave who escaped to the area via the Underground Railroad.

Finally, the calendar of events in this town will hold anyone's interest. Hillsboro stakes its claim as the "Czech Capital of Wisconsin," and every June a weeklong celebration marks local heritage with spirited music and dancing, handmade crafts and Czech fare such as roast pork, sauerkraut and dumplings. The town also hosts a two-day tractor pull around the Fourth of July and the region's largest Labor Day celebration complete with a parade, carnival and softball tournaments.

Whether you come to Hillsboro for a day or a week, be sure to travel its hometown rail-trail as a way to immerse yourself in the flavor of this lively community.

DIRECTIONS

Take WI-33/WI-82 into the town of Hillsboro; Route 33/82 will become Water Avenue; turn left on East Madison Street, then go two blocks; the trailhead will be on your left.

Contact: City of Hillsboro
P.O. Box 447
Hillsboro, WI 54634
(608) 489-2521

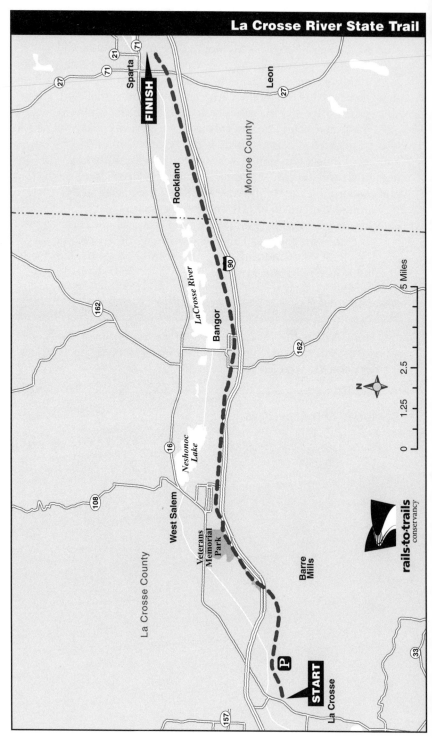

La Crosse River State Trail

The La Crosse River State Trail is a link in a chain of rail-trails that connect more than 100 miles. This 21-mile trail leads you from the industrial river community of La Crosse to Sparta, the self-proclaimed biking capital of the United States. There are seamless trail connections from the 24-mile Great River State Trail (page 315) on the west end and the 32-mile Elroy-Sparta State Trail (page 297) on the east end. All of these trails require a state pass, which can be obtained at numerous places along the trail.

The La Crosse River State Trail follows the old Chicago and North Western Railroad line traveled by Harry Truman during his 1948 presidential campaign. The crushed limestone trail now carries runners, walkers and bikers through beautiful green rolling hills and classic Wisconsin farmland.

Beginning in Medary, right outside of La Crosse, the trail travels east through some nice wooded areas as it

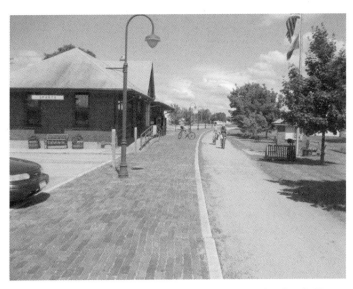

Linking the Elroy-Sparta and Great River State trails, the La Crosse River State Trail hums along beside an active rail line in transportation harmony.

Location
La Crosse and Monroe counties

Endpoints
La Crosse to Sparta

Mileage
21

Roughness Index
1

Surface
Crushed stone

very gently ascends out of the river valley. An active rail line parallels the trail for its entire length. Once you pass under Interstate 90 near the start of the trail, you are surrounded by serene rolling hills that are vibrantly green in the summer and punctuated by orange, yellow and red in the autumn. The flagship Wisconsin silos dot the landscape as far as the eye can see.

A popular feature of this trail is its camping opportunities. Two connecting trails, both within the first 10 miles, lead to campgrounds just north of the trail. These campgrounds are both close to the La Crosse River.

The trail breezes through the small Wisconsin towns of West Salem, Bangor and Rockland. All three of these communities have built pleasant parks along the trail and have quaint Midwestern main streets with all the amenities you might need for a trail excursion.

The trail reaches its end in Sparta, at an old railroad depot that now serves as a central information center for the entire trail system. Here you will find all you need to know while traveling though this trail-friendly region. Sparta is truly a biker's town and the small community is very proud of it. Be sure to check out all the bicycle-themed sculptures around town before you continue your journey on the Elroy-Sparta State Trail.

DIRECTIONS

The Sparta depot, with parking, is on Milwaukee Street. From Interstate 90, take the Sparta exit, travel north for 0.2 mile and turn right on Avon Road. Turn left onto South Water Street and left again on Milwaukee Street.

To reach the Medary trailhead from I-90, take the WI 157 exit (Exit 4), travel south for less than 1 mile and take a right on State Route 16. Take a left onto County Highway B and you will see parking for the trailhead approximately 0.5 mile down the road on the left.

Contact: La Crosse River State Trail, Inc.
111 Milwaukee Street
Sparta, WI 54656
(608) 269-4123
www.lacrosseriverstatetrail.org/main.htm

Military Ridge State Park Trail

The humble beginning of the Military Ridge Trail, at an unadorned highway intersection in Fitchburg, doesn't hint at the beauty of this trail's 40 miles through idyllic farmland and scattered small towns in southwest Wisconsin. Though its first miles parallel the busy road, you will be cheered by summer wildflowers—yellow and white moss rose, chicory, purple clover, thistles and yarrow.

Moving southwest, within 2 miles the traffic clamor is overtaken by birdcalls and rustling branches. You cross the first of 47 bridges, this one spanning a wetland lush and colorful with irises and cattails.

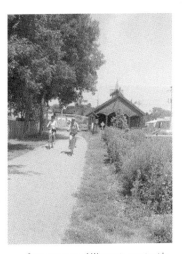

Open expanses of Wisconsin countryside and a dose of local Norwegian history make for a cultural visit on the Military Ridge State Park Trail.

The first town on the trail is Verona. With a population of more than 8,000, Verona has a number of amenities available, though you will have to venture north on Main Street a block or two to reach the heart of the town. Leaving Verona, the asphalt surface changes to stone dust and nature in these lowlands takes over. As the trail gently stretches through the Sugar River Valley, it is sprinkled with open cornfields, wetlands with cattails, weeping willows, birches and gnarly old oak trees. Just past the 10-mile mark a boardwalk takes you out to a marsh teeming with wildlife. Look for sandhill cranes and listen for the leopard toad, which sounds like a finger rubbing across an inflated balloon.

Bring your appetite to Mount Horeb, which has retained elements of its early settlers' Norwegian heritage and possesses a unique and charming trail station. The

Location
Dane and Iowa counties

Endpoints
Fitchburg to Dodgeville

Mileage
45

Roughness Index
1

Surface
Asphalt and crushed stone

327

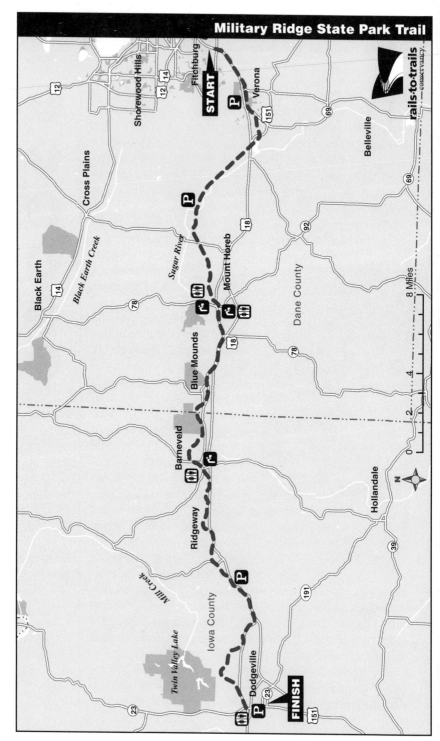

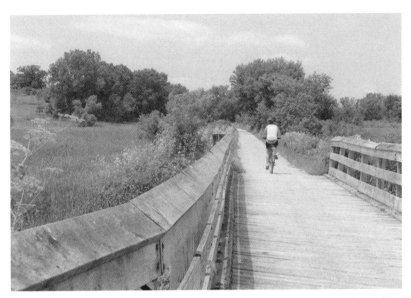

In 45 miles you'll cross 47 bridges on the Military Ridge State Park Trail, making the moments you're on solid ground nearly as unique and exciting as when you're over water.

main street is only one block south of the trail and has convenient and delicious eateries.

From here the trail traverses the top of Military Ridge (a name derived from the Blackhawk Battle between the Sauk and Fox Indians and the U.S. Army and militia over the land in 1832). Later the well-used route became a road connecting Green Bay with Fort Crawford. The trail rises gradually to skirt the southern slope of Blue Mound, its highest point at 1,300 feet above sea level. After the village of Blue Mounds you will see a spur trail on the right to Blue Mound State Park, where the view of the ridge and countryside are exceptional. Also near here is the Cave of the Mounds, with delightful subterranean geology (follow a spur to the left just after the tunnel under Highway ID for about a half mile south.)

Shortly after Barneveld (around 25 miles) and for most of the last 15 miles, tidy dairy farms and Holstein cows pattern the sloping fields in the distance. The trail feels tranquil here and is often sheltered by a dense tree canopy that is cool and refreshing in the high summer.

After curving through miles of lush farmland, you enter the pleasant town of Ridgeway, home to the single remaining active railroad depot on this converted corridor. A nearby community park has restrooms, parking and a drinking fountain.

The trail ends in Dodgeville (settled in 1827 by the first governor of the Wisconsin Territory), but if you're not ready to wrap up this trail trip, head for Governor Dodge State Park, a couple of miles to the east of Dodgeville (mile 38). A paved access trail to the right paralleling County Highway Z leads to the park's miles of trails for hiking, biking and cross-country skiing.

Trail passes, required for ages 16 and up, can be purchased at self-registration stations on the trail or at select parks and private businesses.

DIRECTIONS

The Fitchburg endpoint can be reached from Madison by taking Route 18/151 south to County Highway PD/McKee Road. The trail starts on the southeast corner of the intersection. Parking and trail access are available at Quarry Ridge Recreation Area. Follow County Highway PD west from Route 18/151, turn left on Nesbitt Road and then turn left on Fitchrona Road. The park is about .3 mile on the left. There is a paved path to the Military Ridge Trail.

For the Verona Trailhead take Highway 18/151 south to Exit 92 for County Highway PB. Go north on Old Highway PB for 1 mile. The trailhead with parking is on the left.

The Dodgeville trailhead is on County Highway YZ, 1.5 miles east of Highway 23 at the Department of Natural Resources Dodgeville Service Center.

There are also numerous access points and trailheads in the towns along the 40-mile route.

Contact: Military Ridge State Trail
P.O. Box 98
Blue Mounds, WI 53517
(608) 437-7393

Friends of Military Ridge State Trail
P.O. Box 373
Mt. Horeb, WI 53572
(608) 437-7393

www.dnr.state.wi.us/org/land/parks/specific/
militaryridge

Muskego Recreation Trail and City of Franklin Hike and Bike Trail

This is the story of two trails in two counties that serve up one seamless connection between the communities of Muskego and Franklin. The corridor was previously the Milwaukee Electric Railway & Light, an interurban railroad in southeast Wisconsin. Wisconsin Electric Power Company, now known as We Energies, acquired the corridor, which explains the power lines draping much of the trail.

The 5-mile Muskego Recreation Trail starts in a residential community just across from the entrance to the Muskego County Park and is marked with a sign at the trail entrance. The trail's crushed stone surface cuts a bright white swath through the surrounding greenery. This trail runs directly west to east and maintains an easy, level grade throughout. Although the first 2 miles take you through the residential community of Muskego in Waukesha County, after crossing Mystic Drive you are immersed in farmland and woodland scenery.

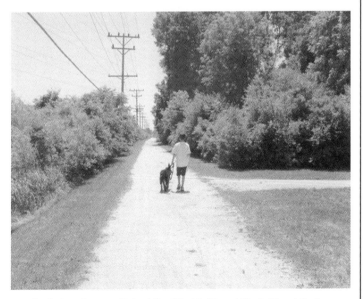

The Muskego Recreation Trail and City of Franklin Hike and Bike Trail is an intimate neighborhood connector and much-used green space.

Location
Milwaukee
and Waukesha
counties

Endpoints
Muskego to
Franklin

Mileage
6.5

**Roughness
Index**
1

Surface
Crushed stone

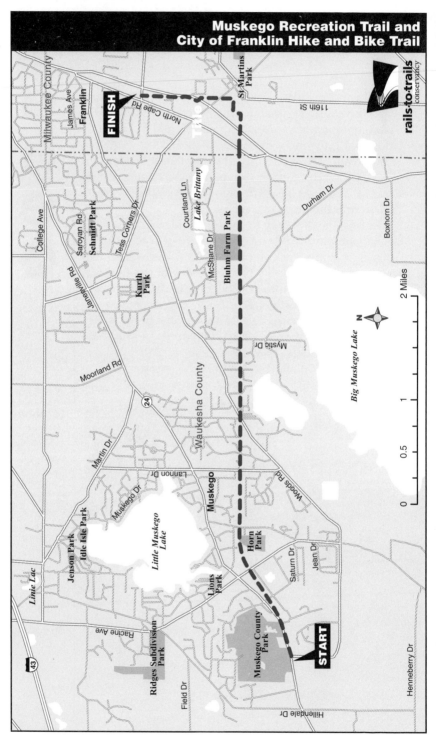

Muskego Recreation Trail and City of Franklin Hike and Bike Trail

From the Muskego Recreation Trail, you arrive at the 1.5-mile City of Franklin Hike and Bike Path in Milwaukee County. The transition is smooth and is marked by trail signage indicating that you have joined this trail segment. The trail continues cutting west through farmland until the last 2 miles, when it abruptly veers north after crossing Forest Home Avenue. The final stretch of the trail returns you to suburban Franklin, where playgrounds and residences flank the route.

While in Waukesha don't miss Little Muskego Lake—which at 506 acres isn't so little—and its public access for boating, water skiing and fishing. This lake is home to the Muskego Waterbugs, a talented group of water skiing performers, entertaining crowds every Wednesday evening throughout the summer. If wetlands are your thing, check out Big Muskego Lake with 2,260 acres of cattail marsh.

DIRECTIONS

To access the Muskego Recreation Trail take Racine Avenue (County Road Y) south to Janesville Road. Turn right on Janesville Road; Muskego County Park is on your right. There is parking available in the park; the trailhead is immediately across the street from the county park entrance.

To reach the City of Franklin Hike and Bike Path, take US Route 45/100 north from Franklin to West Rawson Avenue (County Road BB). Turn left on West Rawson and cross Forest Homes Avenue. The trailhead is on the left between Forest Home Avenue and South North Cape Road. There is no public parking at this trailhead.

Contact: Waukesha County Department of Parks and Land Use
Park System Division
1320 Pewaukee Road, Room 230
Waukesha, WI 53188
(262) 548-7801
www.midwestroads.com/craigholl/bike/muskego.html

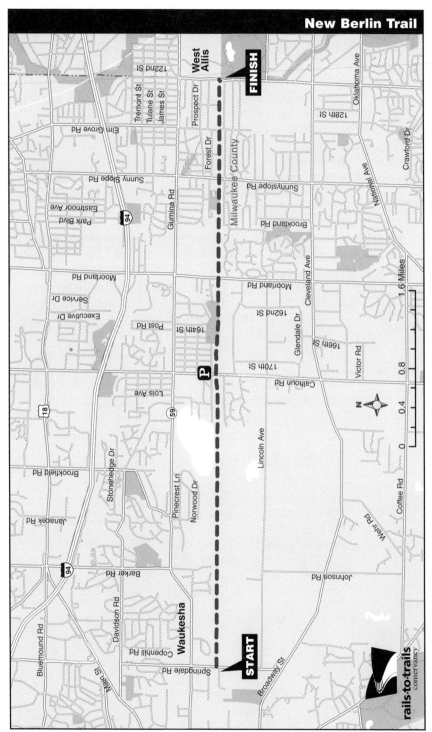

New Berlin Trail

New Berlin Trail

The communities of Waukesha, New Berlin and West Allis were sleepy outposts of Milwaukee in the late 1800s. Although the Chicago and North Western Railroad serviced the area, a critical turning point for growth came with the state of Wisconsin's 1892 selection of West Allis as the official location of the annual state fair. Increased rail service was established to bring residents of Milwaukee to the fairgrounds. In 1894 the Milwaukee Street Car Company again expanded service to the fairgrounds in West Allis and these communities began to thrive.

The legacy of the railroad continues today with the New Berlin Recreation Trail. The 7-mile paved trail runs directly west to east from Waukesha through New Berlin to Greenfield Park in West Allis. You will find a very smooth, flat trip with a slight downhill advantage if you travel west to east. The first 5.5 miles of the trail are in Waukesha, with wide-open spaces and a rural

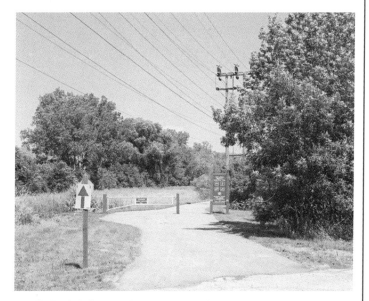

The New Berlin Trail serves Waukesha and West Allis communities as a useful transportation corridor.

Location
Waukesha County

Endpoints
Waukesha
(Springdale Road)
to West Allis (South
124th St.)

Mileage
7

**Roughness
Index**
1

Surface
Asphalt

335

environment. As you approach New Berlin and continue into Greenfield Park, parks and residential areas flank the trail. There are a few major road crossings that require caution.

This is not a particularly beautiful trail; the Wisconsin Electric Power Company owns the right-of-way and power lines rather than trees provide cover. What it lacks in scenery it makes up for in location. Though mainly a community path, the trail provides an important link in the system connecting the Oak Leaf Trail (page 337) and the Glacial Drumlin (page 307) and Fox River trails (page 301). The trail takes you to Greenfield Park, rich in amenities including a golf course, swimming pool, tot lot, concessions, and picnic and ball fields. And don't forget to experience the event to which this corridor traces its origin: the Wisconsin State Fair.

DIRECTIONS

The trailhead in Waukesha can be accessed by following Highway 59 west, which dead-ends into Arcadian Avenue at a traffic light. Highway 59 goes left, but go straight and follow Arcadian Avenue. Take a left on Springdale Road. The trail entrance and parking lot are on the left. From here the trail continues to the right; however, it only goes 0.2 mile into the Cooper Power Systems Plant parking lot. From here 2 miles of on-road connections will take you to the Glacial Drumlin and Fox River trails.

The trailhead in West Allis is in Greenfield Park, at the intersection of Highway 59 and 124th Street. You'll find the trailhead adjacent to the main parking lot, across from the Greenfield Park Pavilion.

Contact: Waukesha County Department of Parks and Land Use
Park System Division
1320 Pewaukee Road, Room 230
Waukesha, WI 53188
(262) 548-7801
www.waukeshacounty.gov/page.aspx?
SetupMetaId=10888&id=10932

Oak Leaf Trail

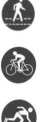

The Oak Leaf Trail (a.k.a. the Old-76 Bike Tour) is the jewel in the crown of Milwaukee County's extensive trail system. The 96.4-mile trail meanders in and around the city of Milwaukee on a changing terrain of flat rural plains and hilly city streets. Nearly a quarter of the trail hugs the beautiful shores of Lake Michigan.

The trail is mostly smooth asphalt, with dozens of easily accessed connections that take you just about anywhere in the Milwaukee Metro Area. (Milwaukee has more than 2,000 bike parking racks, with more installed every year.) Three miles of the trail follow the route of an old Chicago and North Western line that was part of the railroad company's long-distance passenger service to Denver, Colorado, and the California coast. The railroad's penchant for purchasing much of its equipment secondhand earned it the nickname "The Cheap and Nothing Wasted." The balance of the trail is made up of parkways and city streets.

The Oak Leaf Trail has more than 22 access points in and around the Milwaukee Metro Area. The best starting point is to park next to the Milwaukee Art Museum

Location
Milwaukee County

Endpoints
Milwaukee

Mileage
96.4

Roughness Index
1

Surface
Asphalt

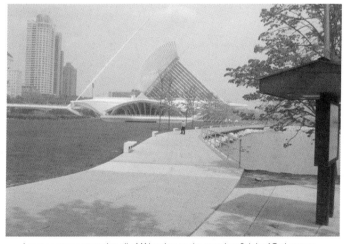

Leave no stone unturned in all of Milwaukee on the sprawling Oak Leaf Trail system.

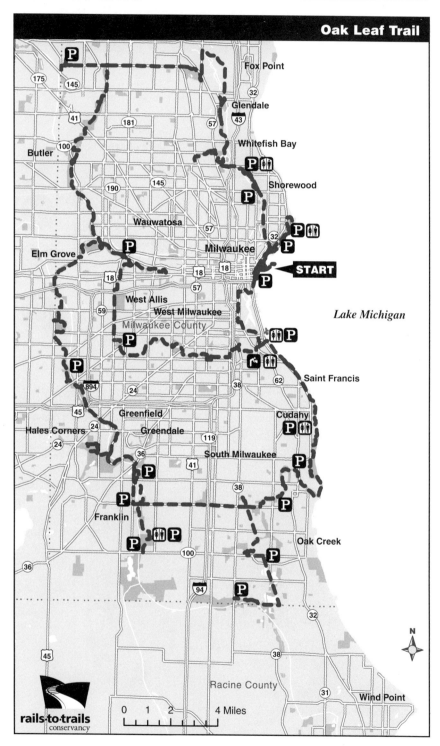

Oak Leaf Trail

Fox Point

175 145

41

181 57

Glendale 43 32

100

Butler

Whitefish Bay

190 145

P

Shorewood

Wauwatosa

57 P

32

Elm Grove

P

Milwaukee START

18

18 18 57

West Allis

59 West Milwaukee

Milwaukee County

P P

Saint Francis

P 894

45 24

24 Greenfield

Greendale

Cudahy

P

Hales Corners 24

119 South Milwaukee

P 36

41

P

38

Franklin P

P

Oak Creek

P

100

36

94

P

32

45

38

31

Racine County Wind Point

0 1 2 4 Miles

N

rails·to·trails
conservancy

and travel either north or south on the trail. Along the entire trail there are rolling hills, parkland and interesting neighborhoods.

In the more remote areas of the Oak Leaf Trail, particularly at dusk, you may spot a coyote or two. Coyotes are common, but they should be treated as the wild animals they are. Keep your pets close and on a leash and talk loudly to scare the coyote away.

Many species of birds can be found on, over and around the trail. Bird-watching is enough of a pastime here that Milwaukee County Parks has developed bird trail maps directing you to prime birding locations.

As the trail draws closer to the city, near mile 10, hilly city streets wind through an eclectic mix of Milwaukee's middle and upper-middle class neighborhoods. You pass three golf courses—the Grant, Warnimont and Lake Golf Course—in short succession. Just south of downtown there is an old warehouse district that has been converted into lofts and condos. Then the trail carries you down to magnificent Lake Michigan and its beaches.

The Oak Leaf Trail has a lot of ground to cover, but it all adds up to a great ride. Several kiosks along the trail advertise refreshments for the hungry and thirsty and you will find ample parking and restrooms. Whether logging just a few miles or canvassing the entire route, this is one trail you are sure to enjoy.

DIRECTIONS

From points north, west and south (I-94 and I-43), take Interstate 794 east and exit at 1E toward North Van Buren Street. Turn left on N. Van Buren, then turn right at East Michigan Street and follow East Michigan Street to the end. From there you will begin to see the Lake Michigan waterfront. The Milwaukee Art Museum/Information Center will be on the left side of the parking area.

Contact: Milwaukee County Park System
Watertown Plank Road
Wauwatosa, WI 53226
(414) 257-6100
www.countyparks.com

Bicycle Federation of Wisconsin
1845 North Farwell Avenue, Suite 100
Milwaukee, WI 53212
(414) 271-9685
www.bfw.org

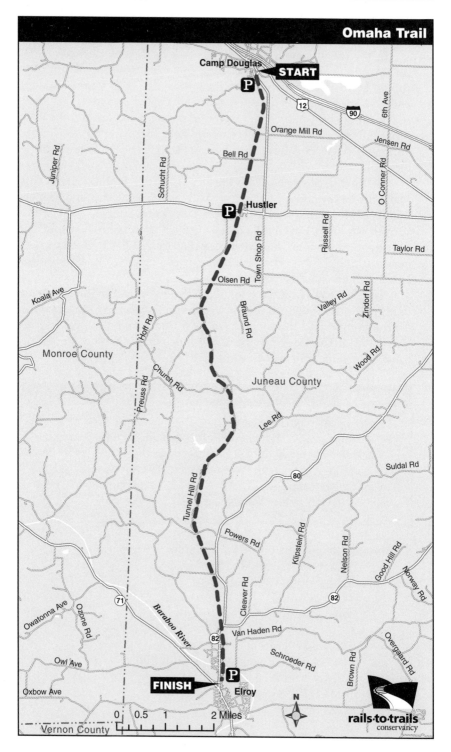

Camp Douglas

START

12

90

6th Ave

Orange Mill Rd

Jensen Rd

Bell Rd

O Conner Rd

Schucht Rd

Juniper Rd

Hustler

Russell Rd

Town Shop Rd

Taylor Rd

Olsen Rd

Valley Rd

Zindorf Rd

Koala Ave

Braund Rd

Hoff Rd

Wood Rd

Monroe County

Church Rd

Juneau County

Preuss Rd

Lee Rd

Suldal Rd

80

Tunnel Hill Rd

Powers Rd

Klipstein Rd

Nelson Rd

Good Hill Rd

Norway Rd

Cleaver Rd

82

71

Baraboo River

Owatonna Ave

Ozone Rd

82

Van Haden Rd

Schroeder Rd

Brown Rd

Overgaard Rd

Owl Ave

FINISH

Elroy

Oxbow Ave

0   0.5   1   2 Miles

N

Vernon County

rails·to·trails
conservancy

Omaha Trail

This 12.5-mile limestone trail is a gorgeous offshoot from a 100-mile continuous trail corridor that includes the Great River State Trail (page 315), La Crosse River State Trail (page 325), Elroy-Sparta State Trail (page 297) and the "400" State Trail (page 365).

The Omaha Trail's gentle surface and superb scenery make it a worthwhile trip. The county-maintained path has several unique features, starting with its surface. The limestone is sealed, making for a smoother ride than the connecting state trails. The trail also passes spectacular rock outcroppings that are not found anywhere else in Wisconsin—or in most of the Midwest.

Beginning at the northern end in Camp Douglas, the trail takes you past farms and though pastures for 4 miles before reaching the small town of Hustler. This tiny community has a pleasant public park right near the trail that provides a great spot to take a breather.

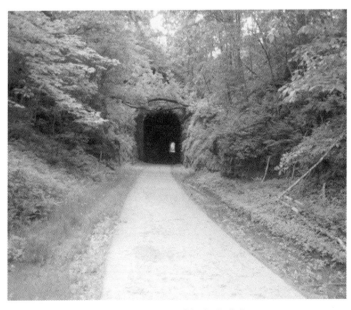

A 300-foot tunnel marks the midway point of the Omaha Trail.

Location
Juneau County

Endpoints
Camp Douglas
to Elroy

Mileage
12.5

Roughness Index
1

Surface
Asphalt and gravel

Leaving Hustler the trail gently rises through scenic bluffs. The type of rock in the stunning outcroppings in these bluffs cannot be found anywhere else in the midwestern United States.

At almost exactly the halfway point, you reach the apex of your climb and the entrance to a 300-foot-long tunnel. This magnificent historic railroad tunnel is one of the highlights of this trip. A small park just before the tunnel's domed entrance provides restrooms and water.

Upon exiting the damp, dark tunnel, it is all downhill to the town of Elroy. The final 7 miles pass through sections of dense forest where you are sure to see white-tailed deer, small mammals and many species of birds. You also shoot past quintessential Wisconsin farms with red barns and grain silos. Use caution crossing the many country roads intersecting the trail as you make your way into Elroy.

The town of Elroy is the endpoint for the Omaha trail, but here you can easily connect to both the Elroy-Sparta State Trail and the "400" State Trail. The town has many cafes and lovely shops and is a great place to take a break while navigating your way though this impressive western Wisconsin trail system.

DIRECTIONS

Get to the Camp Douglas trailhead from Interstate 90 by taking Exit 55 and heading south on County Road C. Take a right on Tomah Road and then turn left on Bartell Street, which becomes Main Street. The trail starts right in the middle of town at the intersection of Main Street and Eddy Avenue.

The Elroy trailhead is located near the intersection of State Routes 82 and 71. From this intersection follow Cedar Street east and the trail will be on the left.

Contact: Elroy Commons Information Center
303 Railroad Street
Elroy, WI 53929
(888) 606-2453
www.elroywi.com

Ozaukee Interurban Trail

The Ozaukee Interurban Trail (Brown Deer Recreational Trail) is an excellent 32-mile path through the communities of Cedar Grove, Belgium, Port Washington, Grafton, Cedarburg, Mequon and Thiensville. The majority of this trail follows an old electric rail line corridor, though there are on-road portions as you navigate through the downtown areas of Port Washington, Grafton and Cedarsburg. The final 2 miles of this otherwise paved trail excursion are on the packed-dirt Brown Deer Recreation Trail at the corridor's southern tip.

Begin your trip—and extend your ride, skate or walk—by starting in Cedar Grove in Sheboygan County, where a new 1.75-mile extension takes you to the start of the Ozaukee Interurban trail in Ozaukee County at County Line K. The section from County Line K through Belgium and into Port Washington is largely farmland. An active rail line runs adjacent to the trail.

Arriving in Port Washington, the trail goes up a ramp and ends on Highland Drive. Bear right at the end of the ramp and follow the bike signs that lead you to a stop sign. Turn right and go under Interstate 43. Turn right again onto East Seven Hills Road and travel a quarter mile, cross to the other side and pick up the trail where it resumes in a field next to a corporate parking lot.

In Port Washington, you must navigate the well-signed roads and some steep climbs before the trail resumes outside of town. Approaching Grafton you have another on-road, unsigned detour. The trail brings you to the doorstep of a residential community, where you turn right and travel down North Street; turn left on 1st Street. Take 1st Street to Washington Street; cross Washington Street and pass Wildwood Park on your right. Several blocks after the park, the off-road trail into Grafton resumes on your right. In Grafton a small half-mile on-street section is well signed and will direct you back to the trail.

The trail from Grafton to Cedarburg crosses many residential streets with scenic views of neighborhoods

Location
Ozaukee County

Endpoints
Cedar Grove to
Brown Deer

Mileage
32

Roughness Index
1

Surface
Asphalt and dirt

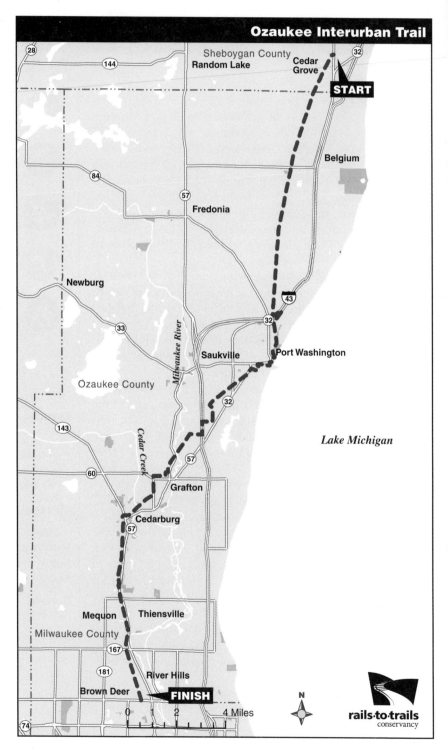

Ozaukee Interurban Trail

Sheboygan County
Random Lake
Cedar Grove

28
144
32

START

Belgium

84

57
Fredonia

Newburg

43

33

32

Saukville

Port Washington

32

Ozaukee County

143

Cedar Creek

57

Milwaukee River

60

Grafton

Lake Michigan

Cedarburg
57

Mequon
Thiensville

Milwaukee County

167

181
River Hills

Brown Deer
FINISH

74

N

0   1   2   4 Miles

rails·to·trails
conservancy

and parks. It only gets better as you enter the charming community of Cedarburg. Historic bridges carry you over Cedar Creek, and you'll be tempted to explore the inviting restaurants and shops.

South of Cedarburg the trail again becomes rural, passing through the communities of Thiensville and Mequon. Halfway between Cedarburg and Mequon the trail crosses an active rail line and provides a model pedestrian crossing and rail-with-trail design. The trail travels alongside the active rail line until the Ozaukee trail ends and the Brown Deer Recreation Trail begins. This short trail isn't much in the way of scenery—it ends at a utility substation—but it makes a nice connection to extend your trip into the village of Brown Deer.

DIRECTIONS

To reach the Ozaukee Trail's northern entrance from Milwaukee, take Interstate 43 north to State Road 32 west, which turns into Union Avenue (County Road D). The trail entrance is on your left as you approach Cedar Grove.

The southern endpoint for the Ozaukee (and the start of the Brown Deer Trail) can be reached from I-43 north; go west on County Line Road Q (at the border of Ozaukee and Milwaukee counties) for approximately 2.5 miles and look for the trail as it crosses the road. The Ozaukee goes north from here; the Brown Deer goes south.

To reach the Brown Deer trail's southern endpoint take I-43 south and then take Hwy. 100 west (Brown Deer Road). The trailhead—also the utility substation entrance—is on your right at the railroad crossing.

Note: There are a wide variety of trail access points but no designated trail parking lots. For a list of parking facilities and amenities go to Ozaukee County's official trail website: www.interurbantrails. us/parking.htm

Contact: Ozaukee County Tourism
P.O. Box 143
Port Washington, WI 53074
(800) 403-9898
www.interurbantrail.us

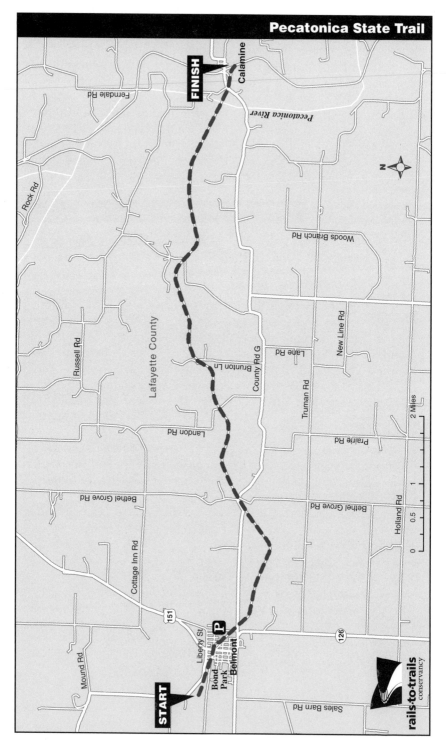

Pecatonica State Trail

Take the Pecatonica State Trail from Belmont to Calamine and you'll travel through some early Wisconsin history. Old Belmont was Wisconsin's capital when it was still a territory. You can visit the First Capitol Historic Site, which includes the two-story white clapboard capitol and adjacent Supreme Court buildings, a few miles northwest of town.

The 10-mile paved rail-trail follows a branch of the old Milwaukee Road railroad corridor that once hauled lead through this valley. The trail twists and turns as it follows the sluggish waters and crooked banks of the Bonner Branch of the Pecatonica River. Take your fishing pole and drop a line from one of the numerous bridges over the river, and you might just catch some sunfish for dinner.

There is parking in Belmont at Bond Park, which has a sheltered picnic area, softball diamond, playground and sand volleyball court. Moving east toward

Location
Grant County

Endpoints
Belmont to Calamine

Mileage
10

Roughness Index
1

Surface
Asphalt and crushed stone

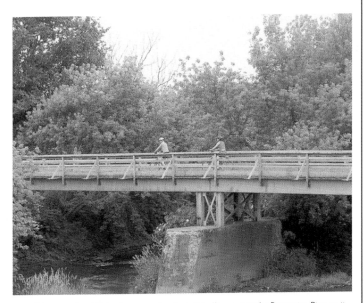

A former railroad bridge is now serving the trail traffic crossing the Pecatonica River as it nears the intersection of the Cheese Country Recreational Trail outside of Calamine.

Calamine the trail passes rolling farmland and tall grasses. Oak and hickory trees shade your way along many parts of the path.

As you take in the beauty of this trail, keep your eyes open for the birds you may be lucky enough to encounter: sandhill cranes, red-winged blackbirds, red-necked grebes, great blue herons and bobo-links.

Near Calamine, at the end of the Pecatonica State Trail, the trail intersects with the 47-mile Cheese Country Recreation Trail (page 291). Both trails require purchase of a state trail pass, which can be obtained at the trailhead or from the Wisconsin Department of Natural Resources website.

DIRECTIONS

The western trailhead is located on East Platteville Avenue (Hwy. G) and South Park Street in Belmont. Parking is available at Bond Park. The eastern trailhead is located at the junction of the Pecatonica and the Cheese Country trails. From Calamine go west on County Hwy. G, just after passing County Road C, turn left and head south for about a half mile to an unpaved parking lot.

Contact: Pecatonica State Trail
Green County Courthouse
1016 16th Avenue
Monroe, WI 53566
(608) 328-9430
www.tricountytrails.com

Pine Line Trail

True to its name, the Pine Line Trail cuts through magnificent stands of white pine on its way from Prentice to Medford. The 26-mile trail maintains an unwavering north-south course, but you will delight in the changes of scenery as dense forests give way to sweeping landscapes of dairy farms and majestic wetlands.

The northern portion of the trail begins in Prentice and traverses Taylor and Price counties. If you start in Prentice, be prepared for a pleasantly challenging journey. Large deposits left by an ancient glacier (called a moraine) create an irregular, rolling topography. The first 23 miles are surfaced with crushed gravel that is well maintained and suitable for walking and bicycle travel from late spring to early fall. The final 3 miles are limestone screening. In the winter months, the trail is primarily used by snowmobiles, the only motorized vehicles permitted on the trail.

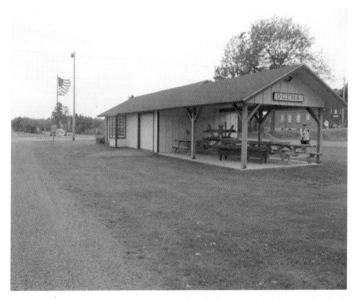

The rest area in Ogema features a useful trailhead and proximity to a local specialty—fried cheese curds.

Location
Price and Taylor counties

Endpoints
Prentice (Morner Road) to Medford (Allman Street)

Mileage
26.2

Roughness Index
2

Surface
Crushed stone

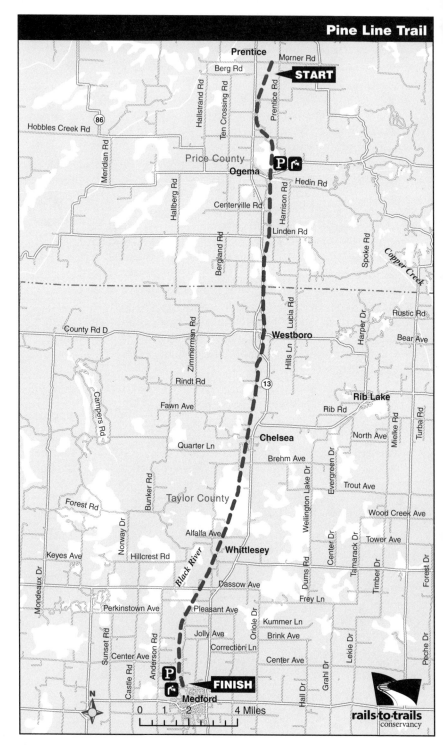

Much of the trail travels through cedar swamps. Be prepared, particularly in warmer months, to encounter large puddles and standing water in boggy areas.

A restored railroad depot provides a welcome rest area in Ogema, approximately 5 miles from the start. If you're hungry, hit a nearby restaurant for some true Wisconsin fare: fried cheese curds.

Moving farther south, the terrain gradually changes from wetlands to picture-perfect dairy farms. This pastoral scene accompanies you on the remainder of your journey.

For more than 100 years, the corridor was used by the Wisconsin Central Railroad to ship large quantities of eastern white pine. Fortunately, enough of these beautiful evergreens remain to color the entire rail-trail with their tall, fragrant, blue-green hue.

DIRECTIONS

Trail access and parking are available in Prentice on Morner Road between County Road 13 and Prentice Road. From downtown Prentice, take County Road A (also called Railroad Avenue) south. County Road A veers right (to the west) and merges with County Road 13. Traveling south on State Highway 13, take a left onto Morner Road. Before Morner Road intersects with Prentice Road, look for the trail on the right.

In Medford, the Allman Street trailhead has a parking lot and a connecting walking path called the East-West Riverwalk. There is a large sign with trail mileage information at the trailhead on Allman Street that points northward toward Prentice. Parking is also available and easily accessible on municipal streets in Ogema, Westboro, Chelsea and Whittlesey.

Contact: Price County Tourism Department
Price County Courthouse
126 Cherry Street
Phillips, WI 54555
(800) 269-4505
www.pricecountywi.net/trails/pineline.html

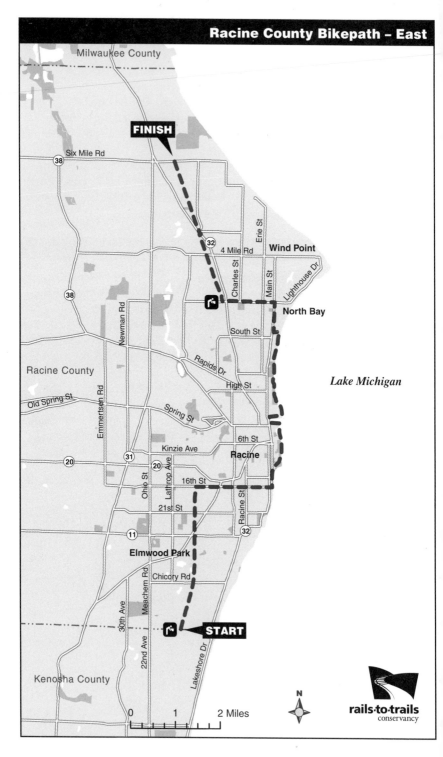

Racine County Bikepath – East

Milwaukee County

Six Mile Rd

38

FINISH

32

4 Mile Rd   **Wind Point**

Erie St

Charles St

Main St

Lighthouse Dr

North Bay

38

Newman Rd

South St

Rapids Dr

Racine County

High St

Lake Michigan

Old Spring St

Emmertsen Rd

Spring St

Kinzie Ave

6th St

31

Lathrop Ave

20

Racine

20

16th St

Ohio St

21st St

Racine St

32

11

Elmwood Park

Chicory Rd

Meachem Rd

30th Ave

22nd Ave

START

Lakeshore Dr

Kenosha County

0   1   2 Miles

N

rails·to·trails
conservancy

Racine County Bikepath – East

Racine County's eastern edge is home to two rail-trails plus a stellar connecting trail. Because the county standardized its signs a few years back, you won't see specific rail-trail names on display (look for Racine County Bikepath signs). But this trip travels the Northshore Trail, Lake Michigan Bike Path and the MRK Trail as it spans 15 miles from the southern county line to just shy of the northern county line. (This route is also known as the Northshore/MRK Trails.)

Start from the Northshore Trail and head north on a crushed limestone surface. (You will also see signs for the Kenosha County Bike Trail that connects here and runs south through Kenosha to the Illinois line.) On the rail-trail, greenery surrounds you, masking residences that border the path. The trail quickly becomes classic Wisconsin farmland scenery. This is an easy, flat and peaceful route for walking or biking. After crossing 19th

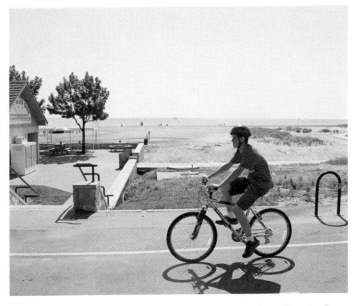

Bicycle by the sandy lakeshores of Lake Michigan on the Racine County Bikepath – East.

Location
Racine County

Endpoints
Racine (Racine County Line Road to Six Mile Road)

Mileage
15

Roughness Index
1

Surface
Asphalt and crushed stone

Street, the Northshore Trail ends, but a seamless connection continues north on the Lake Michigan Bike Path.

The Lake Michigan Bike Path is not a rail-trail, but a connector between the Northshore and MRK rail-trails. It is a series of on-road segments and paved off-road paths along beautiful Lake Michigan, through downtown Racine and its fantastic waterfront and to the famous Northshore Beach Park. There is plenty to do and see on this route, from shopping and dining in downtown Racine to the terrific playground (a fee applies) in Northshore Beach Park.

On the hill above Northshore Beach you will find the Racine Zoological Park. Following the path north, you pass below the zoo and then have a steep climb back into a residential area. Several major street crossings end this section near the Layard Avenue entrance to the MRK Trail.

The MRK Trail (named for the Milwaukee-Racine-Kenosha Railroad that traveled this route) winds up this trip with a 5-mile run to Six Mile Road. This section has an industrial feel to it: An active Union Pacific rail line shares the route and power lines drape the trail. The surface here returns to crushed limestone. You will notice a very gradual incline as you travel north, which makes for a swift trip back to the southern end of this county corridor.

DIRECTIONS

To access the southern terminus of the Northshore Trail, take State Route 32 south from Racine to County Line Road KR. Turn right. The trailhead is on the right about a half mile ahead. No parking is available.

To access the northern point of the MRK Trail, take Route 32 north from Racine. Turn right on Six Mile Road. The trailhead is on the right, a quarter mile ahead. No parking is available.

Contact: Racine County Wisconsin
Public Works Department
14200 Washington Avenue
Sturtevant, WI 53177
(262) 522-6240
http://pw.racineco.com/Biking/Index.aspx

Racine County Bikepath – West

The scenic trail corridor stretching 13 miles south to north from Burlington to Wind Lake actually comprises three rail-trails—the Burlington, Waterford-Wind Lake and Norway trails—stitched into one. (Racine County standardized its trail signs several years ago and the distinct names of the walking paths and biking trails are not specified on the new signs.)

Start your trip in Riverside Park in Burlington, which is located along the picturesque Fox River. You'll find parking, bathrooms and picnic pavilions at this lovely community park. Traveling north from Riverside Park, the 4-mile Burlington Trail section runs along the east side of Highway 36. After crossing Highway 36 you travel west through a pine forest before hitting a short on-road detour. Back on the trail, the path returns to woods and crosses the Fox River. After passing Case Eagle Park, with ball fields, a playground and seasonal restroom facilities, the trail returns to Highway 36, this

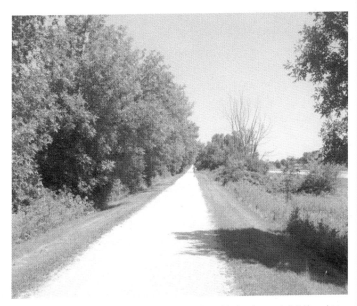

The Racine County Bikepath – West glides though neighborhoods, past ball fields and into pine forests.

Location
Racine County

Endpoints
Burlington to Wind Lake

Mileage
13

Roughness Index
1

Surface
Asphalt and crushed stone

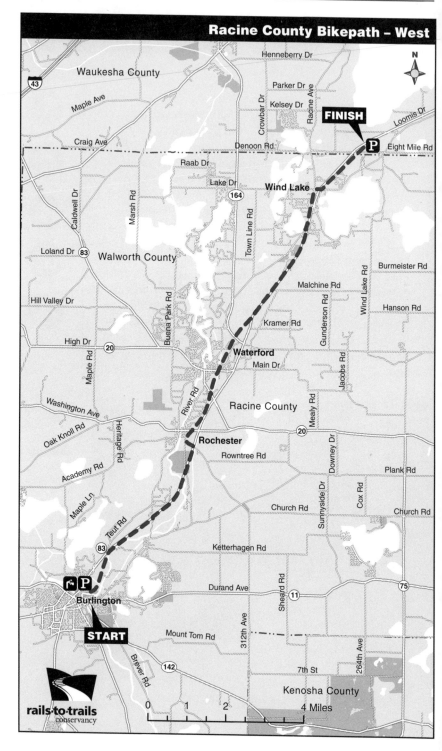

Racine County Bikepath – West

time traveling north along the west side. The highway is a constant until just outside Waterford, where the trail veers into residential and remote sections of this community. There are several street crossings before the end at Buck Road, where the trail seamlessly transitions into the Waterford-Wind Lake section.

The 5 miles of the Waterford-Wind Lake section run mostly along the west side of Highway 36; however, significant tree cover on both sides lets you forget you are close to the road. As you approach the community of Wind Lake, you detour on-road. Turn left at South Wind Lake Road, then right at South Loomis and follow this north until you come to a Y in the road where South Loomis and Racine Avenue intersect. Stay on Loomis and bear right toward the traffic light and cross Highway 36.

The Norway Trail picks up on the east side of Highway 36. Look for the trailhead on your left as soon as you cross the highway. Following this 1.2-mile rail-trail north to the county line, you enjoy remote wetland scenery. When the trail shifts from crushed stone to grass, keep going until the trail dead-ends at a parking lot and boat access for Muskego Canal, providing access to Big Muskego Lake.

DIRECTIONS

To access the northern terminus in Wind Lake, take State Route 36 north (Loomis Road) from Wind Lake to the Waukesha and Racine county line. Immediately after the county line take your first right turn into a gravel parking lot that is designated for boat access to the Muskego Canal. From the parking lot you'll see a grassy entrance to the trail. The official trail with crushed limestone surface continues off the grassy area about 20 feet south.

To access the Burlington trailhead you must start in Riverside Park. Take State Route 11 west into Burlington. Turn right onto Bridge Street (83), go over the bridge and turn right onto Congress Street to Riverside Park. The trailhead is at the end of the park off Congress Street.

Contact: Racine County Wisconsin
Public Works Department
14200 Washington Avenue
Sturtevant, WI 53177
(262) 522-6240
http://pw.racineco.com/Biking/Index.aspx

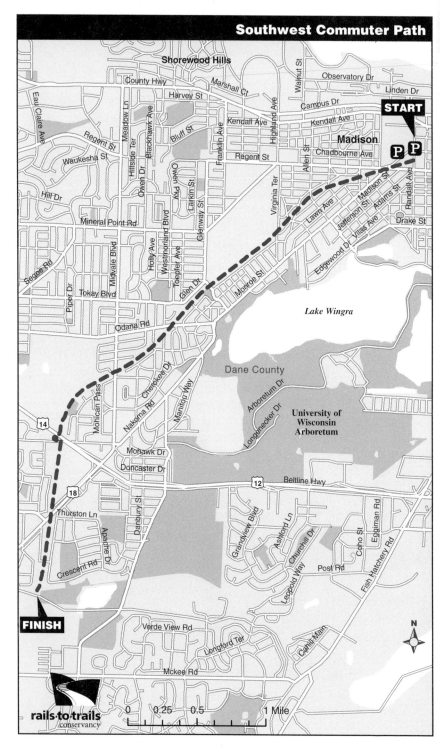

Southwest Commuter Path

Southwest Commuter Path

Aquick trip on Madison's 4.6-mile Southwest Commuter Path (a.k.a. the Badger State Trail) conceals the full scale of this trail. It also serves as the northern segment of the Badger State Trail that, when completed (there are approximately 5.5 miles still to develop), will travel 40 miles to the state line and continue for another 32 miles into Illinois.

Despite its potential for remote reaches, the Southwest Commuter Path is rich in urban terrain and history. The trail takes you over, under and sometimes finds the shortest route across major roads.

Pick up the trail just south of the intersection of South Bedford Street and North Shore Drive as it branches off from the Brittingham Trail that hugs the west bank of Lake Monona and runs through Brittingham Park.

The trail makes a northwest arch and parallels an active rail line until it reaches the historic Milwaukee Road railroad depot. Designed by noted Chicago architect

Location
Dane County

Endpoints
North Shore Drive
to Jenewein Road
in Madison

Mileage
4.6

Roughness Index
1

Surface
Asphalt

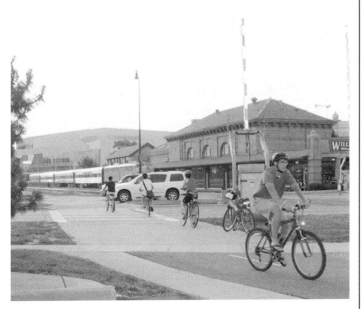

There's plenty to see in Madison, and the Southwest Commuter Path is one of the quickest ways to take in the sights.

Charles Sumner Frost, the imposing 1903 structure is listed on the National Register of Historic Places. Railroad cars of the Chicago, Milwaukee, St. Paul and Pacific railroad line flank the depot.

From here the trail heads southwest, bordered by vegetation and historical homes. Impressive ramping and stairwells connect the trail to the neighboring streets and you are sure to see neighbors grabbing a quick run or taking the kids for a ride. On the last 2 miles of the trail you sail under simple span bridges that artistically display street names and help you stay oriented. Be sure to take a look back toward downtown Madison, as the bridges and greenery frame a perfect view of the capitol dome.

DIRECTIONS

From the south, take State Highway 151 to Madison, turn right on Red Arrow Trail Road and go 2 blocks to Jenewein Road. Street parking is available.

From the north, take Hwy. 151, which becomes East Washington Avenue in Madison. Turn left on South Blair Street, then turn right on John Nolen Drive. Follow the water and turn right on Lake Shore Drive. Street parking is available.

Contact: Friends of the Badger State Trail
101 South Webster Street
P.O. Box 7921
Madison, WI 53707
(608) 325-5607
www.badger-trail.com/friends

Sugar River State Trail

If you can't make it to Switzerland, do the next best thing: Take the Sugar River State Trail to "America's Little Switzerland," New Glarus, Wisconsin. Settled in 1845 by a small tribe of Swiss pioneers, New Glarus today is a living monument to all things Swiss. Chalet-style buildings line the streets, restaurants dish up savory Swiss fare and a chorus of annual celebrations include Polkafest, the Heidi Festival and Volksfest, which marks the Swiss independence day.

Leaving the accordions and bellowing alphorns behind, hop on the scenic Sugar River State Trail at the restored railroad depot in New Glarus. The 23-mile rail-trail crosses the Little Sugar and the Sugar rivers and travels gently rolling hills and meadows through the farming communities of Monticello, Albany and into Brodhead in the southeast.

Less than a half mile into the ride you cross Highway 69. From here, the trail follows the course of the

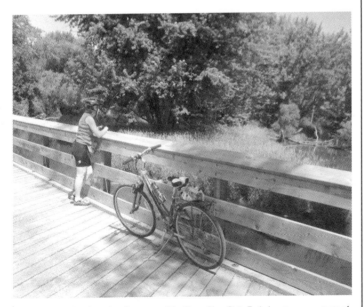

The wooded and gently rolling route of the Sugar River State Trail also gives you a taste of local Swiss heritage.

Location
Green County

Endpoints
New Glarus to
Brodhead

Mileage
23

**Roughness
Index**
1

Surface
Asphalt and
crushed stone

361

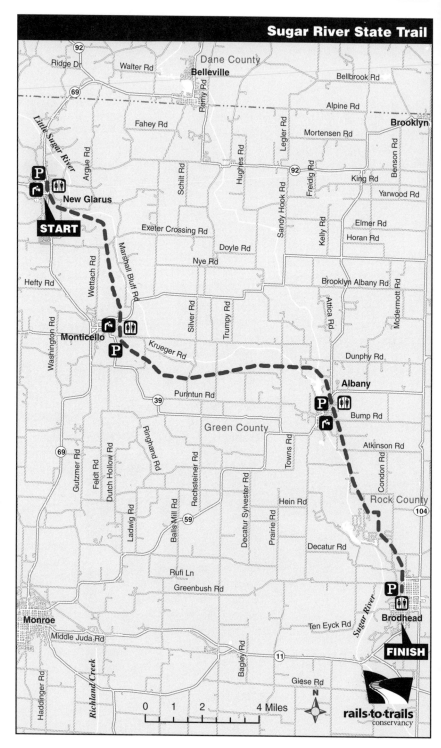

Little Sugar River. Near mile 6, approaching Monticello, you arrive at a brightly painted railroad depot that is not open to the public. Between Monticello and Albany there are five stream crossings with views of scenic farmland. Then, at mile 14, the trail crosses the Sugar River on a long, curving bridge that provides spectacular views of lowlands of cattails and reeds and woods of oak, hickory, walnut, cherry and willow trees. Visitors in June or July will get an added treat in the wild raspberries found sporadically along the trail.

At mile 21 the trail crosses Norwegian Creek on a replica covered bridge built in 1984 from wood supplied by the Wisconsin Department of Natural Resources from demolished old barns and other buildings in the state.

Arriving in the small farming community of Brodhead, named after Edward Brodhead, who was chief engineer of the Milwaukee and Minnesota Railroad, you can hop off your bike and take in the sights. Be sure to visit the Depot Museum, open in the summer, which chronicles the trail's Milwaukee Road railroad days; and the Half Way Tree, located south of the town, designated by Native Americans as the halfway point between the Great Lakes and the Mississippi River. Users of this trail must obtain a state trail pass, which can be acquired from the Wisconsin Department of Natural Resources website.

DIRECTIONS

Get to the northern end by traveling west of State Route 69 on Route 39 (Sixth Avenue) in New Glarus. Go one block and turn right onto Railroad Street and into the New Glarus Depot trailhead parking lot.

At the south end in Brodhead, park at Exchange Street and West Third Street, two blocks west of State Route 11 (Center Avenue).

Contact: Sugar River State Trail
418 Railroad Street
New Glarus, WI 53574
(608) 527-2334 (summer)
or (608) 527-2335 (off-season)
www.dnr.state.wi.us/org/land/parks/
specific/sugarriver/index.html

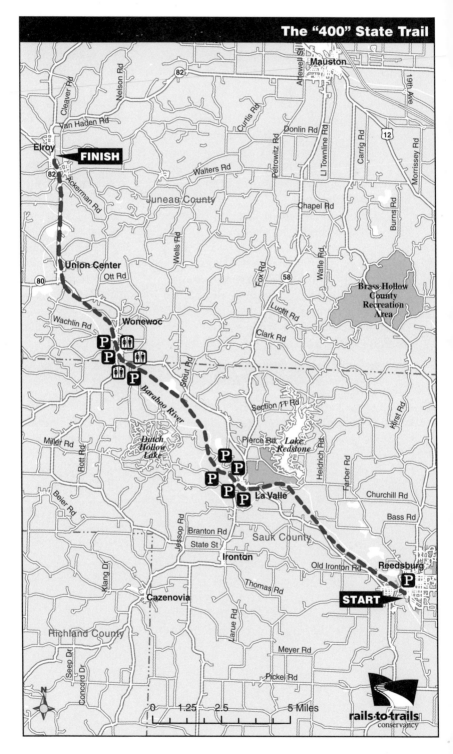

The "400" State Trail

The "400" State Trail

The "400" State Trail travels between Reedsburg and Elroy on 22.3 miles of old Chicago and North Western Railroad line. The trail's curious name has an obvious origin. It is named for the train—Number 400—that traveled 400 miles from Chicago to Minneapolis in 400 minutes.

The trail, which parallels the Baraboo River for its entire run, is really four trails in one. It connects to the Hillsboro, Elroy-Sparta and Omaha rail-trails for a combined total of 95 miles. With a packed limestone surface, plus 11 bridges crisscrossing the Baraboo, the "400" State Trail provides a smooth, flat riding surface. You will see many bicyclists on this trail, although snowmobilers use it in winter months and there is an adjacent, 7-mile equestrian path between LaValle and Wonewoc. Start your ride in Reedsburg near the visitor center in the restored railroad depot. Stop here to purchase a trail pass, or visit the trail's website for other ticket locations. Reedsburg is known for small-town friendliness and city convenience. There are antique shops galore and all variety of restaurants. Spending the night is easy, too, with hotels and bed-and-breakfasts, plus a campground if you want to connect with the area's rich natural surroundings.

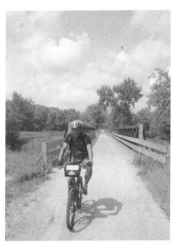

The "400" State Trail is named for the Number 400 train that once traveled 400 miles on this route in 400 minutes.

After 6 miles on the trail you arrive at Lake Redstone. To reach the lake, travel 0.5 mile off the trail itself. This mammoth artificial lake has a public rest area where you can refresh yourself and take in the gorgeous natural scenery. Continuing north, travel through the village of LaValle where you can make a pit stop, visit one of

Location
Juneau and Sauk counties

Endpoints
Reedsburg to Elroy

Mileage
22.3

Roughness Index
1

Surface
Crushed stone

LaValle's local treasures and then pass Dutch Hollow Lake. The lake, clear and inviting, has a sandy beach and campground.

Wonewoc is the trail's midpoint. A campsite and public rest area make it a great place to stop and take in the wooded scenery. Next is Union Center, with another public rest area and the starting point for the 4.3-mile Hillsboro Trail (page 321). Staying on the "400" State Trail for about another 4 miles brings you to its end—and the start of the Elroy-Sparta and Omaha rail-trail (pages 297 and 341)—at Elroy Commons. After 22 miles of riding, you might want to stay awhile and enjoy this quaint town's public library and museum, eat at one of the local restaurants or visit a specialty shop. Or stay overnight and rest up for a journey on one of the other scenic rail-trails in this quiet corner of southwestern Wisconsin.

DIRECTIONS

From Milwaukee, take Interstate 90 to I-94 west to Highway 23, then turn onto Highway 33, which will take you into Reedsburg. Once in Reedsburg, pass four traffic lights and make a left, then go two blocks; the trailhead is on your right.

Contact: 400 Trail Headquarters
Reedsburg Chamber of Commerce
P.O. Box 142
Reedsburg, WI 53959
(608) 524-2850
www.400statetrail.org

Tri-County Corridor

Get away from it all on the Tri-County Recreational Corridor. Pick up this North Woods rail-trail in Superior, where it connects with the urban Osaugie Trail. Spanning the three counties of Ashland, Bayfield and Douglas, the Tri-County trail is a direct west to east shot between Superior and Ashland. Most of the trail is surfaced with crushed limestone and open to a wide variety of uses. (If asphalt is what you're after, head east to Ashland's Central Railyard Park for a short, smooth trip on the trail's 3-mile strip of pavement.)

Bicyclists, hikers and equestrians share the trail with all-terrain vehicles from spring through fall, while snowmobiles dominate in winter. Signs specify that motorized users keep to one side of the trail, which keeps the surface suitable on the opposite side. However, increased ATV traffic—especially on weekends—can make for a bumpy bike ride in some sections due to sporadic patches of loose gravel.

Even though Highway 2 parallels most of the trail and is somewhat visible, the long ride from Superior

Location
Ashland, Bayfield and Douglas counties

Endpoints
Superior to Ashland

Mileage
61.8

Roughness Index
2

Surface
Asphalt and crushed stone

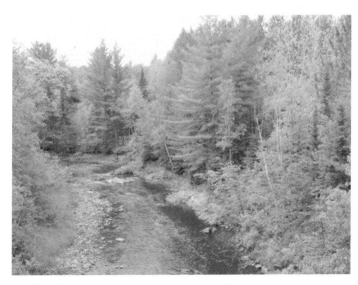

The Tri-County Corridor is a rustic and rural getaway, with stunning lake and river vistas.

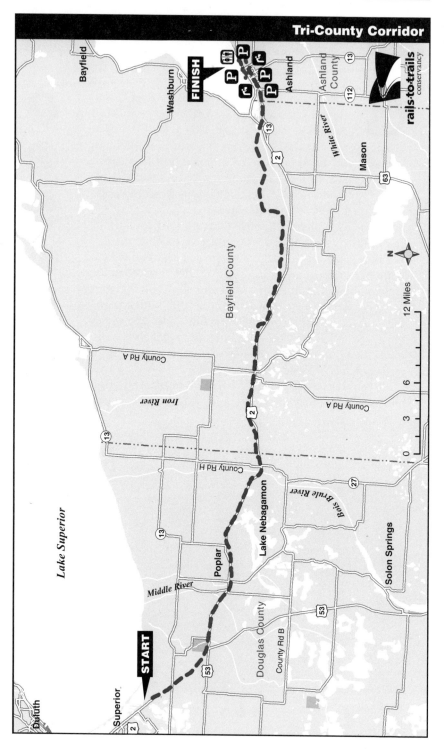

to Ashland feels secluded and peaceful. Wildlife is abundant. Scenic Amnicon Falls State Park, just 7 miles outside Superior, is home to foxes, porcupines and other small animals. Farther along, peer into the beautiful stands of birch trees lining the path to find deer quietly hiding. Bridges and old railroad trestles high over churning rivers and streams create a peaceful respite for bird-watching.

Amenities along this trail are scarce. The town of Iron River, at mile 40, is the first—and last—chance to find refreshments or a restroom (take County Road A south into town) until the trail's end.

Nearing Ashland, at mile 60, the trail becomes a paved backyard path, intersecting sleepy neighborhood streets. This 3-mile section is the only portion suitable for wheelchairs and in-line skates.

Ashland, with beautiful views of Lake Superior's Chequamegon Bay, is the perfect end to this scenic trail. But if you choose to begin in Ashland, bypass the Tri-County trail's official terminus, in an industrial area lacking parking and other facilities. Start instead at Central Railyard Park, where an old rail complex has begun a new life as a thriving community center with playgrounds, gazebos and a skateboard park. There are plans in place to extend the trail to the waterfront, where the lakeside breeze will provide an even more refreshing finish to a long journey.

DIRECTIONS

To reach the Tri-County Recreational Corridor in Ashland from the west, take State Highway 137 east into town. The road becomes West 6th Street. Parking is available at Central Railyard Park across from the intersection of 4th Avenue West and West 6th Street.

From the east, take US Highway 2 west into Ashland, where it becomes Lakeshore Drive East. Turn left on Ellis Avenue (State Highway 13) and right on West 6th Street. Look for parking at Central Railyard Park to your right across from the intersection of 4th Avenue West and West 6th Street.

To reach the trail from Superior, take East 2nd Street south out of town. Immediately after it becomes US Highway 53 south, take a left on Moccasin Mike Road (also 57th Avenue East). Take the first left into a parking lot and the trail will be on your right.

Contact: Tri-County Corridor Commission
P.O. Box 663
Iron River, WI 54847
(715) 372-5959

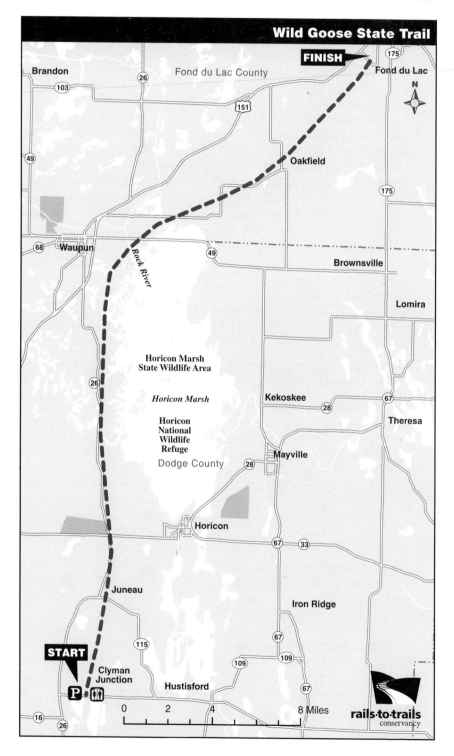

Wild Goose State Trail

Wild Goose State Trail

The Wild Goose State Trail is a premier rail-trail, spanning nearly 35 miles in Dodge and Fond du Lac counties. If you are looking for a peaceful and beautiful place to visit, this trail has it all. Almost the entire trail is tree-covered, very flat and well maintained. The "wild" in the trail name is apt, as wildlife is in abundance. If you are traveling by bike you will want to concentrate on the trail surface: Chipmunks frequently scramble across the path. Throughout the trail there are multiple highway and farm access roads to cross—all are well marked, but use caution.

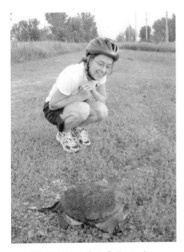

The Wild Goose State Trail puts the "wild" in wildlife.

Starting from the southern endpoint, Clyman Junction, travel through wooded areas and farmland. A horse path parallels the trail for 7.5 miles from Clyman Junction to Minnesota Junction.

Several industrial buildings mark your arrival in Juneau, where you'll find a typical small town with a few restaurants and bars to visit. The trail becomes a bit tricky to follow as it passes through a grassy lot and then resumes. Rule of thumb: Go straight when the trail seems to disappear and you will find it again shortly.

Outside of Juneau the trail quickly returns to farmland. Although the trail skirts the western edge of the Horicon National Wildlife Refuge and Horicon Marsh State Wildlife Area, you will not actually see the marsh. You may, however, see some of its feathered inhabitants: The marsh is home to herons, egrets and hawks, to name a few. A tenth of a mile before you reach Highway 49,

Location
Dodge and Fond du Lac counties

Endpoints
Clyman Junction to Fond du Lac

Mileage
34

Roughness Index
1

Surface
Crushed stone

look for the sign marking the short path to the Marsh Haven Nature Center. Covering 32,000 acres, the Horicon Marsh is one of America's most important wetlands. Tour the marsh on guided or self-directed canoe or kayak tours and don't miss the spring and fall migratory season, when it is estimated that more than 500,000 birds pass through.

Crossing into Fond du Lac County for its final 14.5-mile stretch, the trail again becomes rural, flat and scenic. Trees provide continuous shelter as the trail takes you into the community of Fond du Lac and ends next to a parking lot at a railroad crossing. Fond du Lac is blessed with beautiful water vistas. Make sure to stop by Lakeside Park at the edge of Lake Winnebago for a picnic after your trail visit and sit right at water's edge near the lighthouse.

When the snow flies, skis and snowmobiles (December through March only) hit the trail, followed by the spring migration of birds wintering over in Horicon Marsh. Summertime's expansive green fields and dense tree canopies give way to spectacular fall foliage. Any time of year is a good time to visit the Wild Goose State Trail.

DIRECTIONS

To reach Clyman Junction from Milwaukee, take State Route 41 north to State Route 60 west through Hartford. Continue on Route 60 west past Road M in Clyman Junction. The trail entrance will be on your right; parking is available.

To reach Clyman Junction from the north, follow State Hwy. 26 south through Juneau. Four miles south of Juneau, turn left on Route 60. The trail entrance is approximately 1.5 miles on left.

The Fond du Lac trailhead is accessible from Highway 15 north. In Fond du Lac, turn right at the light onto Rolling Meadows Drive. After passing a golf course on the right, go approximately a quarter mile. You'll find the trailhead, with parking, right before the railroad crossing on your right.

There are parking lots at both trail endpoints at Rolling Meadow Road in Fond Du Lac and off State Route 60 in Clyman Junction. The trail cuts through the city of Juneau; there is ample parking in the community. There are official trail parking areas off State Route 33, Road B in Burnett and at the Marsh Haven Nature Center entrance off Highway 49.

Contact: Dodge County Land Resources and Parks
127 East Oak Street
Juneau, WI 53039
(920) 386-3700
www.co.dodge.wi.us/landresources/recreation/index.html

STAFF PICKS

Popular Rail-Trails

When Rails-to-Trails Conservancy staff members traveled through the Midwest: Great Lakes region to ride on, map and write about great rail-trails for this book, these were the ones that stood out as their favorites. Short or long, city or country, these are the rail-trails not to miss.

Illinois
Fox River Trail
Great River Trail
Illinois Prairie Path
Tunnel Hill State Trail

Indiana
Cardinal Greenway – Marion Section
Cardinal Greenway – Muncie Section
Monon Trail

Michigan
Fred Meijer Heartland Trail
Hart-Montague Bicycle Trail State Park
Pere Marquette Rail-Trail
White Pine Trail State Park

Ohio
Holmes County Trail
Kokosing Gap Trail
Little Miami Scenic Trail
Slippery Elm Trail

Wisconsin
Bugline Recreation Trail
Capital City Trail
Elroy-Sparta State Trail
Glacial Drumlin State Trail
The "400" State Trail

ACKNOWLEDGMENTS

Each of the trails in *Rail-Trails Midwest: Great Lakes* was visited by Rails-to-Trails Conservancy staff and volunteers. Maps, photographs and trail descriptions are as accurate as possible thanks to the work of the following contributors:

Andrea Maguire
Barbara Richey
Barry Culham
Ben Carter
Bev Moore
Brian Ullmann
Carol Beckman
Catherine Herron
Cindy Dickerson
Dave Rumohr
Dick Westfall
Elton Clark
Eric Oberg
Frederick Schaedtler
Heather Deutsch
Ira Weiss
Jamie Pallay
Jane Brookstein
Jeff Adams
Jerry Dobbs
Jessica Leas
Jim Barrett
Judy Culham

Judy Dobbs
Kathy Weiss
Kelly Cornell
Kelly Pack
Ken Adams
Kevin Heber
Kirt Livernois
Lee Rumohr
Mark Fritsma
Matt Cline
Matthew Hoehn
Melissa Lott
Nancy Krupiarz
Peggy Portier
Ralph Portier
Roger Storm
Ryan Phillips
Sandra Lach
Steve Haddad
Susan Wedzel
Tim Kelley
Tom Krupiarz
Tom McCain

And, with fond remembrance, Rosann Sternberg

Additional assistance was provided by:

Michigan Trails
and Greenways Alliance
410 South Cedar Street, Suite A
Lansing, MI 48912
(517) 485-6022
www.michigantrails.org

INDEX

BECOME A MEMBER OF
RAILS-TO-TRAILS CONSERVANCY

As the nation's leader in helping communities transform unused railroad corridors into multiuse trails, Rails-to-Trails Conservancy (RTC) provides vital technical assistance to communities throughout the country, advocates for trail-friendly policies at the local, state and national level, promotes the benefits of rail-trails and defends rail-trail laws in the court. RTC depends on the support of its members and donors to help support programs, projects and services that have helped put more than 15,000 rail-trail miles on the ground.

Join RTC in "inspiring movement" and receive: new member welcome materials, including *Destination Rail-Trails,* a sampler of some of the nation's finest trails; a subscription to RTC's quarterly magazine, *Rails to Trails;* **discounts** on publications, apparel and other merchandise, including RTC's popular rail-trail guidebooks; and the **satisfaction** of knowing that your dollars are helping to create a nationwide network of trails.

Membership benefits start at just $18. Join online at **www.rails totrails.org** or by calling (866) 202-9788. Join by mail by sending your contributions to Rails-to-Trails Conservancy, Attention: Membership, 2121 Ward Court, 5th Floor, Washington, DC 20037.